your
preschooler
BIBLE

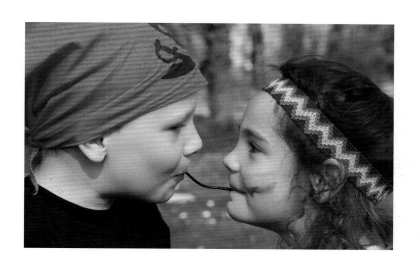

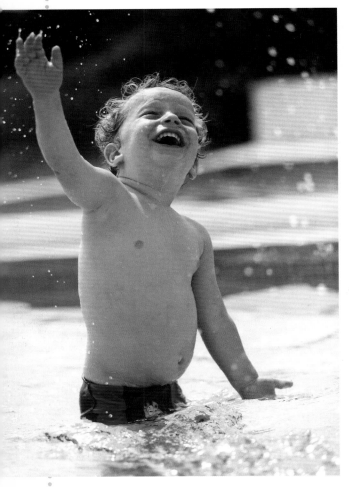

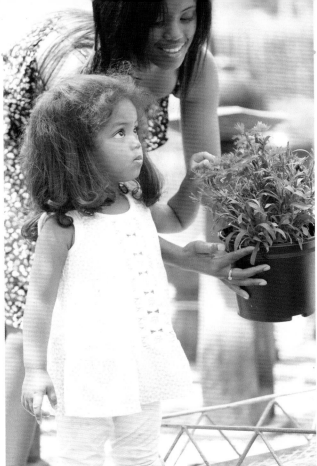

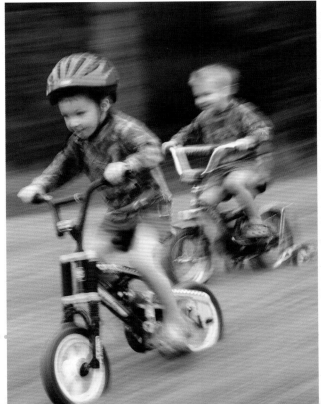

your
preschooler
BIBLE

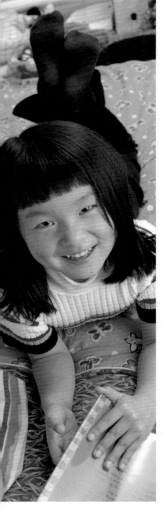
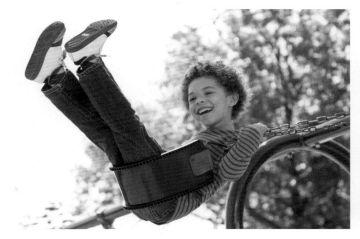
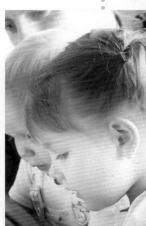

Consultant and chief contributor
Dr. Richard Woolfson
PhD, PGCE, MAppSCi, CPsychol, FBPsS

hamlyn

Contents

First published in 2014 in Great Britain by Carroll & Brown

This edition published in 2016 by Hamlyn, a division of Octopus Publishing Group Ltd
Carmelite House
50 Victoria Embankment
London EC4Y 0DZ
www.octopusbooks.co.uk

A Hachette UK Company
www.hachette.co.uk

Distributed in the US by Hachette Book Group
1290 Avenue of the Americas, 4th and 5th Floors
New York, NY 10020

Distributed in Canada by Canadian Manda Group
664 Annette St., Toronto, Ontario, Canada M6S 2C8

ISBN 978 060063 219 1

Printed and bound in China
10 9 8 7 6 5 4 3 2 1

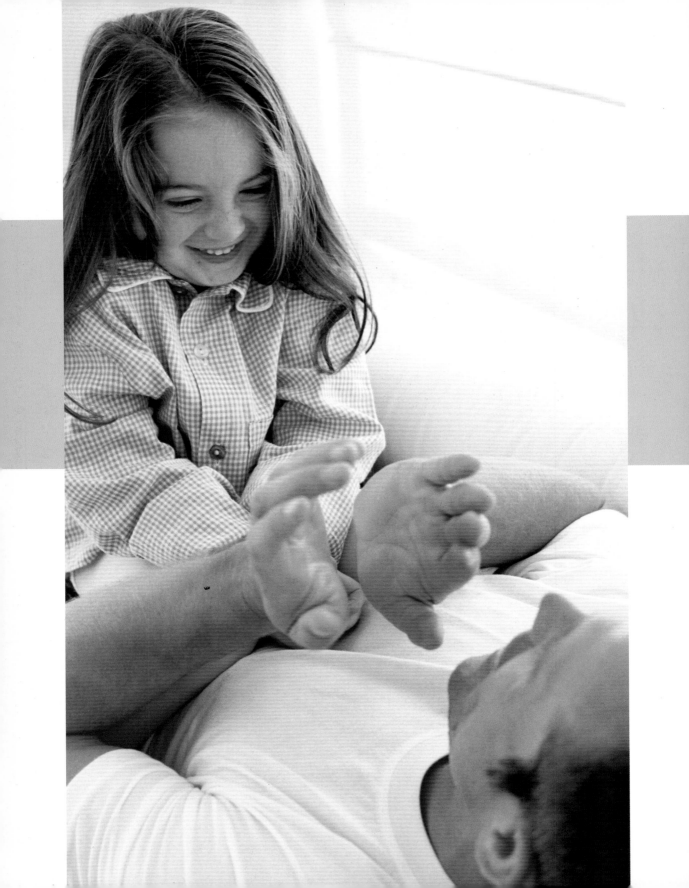

CHAPTER 1
YOU AND YOUR PRESCHOOLER

Once your child reaches the age of three, she has left babyhood behind and is on the brink of becoming an independently minded individual with a recognizable personality. Your task over the next few years will be to equip your child with the skills necessary to go to school and become a welcome member of a larger community. But it's not all going to be hard work! In fact, the preschool years can be the most fulfilling time for you both. Unlike when she was a baby, your child is now old enough to appreciate your care and attention but not so old that your influence will be eclipsed by her peers. To find out what's in store, read on. At this age, development is subject to advances and seeming retreats, and the "snapshot" of your child at various stages will cover the expected highs and lows.

Sharing your life with your preschool child

You probably can't remember a time when you didn't have a child in your life. That phase seems just a dim and distant memory from long ago, a surreal time when you had nothing to think about except yourself and your partner, a time when you could do exactly what you wanted exactly when you wanted. Learning to share your life with your child has certainly been challenging up until now, though you have probably adapted to it better than you expected. In the first year or so, you had to adjust to focusing your time on your baby instead of solely on yourself and your partner, you had to adapt to a change in routine in which your baby's needs came before your needs, and you had to learn to carry out babycare tasks when there were moments that all you wanted to do was to stay in bed and hide under the covers. A young baby becomes so much a part of your life—it's not that you share your life with her, it's that your two lives become intertwined to such an extent that some days you feel she and you are completely at one together.

Then came along the toddler years, with that wonderful explosion of development, in which your child started to speak, walk, to have ideas of her own, and to show her sense of humor. Suddenly, the calm at home was disrupted as your toddler made it clear that sharing your life with her had entered a new and more challenging phase altogether, one marked by tantrums, determination, and a strong desire to be independent. But once again you both gradually adapted to each other, learning when to insist and when to compromise, when to follow the rules, and when to be flexible.

That type of sharing is a normal part of parenting, and is a natural process that usually takes place without any actual deliberate thought or planning. The very fact that you chose to become a parent in the first place meant you were ready to share your life with someone else. Yet just when you thought you had it all worked out, just when you and your toddler had meshed into a way of sharing your lives together that suited you both, she has now become a preschooler, with strong ideas of her own, an insatiable curiosity to discover how the world works, a much greater use and understanding of spoken language, and a very distinctive personality and temperament. Sharing your life with your preschooler will be new, exciting, and altogether different.

There are several reasons, covered in more detail below, why your child's feelings and behavior change significantly during preschool years, and all are linked to progress in her psychological and physical development. Because of them, sharing your life with your preschooler usually will be a combination of

TIME MANAGEMENT

Through the preschool years, your child will require less hands-on attention from you. She will still need you to attend to or supervise her personal care, to spend individual time with her—either talking or reading, playing or teaching her things—and to watch over her while she plays outdoors. However, there will be more things she can do on her own with less supervision (though still within sight or earshot), such as playing by herself or with others, using the computer, or watching TV or a DVD. This means that in a 24-hour day, your
- 3-year-old child will require about 6½ hours,
- 4-year-old child will need about 6 hours,
- 5-year-old child will require about 4 hours of your time.

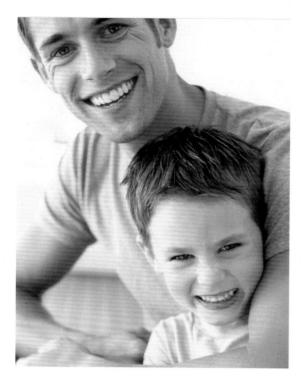

emotional highs and lows. Sometimes everything will seem to go so smoothly and yet other times you will feel that you and she are completely out of sync. You may even feel aggrieved that your child takes more than she gives back, and that you hadn't imagined your life would be like this during these precious preschool years.

Your partner is sharing, too

Decisions were much simpler when your child was younger, for instance, choosing whether she wore the striped or single-color sleepsuit, or which brand of formula milk she would drink during weaning. Even if important, such decisions were unlikely to be a source of controversy between you and your partner.

When your child became a toddler, decisions grew more complex. For instance, you and your partner had to reach an agreement about how to encourage your child's behavior in positive ways and how you would ensure she followed rules. Somehow, though, these decisions were reached reasonably quickly. During the preschool years, however, you have to make decisions that will have a significant impact on your child's

future development, such as the type of day care you use for her when you return to work, or the type of nursery school you want her to attend. Then there are her friendships, some of which you'll be pleased with and others you would prefer her not to have. And toward the end of the preschool phase, you need to select a school for her—perhaps one of the most important decisions of this life phase.

No wonder then that the preschool years can be a time of tension and disagreement between partners. Sharing your life with your child also involves sharing major decisions with your partner. It is not about making choices and then informing your partner after the event as a *fait accompli*.

Whenever engaging in discussions about aspects of your child's future, think through all the pros and cons very carefully. Consider all the advantages and disadvantages of each option before coming to a conclusion. Be prepared to shift your initial opinion if necessary. After all, your partner's view may be right, even if your original idea was different. A couple is more likely to support a strategy for their child when they have reached a joint agreement, and that makes it more likely to work effectively.

Adapting to your changing child

Sharing of any kind involves giving something of yours to someone without any guarantee that you'll get anything back in return; that's why sharing is so difficult for young children. And sharing your life with a constantly changing and growing preschooler will be especially demanding for you because she will seem to ask constantly for so much from you—and will often seem prepared to give so little back. However, you are the parent and she is the child. You can't reasonably expect your child to be sensitive and responsive to your needs in the same way that you are to hers.

Over the next couple of years, she will become less self-centered and focused on what she wants, and more empathic and focused on what you want as well. When she reaches school age, she will be much easier to be with. In the meantime, however, she's finding her way in her own little world, testing out the limits of her strengths, talents, and abilities, and is determined to assert her independence.

Sharing your life with a child during the preschool years, therefore, involves recognizing that she is trying to develop a view of herself and who she is and that she achieves this through trial and error. She learns by example and also by her mistakes. This means you will find yourself in role of rule-setter and rule-enforcer, perhaps when you'd rather be sharing songs, games, and fun activities. It also means you will find yourself in the role of peacemaker and soother when your child has a temper tantrum, perhaps when you'd rather be relaxing by yourself or enjoying a day out together. That is what sharing your life with a child means.

Keep things in perspective, however. True, your preschooler will be more demanding, challenging, confrontational, and volatile than she was when younger but she's also more communicative, physically affectionate, interesting, curious, and fun to be with. Don't lose sight of the positives just because you also have difficult moments. Concentrate on the times when things go well. Learn from the more challenging episodes and try to avoid repeating negative incidents in the future. Sharing your life with your preschooler can be very fulfilling as you both adapt to each other's changes needs, interests, and feelings.

STEP-PARENTING A PRESCHOOLER

Whether your partner's preschooler lives with you or stays on a regular basis or even if the child is an infrequent visitor or remains with her other parent, it will have an impact on your relationship with your partner. Be prepared for complications! No matter how you relate to your step-child, the vital thing is to keep the lines of communication with your partner open and to ensure that he/she takes the leading role. Most importantly, you need to agree about the rules you set your child and when and how to discipline her if they are transgressed, the level of child care you provide, and how you relate to others, particularly her other parent and grandparents.

As a rule, it's easier to be a step-parent to a preschooler than an older child but that doesn't mean it's easy. Young children (younger than nine years) are more accepting of step-parents and can more readily adapt to having two homes, though it's best if daily routines are kept the same in both. But, of course, they also require more care and attention.

Key to creating a relationship with your step-child is not to be overly ambitious in expecting her to love or even like you, but to take your time and cues from your child. Some children need a while to accept change—particularly if circumstances have been traumatic—so it's important to set realistic expectations. Even if your preschooler will live with you all the time, it's best not to think of yourself as her "new" mom or dad. You can be a significant other but your step-child's biological parent will always have a particular place in her heart. Similarly, don't expect that your "new" family will be better or even similar to what she had previously, only that it will be different. One thing that can build bridges, is to share a particular activity that both of you like—maybe creating a scrapbook of found items from your nature walks or even watching favorite DVDs together.

Often, step-families have problems not because of the children but because the adults in the family become jealous or resentful of the biological parent's attachment or feel rejected by the child and her other parent or even guilty about breaking up the former family in the first place. So, if you suffer from any of these emotions, it's important to discuss them with your partner and if he or she can't resolve them, seek help. Organizations such as the National Stepfamily Resource Center (www.stepfamilies.info) offer a free online step-parenting toolkit and other types of support.

Preschool twins

As you have already discovered, twins are twice the usual work—but twice the usual fun as well. Happily, most parents of twins find that their workload decreases through the preschool years since their children begin to eat by themselves and no longer need diapers and, luckily, there's always a willing playmate on hand. On the downside, it can be more of a challenge to keep two children of the same age safe from harm (see chapter six).

There are particular parenting challenges for parents when it comes to twins, simply because of their closeness in age, their special relationship (which is often more intense than normally found between siblings), and their underlying need to develop as distinct individuals despite being part of a tightly knit twosome. You have to find a way to balance their similarities with their differences in order to ensure that each of them is allowed to become a unique individual. Bear in mind, too, that if you have boy/girl twins, girls generally develop more quickly, reaching milestones at an earlier age, which can be discouraging for their brothers. Moreover, boy/girl twins' behavior may be less sterotypical than singleton boys and girls; your son may be less boisterous and aggressive than his peers or your daughter more of a tomboy.

The practicalities of looking after and stimulating two preschoolers is demanding for even the most competent parent. So be willing to ask for help, whether from your partner, relatives, or friends. And if you are lucky enough to receive spontaneous offers, take them. That doesn't mean you can't manage on your own, it's simply a very practical solution to help you juggle the continuous child-care demands. Don't wait until you feel totally overwhelmed by everything because that's leaving it too late.

Same, but different

Bear in mind that even if you have identical twins who look alike in every way, they will each have their individual characteristics. For instance, one twin might enjoy imaginative play while the other might prefer problem-solving play with shape-sorters and other basic puzzles. Or perhaps one prefers

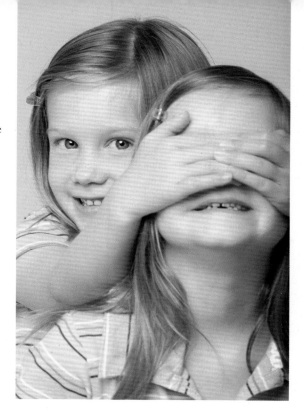

rough-and-tumble play while the other is more comfortable with quieter activities. Try to provide appropriate play opportunities that meet these different interests, so that their individuality is allowed to develop.

You may find that while your twins are good at playing together as preschoolers, even having a shared, private language, they are not so good at playing with other children. You may need to give them a helping hand with this. As well as affording them experience of sharing, taking turns, and playing games with rules at home, make a special point of letting them play with their peers. This gets them used to being with others their own age. Since their initial reaction might be to stick together, encourage them to interact. It can be a good idea to take them to play groups or twins' clubs.

Of course, time is tight when you have two preschoolers the same age to look after. Whatever time you have during the day, however, make an effort to spend some moments alone with each twin, instead of only spending time with them together. All it takes is a few minutes each day playing with one of your twins, while the other is either cared for by someone else or is engaged in his or her own activity. And when you do spend time stimulating them, focus on language-based activities. Twins often develop speech and language skills at a slower rate than nontwins, probably because they often construct their own shorthand system for communicating with each other. That's why a broad range of language activities is so indispensable for your twins. Talk to them throughout the day as they progress through their routine activities. Read them stories, sing them songs, and recite poems and nursery rhymes when you can.

Having a fair discipline system isn't always easy. For example, when something goes wrong, you might not be sure which of the two misbehaved, and the true culprit is unlikely to confess. Instead of punishing them both, try to identify the one who really was at fault.

Likewise, one twin could be harder to handle than the other, and therefore may require firmer limits. Recognizing and responding to your twins' individual behavior patterns by having different ways of managing them is perfectly reasonable. If you simply treat each twin the exact same way, they might actually end up feeling hard done by.

It maybe they both enjoy music or dance "classes" but, more likely, one twin could be interested in dressing up and play-acting while the other is more fond of sports. If they are forced to follow the same interests, at least one of them will feel thoroughly miserable. True, encouraging your twins' individual interests in this way is not entirely convenient for you and may not be cost-effective, but that applies to all parents who have two children close in age, not just to parents of twins.

Point of separation

One of the key decisions you have to make about encouraging the individuality of your twin preschoolers arises when they start nursery school or kindergarten. Assuming they both attend to the same school, should they go into the same class or should they join separate classes? Or maybe you'd like them to attend the same nursery school but different schools later on. There is no easy answer.

8 ways to encourage your twins' individuality

1 **Dress them differently** or if they want to dress similarly, make sure they have different haircuts. This will make it easy for people to tell which child is which.

2 **Make sure they have their own possessions** as far as possible, and don't just share things from a general pool.

3 **Afford them time alone with you or friends.** Make sure each twin spends individual time with you and that each has the opportunity to play with other playmates.

4 **Tailor your shopping excursions:** just because one needs new shoes doesn't mean they both do.

5 **Teach your children to say their names** and to correct anyone who calls them by the wrong one.

6 **Speak to your children individually.** Address each by name. When speaking to others, talk about them individually rather than as a duo.

7 **Take individual photographs** as well as joint ones and put them on display at home.

8 **Make each twin a cake on his/her birthday** and ensure family and friends give each child a separate present and card. You could also appoint other days in the year, which each child has as his/her own special day.

The advantages of your twins being in the same class—whether in nursery or elementary school—is that they could support each other, could help each other when minor problems arise throughout the school day, and would each have a ready-made friend in the school playground. But a potential disadvantage is that they might be treated like two peas in a pod, not just by the nursery school or teaching staff but by their classmates as well. (In fact, if you've downplayed their twin status at home, you may need to explain about twinship because their new schoolmates or teachers may refer to them as "the twins" instead of by their names.) In other words, they might be expected to fit into people's stereotyped expectations of twins, which would then constrain their individual differences from emerging.

In contrast, going into separate classes would have the advantage that each twin would be more likely to be accepted as an individual, without constant daily comparisons with her twin. This allows for more individual growth and expression. Yet temporary separation from each other during the school day could leave them feeling lonely, isolated, and perhaps even afraid. Consider the pros and cons very carefully before making your choice.

Discuss this with your twins in order to find out their feelings on the matter. Talk to nursery school or teaching staff as well. Even though your children are more likely to develop their individual interests if placed in separate classes, sensitive teaching can still encourage their differences even if they are in the same class. The choice is yours.

Some parents are so determined to allow each twin to develop individually, that they enroll them in different schools after finding ones that suit their children's specific individual blend of talents, abilities, and personality. However, that is a rather extreme strategy; generally, twins don't need to be separated entirely, they just need to be allowed to have their own opportunities.

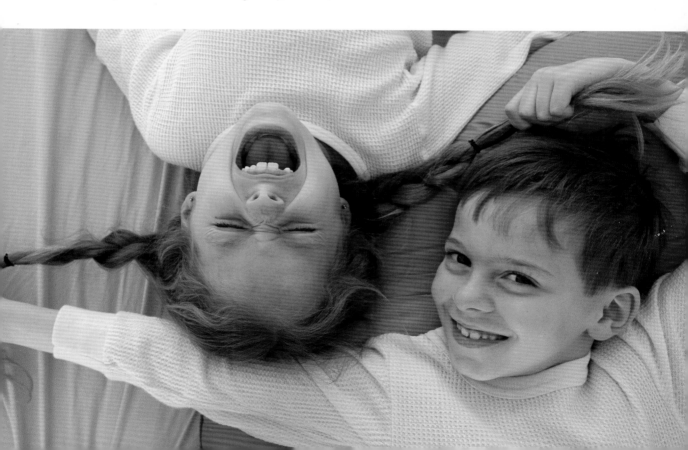

How your child changes during the preschool years

As your child's individual blend of temperament, skills, interests, abilities, emotions, and thoughts continue to emerge and develop, he will change in many exciting and fascinating ways. He will become much more of an independent free-thinker with very clear ideas about what he likes and dislikes, what he wants to achieve, and with whom he prefers to spend time. In many ways, living with your preschooler will become much more dynamic than during earlier years because in comparison to babyhood and infancy, he can do more, communicate more effectively, think more maturely, and has a better sense of humor. But, of course, these personal "highs" can also be matched with personal "lows," such as shyness, temper outbursts, and even sagging self-confidence. It's the combination of all these characteristics that makes your preschooler a wonderfully unique, special person.

Growing independence

Your child has two conflicting yet complementary urges that develop strongly in this phase. On the one hand, your child has a natural, inborn desire to be able to do more for himself without any help from you, and this intensifies. It happens because not only does he continue to want to be independent but he now believes he has the ability to cope on his own. His improved physical skills contribute to this belief. On the other hand, your preschooler still needs you to be beside him whenever he wants. You are the one who guides him, helps him, loves him, and makes him feel valued and important. In other words, he still needs you as his parent as much as ever.

The challenge for your child is to balance those competing psychological forces by improving his independence skills (physical abilities and emotional self-reliance) while at the same time keeping close emotional ties with you. Sometimes this results in confusion for him (and can be trying for you),

especially in situations when his ambition outstrips his ability, for example, when he moves bravely and confidently upward on the climbing frame on his own, only to burst into tears and call out for you seconds later when he realizes he is stuck halfway. Or, when he insists on putting on his shirt without help yet dramatically bursts into tears when he discovers it's inside out. Ironically, you will think it was easier and quicker for you when you did everything for him.

Greater ability to communicate

Listening to your child now, it's hard to imagine that he was once a baby with no words, phrases, sentences, questions, or arguments. His language and

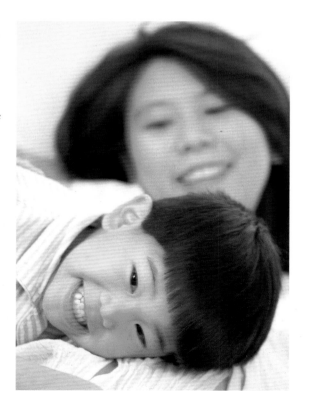

communication skills lift off at a rapid pace during the preschool years. It's not just that you see a huge increase in the number and range of words your child uses to express his thoughts and feelings, it's also the way he uses these new language features that make him so much more interesting. Words and questions are used to challenge and explore the world around him. If he wants to know more, he just asks, whether or not you feel in the mood for a detailed discussion; the endless chatter of a talkative four-year-old can be draining and giving him looked-for explanations will take up much more of your time than previously.

Your preschooler can also give a more accurate account of his experiences when he isn't with you. Conversations between you and your child start to have adultlike qualities and you can begin to reason with him when you have a disagreement. Favorite words at this age are usually "No," "I don't want to," and "Why can't I do that?", so brace yourself for living with a child who is able and willing to voice his opinions. These sophisticated communication skills also reflect his better understanding of the world around him and of his relationships with the people in his world.

Wider sociability

Friendships start to matter to your child now. He wants to have lots of buddies and to be popular, though he might not have the necessary social skills to achieve this target. He's at the age when children learn how to cooperate in play with one another, to share their toys, and to play games with rules, especially as they near school age, but there can be a steep and difficult learning curve. Some children are more outgoing and make friends more easily than others.

One of the features of peer group relationships at this age is that they are often quite fragile—a best friend one week might be a forgotten memory by the next. And because preschoolers aren't always effective at resolving conflict peacefully, minor bickering is common even among friends. So the social life of a preschool child can be full of ups and downs.

Another social dimension that often emerges is shyness, as when your normally outgoing child suddenly freezes, say, as he is about to enter his best friend's party. In an instant, he bursts into tears and claims he doesn't want to go inside with the others even though he knows most of the children there. This type of unexpected shyness is common but fortunately, the frequency of such episodes steadily diminishes over the next couple of years.

Your life, too, changes since more than before, you spend time organizing and implementing your child's social diary, driving him from one social encounter to the next, and dealing with any friendship squabbles.

Increased confidence

Your child's self-confidence is very important because if he feels good about himself, he will have the courage to try everything at least once. There are new social, learning, and relationship experiences every day, and your child needs the confidence to tackle them effectively.

A child with low self-confidence is easily discouraged when facing a new task; the challenge can seem insurmountable to him. You know what it's like when you are trying to learn a new skill, such as striking a golf ball so that it travels a long distance. At first you think you'll never do it because every time you swing the club you miss the ball. Then comes that sweet moment of success, when you feel the club and ball connecting in the way they should. It's a great feeling—and your child feels the same when he achieves something. His self-confidence is highly variable and can be extremely fragile. One day he might show you how he can dress himself yet the next day he'll insist he can't put his clothes on without your help. Or perhaps he jumps wildly and happily on a trampoline then suddenly demands to leave because he is afraid of injury. He may try to avoid difficult tasks for fear of not mastering them. But the more success he achieves in any area of his life, the stronger his confidence will become.

Emotional control

Regulating feelings and developing sensitivity to others ("emotional intelligence") will be an on-going internal struggle. Your child has been used to expressing whatever he wants whenever he wanted. When he was

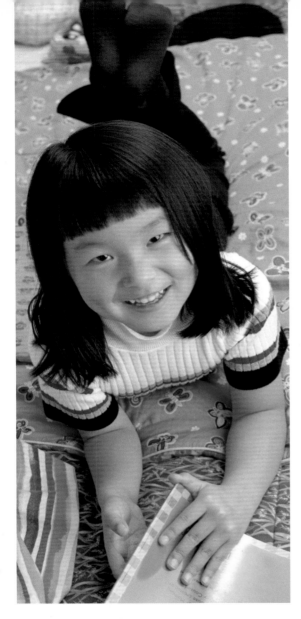

some children have difficulty with this. A preschooler's outburst of temper can easily intensify to explosion point. Tantrums occur when a child's temper flares to such an extent that he loses all control of his rage. While most children manage their anger effectively by the time they start school, dealing with an enraged preschooler can keep your hands full.

There is no doubt that a child who manages to regulate all his emotions (positive and negative) effectively and who shows empathy to the emotions of others generally has a more enjoyable life experience. A child who has little emotional regulation experiences exhausting emotional extremes. You'll see moments when your child will struggle to keep control because, even though he would rather do and say exactly what he wants, he successfully manages to keep his intense feelings in check.

Learning gains

Many children spontaneously learn early reading and number skills. For instance, they can recognize their written name and can complete very simple additions. Others need more help to achieve this. Every child is different in his rate of learning. Whatever your child's natural talents, however, tackling the early stages of literacy and numeracy becomes an important factor in his life.

As your child grows and thrives throughout the preschool years, the influence of these changes will become ever clearer. The way your child deals with those influences will affect the type of person he develops into. If he can build a solid emotional base during this phase of his life, he will be secure, confident, and psychologically ready to start school.

a baby, he cried when he wanted feeding without a thought for anyone else. When he was a toddler, he had a tantrum when he couldn't get his own way. In other words, he vented his emotions at the time they arose, without making any effort to control them or without thinking of the impact they had on others around him. That changes now. Your preschooler will see, for example, that his friends back away from him when he loses his temper, or that you become upset when he won't do what is asked of him. As a result, he will try harder to gain control over his feelings, though

What you need to do

There are many specific ways you can help your preschooler maximize all aspects of her potential and these are dealt with in subsequent sections of this book. However, here are some general parenting strategies, which will be needed to support your growing child throughout the preschool years.

Provide structure, stability, and consistency

Children thrive best when they grow up in a stable and predictable environment. It's not that they are resistant to change—in fact most preschoolers find small changes in their lives exciting—it's just that they need to feel emotionally secure in their surroundings. For example, your child takes for granted that her bedroom will look the same tonight as it did last night, and that she will go to the same nursery school tomorrow as she did today. Stability boosts her confidence, enhances her sense of well-being, and makes her feel safe and secure.

The same should apply to your parenting. Your growing child knows the type of parent you are and expects you to behave in certain ways. When it comes to discipline at home, she understands the family rules and expects them to be applied consistently. Once she knows your expectations of her behavior, she will do her best to conform, at least most of the time anyway. If family rules or your expectations of her change unpredictably, she will become confused and disoriented. That's why consistent parenting is crucial for your preschooler's psychological development. A child raised in uncertainty and constant change is likely to feel emotionally unsettled.

However, that doesn't mean everything has to stay exactly the same all the time. There will be times when you bend the rules, for example, when you allow her to stay up late one night as a special treat, or when you don't allow her to play outside because of bad weather. She will adapt to small irregular changes like that, as long as she experiences overall structure and stability within a background of consistent parenting.

There may also be major (possibly unplanned) changes in your family life, for instance, if you move to a new home, change your child carer, separate or divorce, or a grandparent dies. Don't fall into the trap of thinking that because she's young, change doesn't matter to your child—it does. Each preschooler reacts to change in her own way. You may be able to tell just by looking at your child that something is troubling her, and if a major change has just occurred in her life—for instance, her dad has just moved out—then you can reasonably make the connection. But distress at change can show in more subtle ways.

For instance, ten minutes before going to spend the morning with her new child carer, your child complains that she has a sore tummy. Or your outgoing preschooler suddenly becomes sad and withdrawn. The better you know your child, the more sensitive you'll be to her reactions.

You can help your child adapt to major (and unwelcome) changes in the structure and stability of her life by acting with sympathy and understanding. If you are moving to a new home, for example, the chances are that you are also having difficulty with the change (after all, moving is a stressful time for you, too) and you may find your preschooler's negative reaction frustrating. Try not to get angry with her, despite the pressure it puts you under. Give her lots of reassurance. True, you can't guarantee that life will be marvelous after a marriage split or that your child will be able to see both of you each day. But reassure her anyway. Tell her that she'll be fine, that everything will work out well, and that in time she'll be just as happy with the new arrangement.

Good communication

Communicating well with your child doesn't happen by chance—you need to work at it, especially with

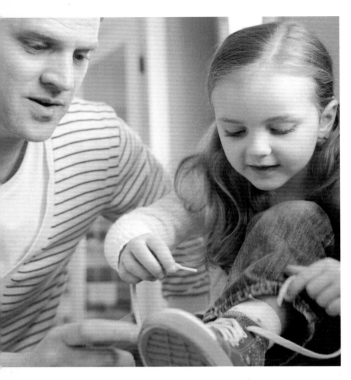

go for a walk—it's the shared time with each other that counts. Communication flows better when you and your child are used to each other and feel relaxed in each other's company—the more you do it, the easier it gets. Give your child your full attention, ignore all distractions, and avoid all interruptions. Instead, let her speak to you without you butting in, so that she feels you are genuinely interested in her comments.

Do your best to ensure that enthusiasm for communication is two-way. Encourage your child to approach you whenever she wants to express something—she should understand that she can talk with you at any time, not just at mealtimes or those special moments when you are together. And when she does reveal a recent experience that upset her, or she tells you her latest exciting news, give her a big hug and tell her how pleased you are that she told you about it. Establishing good communication habits at this age sets the foundation for a continued close connection between you and your child for the rest of her childhood.

Positive parenting

Raising your preschooler has many wonderful moments, but it's also hard work. The constant running after him, dealing with his moods, taking him from here to there several times each day, and making his meals can be very demanding. If you are not careful, the pleasure of parenthood can slip away letting a more pessimistic viewpoint take over. When that happens, in fact, before that happens, turn the situation around and instead make yourself a "positive parent"—one who has an optimistic outlook in life. Positive parenting is not simply about pretending that everything in the parenting garden is rosy (because it isn't). Instead, it's about developing strategies for managing your child and your role as a parent in an effective way, so that you feel good about yourself. And if you feel good about yourself this benefits everyone in your family. Positive parenting is about taking the initiative, planning ahead, and keeping control of your life.

all those other attractions that compete for her time. That's why you need to keep communication high on your parenting agenda. There will always be a thousand other things that you could do instead of spending time with your child—and likely a thousand other things she could do as well instead of spending time with you—so if you don't make communication a priority it won't happen by itself. Try to build "communication opportunities" into your weekly (and daily) routine. Perhaps the most effective strategy is to organize a traditional family meal at which you and your preschooler (along with all other family members) sit down and eat together at the table. Communication works best in face-to-face situations, not when you are in separate rooms, at separate times, engaged in separate activities. Do your best to have a family meal together at least a couple of times a week.

In addition, set aside ten or twenty minutes every day for the specific purpose of spending that time with your child. It really doesn't matter what you do during these minutes, whether you play or watch television together, talk about school or friends, or

10 techniques that encourage positive parenting

1 **Reflect.** The problem with being a parent is that you are so busy doing things you rarely have time to think about them. So take a few minutes to consider your routine. Maybe you don't have to do absolutely everything. Your house will survive if you don't take all the papers to the recycling this week. Be prepared to drop some of the less important daily tasks.

2 **Take short breaks.** Try to organize your day so that you are able to put your feet up for 10 minutes. This could be when your child goes to nursery school, or when he watches his favorite TV show. Tell yourself that you need a short break, that you deserve it, and that it must be a priority for you each day.

3 **Monitor "nagging."** Nobody likes to think that he or she is negative toward his or her child, but it is easy to fall into this trap. Think about the number of times you have reprimanded your child today—maybe you could have ignored some of these instances or perhaps made a more positive remark to him.

4 **Focus on good behavior.** When you see moments of good behavior—for instance, when your child plays quietly with his toys in his room—make a big fuss of him. Let him know how pleased you are with his actions. This helps both of you realize that there are good moments too, and that there aren't arguments all the time.

5 **Ask for/accept help.** The chances are that your partner, relatives, and friends are more than willing to look after your preschooler once in a while so that you can have time to yourself—even if you have to ask. Take advantage of these offers. A short break on your own for only, say, an hour will enable you to recharge your batteries so you'll feel more positive.

6 **Structure your day.** Try to have a reasonable idea of what each day will hold—a schedule of activities for you and your child. Even though you probably won't be able to follow the schedule to the letter, having a plan keeps you in control of your life. You are in charge of what you do, and it's not just down to chance.

7 **Praise yourself.** Tell yourself each day that you are doing a good job. Reflect on at least one incident that day that you handled really well. Be proud of yourself as a parent. Other people may not think to praise you or give you encouragement, so give yourself a pat on the back every day.

8 **Enjoy your child's achievements.** Your child may be annoying at times when he whines and complains, yet he's also an amazing child who does new things every day. You can't fail to notice the new skills he acquires as he progresses through the preschool years. Be proud of his progress, maybe even keeping track of each new stage in a diary.

9 **Have realistic expectations.** Positive parenting also means that you need to recognize your own limitations as a parent. Everybody wants to be the best parent in the world but that title can only go to one person. Set yourself attainable goals instead of creating a set of overly high expectations of yourself that are totally unrealistic.

10 **Give lots of hugs and cuddles.** No matter how strained your relationship with your child might become at times, make sure to be generous with the hugs and cuddles. Loving, physical contact of that sort helps melt away the negatives and puts you both in a positive, caring frame of mind. A good hug will cheer you both up.

The importance of routine

A regular routine provides your preschooler with stability. He likes the world to operate according to routines and has an underlying need for a predictable structure in his life. In the same way that unexpected events might make you feel uneasy and momentarily insecure, an unstructured pattern to the day unsettles your child. Most children this age like to know, for example, that they go to nursery school three days a week, that they go to the swimming pool another day, and so on. This sort of structure enables your child to plan ahead and to organize his life in a limited way. However, he may not fully realize that routines are there to help him rather than enslave him, or that a change in routine can be positive. When he is older, he'll be much more able to organize himself if he has had experience of doing this during the preschool years.

Another benefit of routine is that it gives your child some control over his life. He enjoys feeling in charge. He's only young, but at this age he still wants to be firmly in the driving seat. Your child prefers to be the one to decide when he should eat his dinner, what television show he should watch, and what time he should go with you to get the groceries. His need for control is very strong, and becoming familiar with daily routines satisfies this need. Bear in mind that most young children are not very adaptable. Flexibility usually improves with age; as your child's confidence grows over time, he will learn that minor changes can make life much more interesting, but for now he just likes the security of fixed routines.

The importance and significance of routines in your preschooler's life becomes even clearer when the established pattern is broken. For instance, he might become furious with you because he can't play in the park one Tuesday and yet he always plays in the park on that day. The fact that the family car has broken down, or that it is raining heavily, will make no difference to him. Routine leads him to expect the same to happen each time, and he will become distressed and angry when there is a break to that routine, whether that involves changes of food, mealtimes, or activities. Suggesting something different may produce a confrontation.

Your child is more likely to enjoy the security and comfort of routines when he understands their purpose. So explain them to him. For instance, it's

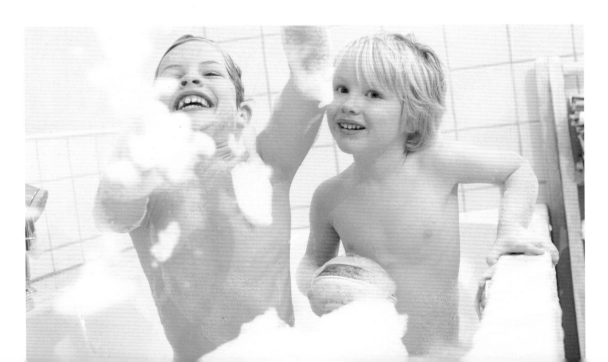

better to tell him "I'm not going to read you another story now because you are tired and I am tired, and we both need our rest" than to say "You're not getting another story now because I say so." Likewise, you can help him adapt to routines by reminding him of the next step. When you are out shopping in the afternoon, for instance, tell your child, "I bet you can't wait to get home so that you can play in a lovely warm bath." This will encourage him to anticipate what's coming next, and to look on it positively.

But make sure you avoid lengthy periods without any change in routine; the longer a routine is fixed, the more your preschooler wants it continue without alteration. That's why he might argue furiously with you because he has taken a bath in the morning for as long as he can remember and now you have decided bathtime should be moved to the evening. Well established routines are hard to break and discourage flexibility. When you anticipate a break in routine, therefore, warn your child in advance. You won't always know ahead of time that you need to change his routine (for instance, if his friend suddenly gets sick and can't play with him that day), but if you are aware of an alteration, let him know as soon as you can. A sporadic break in your normal routine is a positive occurrence, and is usually as exciting for your preschooler as it is for you. Turn it into a special treat.

Likewise, be prepared to change routines if you feel they are too tiresome. For instance, if you find that putting your child to bed at seven in the evening is difficult because that's the exact time when your partner comes home, then change bedtime (or other task) for earlier or later. The less demanding the routine is for you both, the more likely you are to enjoy the activities together. Think about the routines you have at the moment. Perhaps you'll discover that they can be altered to make life less stressful and more fun.

Formal schedules

By the time your child is aged four or five, you can consider creating more formal schedules, to transfer some of the responsibility of setting routines from

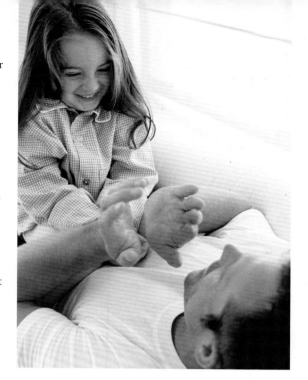

you to your child; this also will help him organize his time more effectively. The schedule can be activity-focused; for instance, your child may have a specific task to complete each day, such as tidying his room, and he could draw up a plan in which he decides to do this as soon as he returns home after nursery school. It can also be time-focused; in this instance, your child could have a specific time each day in which he's allowed to watch TV or a DVD. If he is not well organized, start with an activity-based plan since a time-based schedule is probably still too overwhelming for him. Pick one activity and begin to draw up a schedule for that.

A schedule will only be effective if your child feels committed to it—if he doesn't, he will feel it is imposed and will make no attempt to stick to the arrangements. An effective way to engage your child with a schedule is by involving him in decisions about the way it is compiled.

Whatever the focus of the schedule, talk to your preschooler about this. Discuss with him the difficulties he experiences at present (for instance, he is always rushed, he feels irritable when doing things, there are many other distractions) and point out the advantages a schedule would bring.

Likely flashpoints

During the preschool years, there are likely to be occasions when you and your child clash. Here are some common areas of conflict, with suggestions about how you could deal with them positively and effectively.

"I don't want to eat that."

Many children go through a phase of picky eating, when they insist that they will only eat certain foods. This can happen for several reasons, including your preschooler's desire to assert his independence, a genuine change in his tastes, his realization that refusing to eat is a great way to get your attention, or even his dislike of having to sit at a table to eat.

Deal with it by staying calm. Bear in mind that you cannot force your child to eat no matter whether you cajole, threaten, or beg him. He will only eat when he wants to. So when he insists he doesn't like anything on the plate in front of him, avoid an argument. Instead, talk to him about something else, and when you have finished your meal, remove his plate. He won't starve. You'll find that the less attention you pay to your picky eater at mealtimes, the less fuss he makes. And try to make the eating experience pleasant by providing child-sized cutlery and good seating for him, and by sitting with you child so that you and he eat together.

"I don't want to do that."

Your preschooler will have more ideas of his own and is willing to challenge your decisions because he thinks he knows better than you. When he can't get his own way, his temper will start to rise. Your child completely believes that he shouldn't be told by anyone

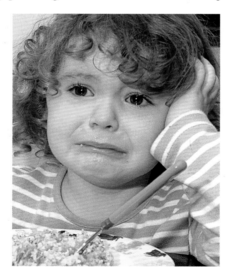

what to do, especially when he is enjoying himself doing something else.

Deal with it by standing your ground. Without losing your temper with your infuriatingly challenging preschooler, simply repeat that you want him to do what you asked. You can give him a brief explanation of why you want him to do this (for example, he should stop playing now because it is time to tidy up) but avoid a long discussion. If you allow him to ignore your request because he has a tantrum or is tearful, you'll soon discover that the frequency of his tears and outbursts increases. If he makes no attempt to do what you asked, lead him gently toward the task you asked him to complete. Praise him when he responds positively.

"I don't want to go to bed."

Life is so exciting for your preschooler that it is hardly surprising he wants to savor every precious waking minute. He enjoys bedtime and being tucked up under the sheets, but he'd still rather be awake for the time being. Refusal to go to bed usually happens when he is busy with an exciting activity or watching an interesting DVD.

You should be prepared to make an exception to his normal bedtime occasionally, but most times you'll tell him he has to go to bed now because he needs the sleep. If he resists and starts crying, take him to bed anyway. You can help minimize this flashpoint by having a predictable bedtime routine every evening (for instance, bath, pajamas, drink), giving him plenty of reminders that bedtime is fast approaching, making sure he only plays quietly or watches a short DVD shortly before, and by making bedtime interesting (for instance, by reading him a story before he goes to sleep).

"I don't want to go to nursery school."

As far as you are concerned, nursery school (or your child carer) is perfect for your child. He always enjoys himself there and talks excitedly about it when you pick him up. Yet he can be easily discouraged, perhaps by a small incident in which he was mildly reprimanded or if he has a minor argument with one of the other children there.

You should tell him that he is going anyway, but add that you are surprised he doesn't want to go because he likes it there so much. Listen to what he says in response. Sometimes a child this age isn't able to verbalize his feelings clearly so he might not be able to say why he is reluctant to go. See if you can discover what's troubling him by talking it through with him. Certainly you should speak to the nursery school staff (or his carer) and explain his reluctance to attend. Ask them if something has happened to unsettle him recently. Even if there is nothing obvious, it's good for you and them to keep an extra close watch on your child for the next few days.

"I want that toy."

Children have an insatiable desire for new and interesting toys. No matter how many toys your child already has, or how many he gets as presents, there will always be something else he desires. He sees new toys on television, at his friends' homes, or when he goes shopping with you. He is as much a consumer as you are.

Pester power can be very strong, particularly if you are in a crowded supermarket with your preschooler and you fear that your refusal will result in an embarrassing tantrum or raging argument. However, be prepared to say "No, not on this occasion." Like it or not, your child has to learn that you have limited resources and that he can't have everything he wants. Point out to him all the wonderful toys he has already, many of which he probably hasn't actually touched in months. In addition, suggest to him that he could ask for that

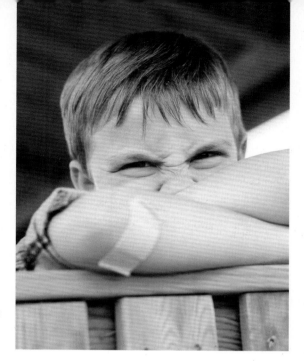

toy for his birthday or another present-giving occasion; by that time he may lose interest anyway.

"I can't do that."

You will know what your preschooler is capable of, so you are certain to be surprised when, say, he won't try a new jigsaw because he insists it will be too difficult. There will be times when your child will have a crisis of confidence because he fears that a challenge facing him is beyond his ability. He will prefer to refuse to attempt it at all, than to try it and fail.

Reassure your child that whatever activity he backs away from (the jigsaw, for example), he will be able to do it. Remind your child that he has solved similar puzzles in the past and point out that you won't be annoyed or angry with him if it turns out to be too difficult for him. To get him started, you could also offer to share the challenge jointly, giving him occasional help when necessary to enable him to move onto the next stage. Explain that you can't do everything you try, and that you just want him to do his best. You'll be happy as long as he makes an effort, rather than giving up before he starts.

3 YEARS OLD

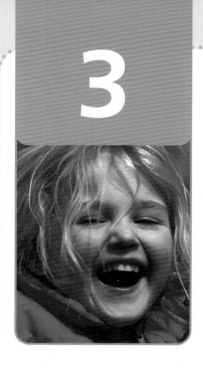

✓ *happy*
✓ *loving*
✓ *giving*
✓ *eager to please*

Your turbulent two-year-old matures into a more relaxed three-year-old—a child who is a better master of his abilities, more eager to share and to learn from others, and calmer emotionally. He's learning a lot and his challenge is to make sense of new things—real or imagined—which may explain why he may be prone to fears (of the dark, for example). His newfound awareness of things can lead to rapid changes of mood or may be expressed as physical and emotional sensations—he may suffer from a tummy ache if told off or become excited and run wild when given a gift.

Language becomes increasingly important and your child will love to talk with you—and often to himself. If you want to know what he is thinking and feeling, it's a good idea to listen to him or perhaps ask him to tell you a story. Much of his conversation is self-initiated—calling attention to himself or asking questions or for information—but he may occasionally respond to something you ask him. He will know his name and be able to repeat it, and it is also a good thing for him to learn to repeat his address. His command of

language should be sufficient so that he is able to express his thoughts, wants, and needs but, if not, he'll be prone to whine. He will be able to use time concepts such as "yesterday" and also times of day, and can learn some numbers. He will also know the difference between large and small, singular and plural, and can identify colors and match shapes. He'll begin to name items in books but he also will use language in "silly" ways, such as repeating funny, made-up words or deliberately mispronouncing them.

Physically, he is more sure of himself when walking and running and riding a tricycle or scooter. This sureness with motion means he very often moves with abandon so it's important to make sure he doesn't become overtired and exhausted. He will love playing outdoors. His hand–eye coordination is much improved and he is better able to build clay models and work with blocks, draw and paint within boundaries, and perform the fine movements necessary for self-help skills; he should be more adept with his fork, pour from a pitcher using two hands, be able to button and unbutton his clothing when dressing and undressing, and wash and dry his hands. He can probably go to the bathroom by himself and wipe himself. Though he will be clean and dry most of the time, there will be plenty of accidents. His increased skills, and his liking to do things unaided, means he can assist you by putting away his toys and clothes and helping to set the table; he even may be able to pour out his own cereal. Make chores fun and when he does well, praise him afterward; if helping becomes routine at this age, there will be less resistance to doing so when he is older.

He enjoys playing with others—both real children and imaginary friends. With friends, he is beginning to play with them instead of, as previously, alongside them, and is starting to share some (less treasured) possessions. He may understand that he has to take turns on the swings or slide and acknowledge that others also have feelings. His happiest times, however, will still be with his parents—just being close to them as well as helping them with tasks, accompanying them to go shopping, and playing with them.

Play at this time also becomes more imaginative whether it involves dolls or role-playing games. Books and music should also feature largely in your child's daily life. Your child may want to hear the same story read over and over again (with no changes) and may occasionally "read" to himself. Music can be the accompaniment to more active play as well as self-created rather than just something to listen to or sing along with.

He will generally adhere to family "rules" but as far as routines are concerned, keeping your child in bed can become something of a challenge as can mealtimes if your child starts to develop fussiness over food—although most three-year-olds eat anything and everything.

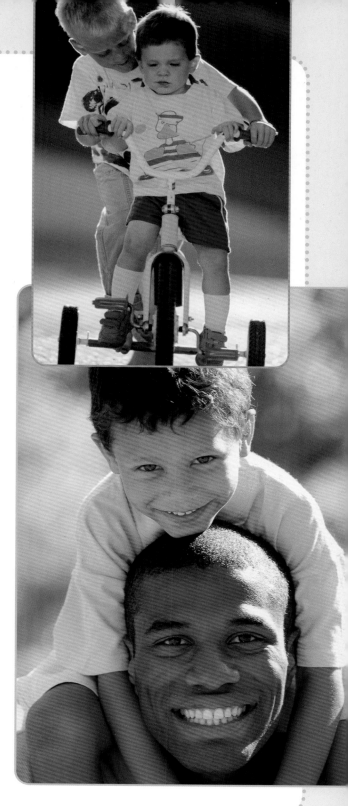

3½ YEARS OLD

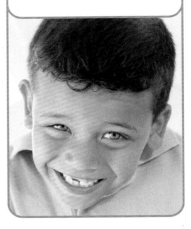

✔ *rebellious*
✔ *determined*
✔ *inconsistent*
✔ *anxious*

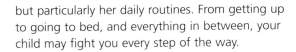

While six months previously, your child was calm and conforming, a sea change is occurring and insecurity will replace stability. She becomes hard to please and hard on the person who tries to please her. She is also struggling emotionally because she wants to be mistress of her surroundings but doubts her ability to do so, and this leads to frequent battles over almost anything but particularly her daily routines. From getting up to going to bed, and everything in between, your child may fight you every step of the way.

Parenting a three-and-a-half-year-old can be tough, so it's extra important for your child to feel loved and appreciated even when you find it most difficult to handle her. Your child is mainly interested in provoking you, as her chief carer, rather than adults in general, so it can be a good idea to have her attend nursery school or be with a child carer some of the time, particularly if you're going shopping or doing errands. When she is in a good mood, make the most of it by talking and playing together. She will commonly be beset by fears and anxieties and feel timid. Instead of belittling her worries, take care of her emotional fragility by giving her "weapons" to combat them or by suggesting alternative activities when she refuses to budge. Distraction rather than confrontation should be your aim.

The reason for all this turbulence and trouble is normal disequilibrium, brought on by a marked

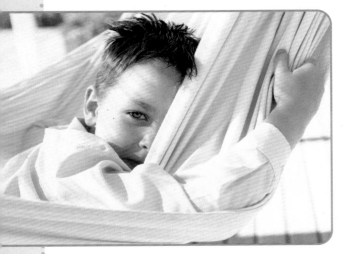

spurt in development that can prove too strong for your preschooler to control. Such a lack of control can prove unsettling and can be exacerbated by a desire to dominate, so that your child becomes prey to a great deal of stress and strain. Even though she can speak more fluently and effectively, she often may stutter; when she walks, she may stumble or fall; and when she manipulates items, she can tremble and be uncoordinated. She will be quicker and more vigorous in her actions but this can mean she may all too easily burst into tears when things don't go her way or swipe another child's toy from under his nose. Whining and tension-relieving actions such as nail biting, thumb sucking, nose picking, etc., become more prevalent.

But the developmental changes at the bottom of her insecurity mean that in spite of her frequent ineptness, she will be more active and willing to challenge herself. She'll be more skilled and effective in physical activities, such as jumping and balancing, riding a scooter, and reproducing drawings or models based on a pattern (instead of copying what you do). She can string beads or dry pasta and arrange them by color and shape.

Language becomes more advanced and she frequently asks questions, can follow more complex directions more accurately (discriminating between under and over, beside and between, for example), and uses language in her play. She can also use her voice to express emotions, hence she will whine when anxious or whisper when fearful, and has many ways of saying "No."

Your child will be happy to play in small groups and will become much more interested in her playmates. While there will be more cooperative play—more sharing, more give and take, less arguing—there will also be more excluding. In fact, your child's "group" can define itself by those whom it won't allow in! Your child and her friends will find shared humor in accidents, incongruous behavior, or by being aggressive.

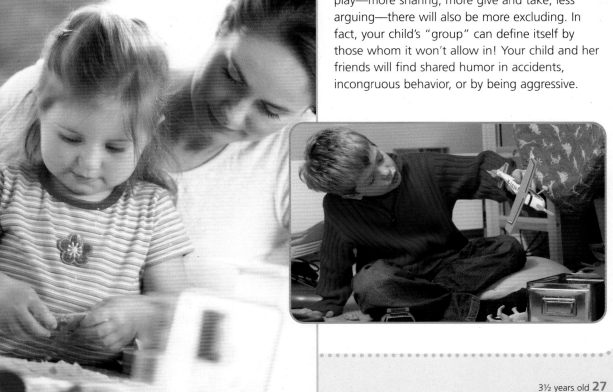

4 YEARS OLD

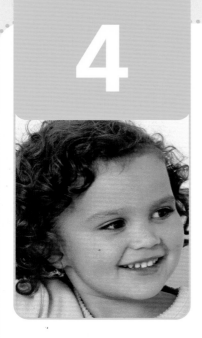

✓ *exuberant*
✓ *adventure-loving*
✓ *emotional*
✓ *imaginative*

The average four-year-old can best be described as "wild and wonderful." She is excited by the new—people, places, games, playthings, and activities —but along with versatility, demonstrates extreme emotions. A child of four has great drive and a fluid imagination.

Your four-year-old will be constantly in motion—hopping, jumping, running, or trying out new stunts—both indoors and out. Her fine motor abilities have strengthened and she enjoys playing games that require complex motor skills, such as activities in which she has to manipulate many small pieces, such as constructing models out of Lego®. She can draw, color, and paint with more detail, using her whole arm to do so, and should be able to dress and undress with very little help.

All fours love to talk loudly or in a whisper and do so constantly. Your child will probably be better at talking than listening; for example, she will ask many questions, but will not be interested in long answers. Her exuberance and liking for all things new will manifest itself in language by her use of big words and her liking for silly sounds and nonsense rhymes, while her emotionality reveals itself in name-calling, swearing, boasting, being a tattletale, and talking back. She demonstrates imagination by telling tales but, in fact, has trouble distinguishing fact from fantasy.

Her memory skills have increased, so not only can she talk about something that happened in the past—a movie she saw and enjoyed—she will also enjoy counting by rote (probably up to 20), repeats nursery rhymes with few mistakes, and, if taught, will know her address along with her full name. She is beginning to understand the concept of numbers and certain grammatical patterns.

Her vivid imagination is also displayed in dramatic play—she loves pretending she's in a dangerous situation—and she relishes scary fairy tales. She remains an avid reader, particularly of humorous books but now appreciates those with complex illustrations. She enjoys playtime with other children, and is most interested in simple games and activities that combine singing and

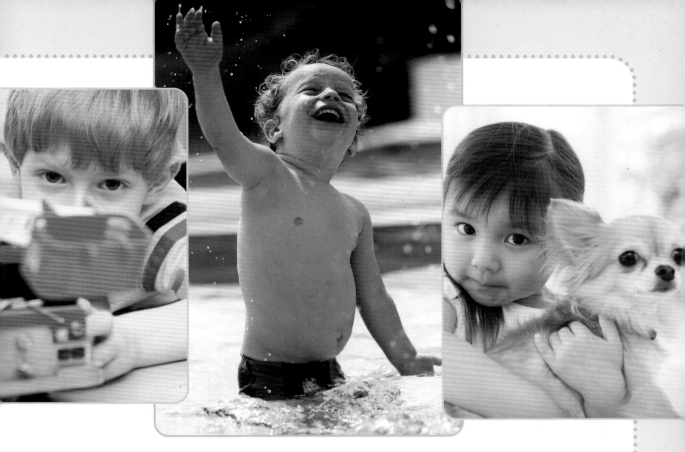

movement. She plays cooperatively, though she often changes the rules. While joining in with others' laughter, she also will cry loudly and may hit, kick, or spit when things don't go her way.

In addition to her liking for silly sounds and rhymes, she also demonstrates a sense of humor in her activities along with greater sensitivity to the feelings of others. She tries to figure out what is the "right" and "wrong" way to act.

Four-year-olds enjoy new adventures, so make the most of this characteristic by both creating and sharing adventures with her. Plan excursions and activities that will interest her (a science or wildlife learning museum with hands-on activities will be preferred over an art exhibit) and encourage her to point out things of interest en route. Show her you enjoy her exaggerated stories or silly rhymes by offering ones of your own.

It's important not to worry too much about your child's overall exuberance—even if she occasionally goes out of bounds. This is totally natural for this age. Instead, make every effort to enjoy your amusing, lively, and enthusiastic preschooler, even if you don't approve of everything she says and does (and don't blame behavior that you don't like—exhibitionism, bad language, sex play, etc.—on her playmates!).

Nor should you try too hard to motivate her if she becomes uninterested or inactive, or feel you can increase her intellectual abilities—these are things that come naturally with maturity or are inborn. By all means provide books and stimulating activities but don't force her to make use of them. Even if she is still sucking her thumb or wetting her bed, this may not be the time to try and put them to an end; she may need a few months' more maturation for them to stop naturally.

4½ YEARS OLD

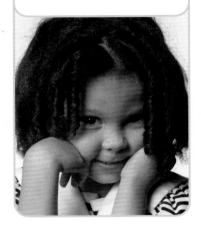

- ✓ *unpredictable*
- ✓ *confused*
- ✓ *demanding*
- ✓ *reality-based*

In maturing from four to five, children appear a little confused and highly unpredictable as they move into a stage of fitting things together. In particular, you will find that your child is now more demanding and is less easily shifted than he was six months previously. Instead of being distracted with humor when he insists on having something he's not permitted, he may become obnoxious, make faces, and stick out his tongue. But in many other ways, he is quieter (though still physically active he has calm periods), becoming better able to withstand frustration although he will still be highly emotional. Very often, having just had a good laugh at something, he will become suddenly tearful.

Your child will love learning new information— and this is the top age for questions. He'll endlessly ask you "why" and "how," not only to gain knowledge, but just to keep the conversation going—and occasionally to be obstructive. He will demonstrate a strong interest in whether things, such as stories in books or that you tell him, are real or not and this is because he is beginning to differentiate fantasy from reality. He may even become scared by same kind of wild stories he loved at the age of four.

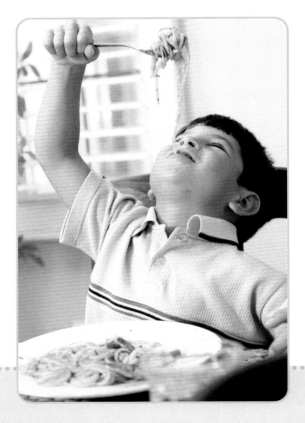

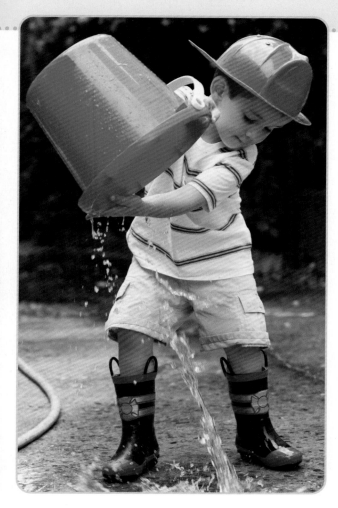

while others may be very willing to follow another child or have intense likes for a particular friend. Even though your child will continue with imaginative play, he will prefer reality in his activities, often suggesting the use of real objects—"Let's put some windows on the house"—when's he's constructing things.

He's also likely to cooperate more with family members, if he's not feeling overly challenged or rushed, and is less likely to push limits. He may even set the table, if asked. At 4½, a child is becoming aware of authority—you may see some fear as well as intentness in his expression when you reprimand him—so bargaining can prove an effective ploy in changing behavior. You give a little and your child may be willing and able to give a little in return. Moreover, you can appeal to his sense of adventure by suggesting a change in routine; if he absolutely refuses to eat his lunch, you can occasionally allow him to have his dessert first (as long as its something healthy). This is an age when praise and compliments work wonders, so feel free to compliment your child extravagantly when he does something well.

Although it's a good idea at any age to avoid situations that you know will be troublesome, it's particularly relevant now. One example is telephone conversations or texting; children of this age hate it when their parents spend "hours" on the phone and generally respond by behaving badly, and invariably they end up being yelled at and possibly punished. It's therefore better if long, chatty phone calls and texting are restricted to times when your child is busily engaged doing something else or is out of the room. Your child loves to talk, and he mainly likes talking to you and having your full attention. Talking to him will ensure that you know what's on your child's mind, and it's this that can help you get through the day.

Self-motivation is more evident and he'll need less adult supervision with tasks; in fact, he'll demand his independence. As well as gathering new information, he will perfect old skills, tending to stay on task with activities that he likes better than before, though his unpredictability is evident in the lack of interest he shows in expanding his skills. He will, however, like to call attention—often dramatically—to his own performance.

Your 4½-year-old considers friends very important and is starting to play collaboratively, although his level of cooperation is unpredictable. At this age, some children demonstrate leadership capabilities

5 YEARS OLD

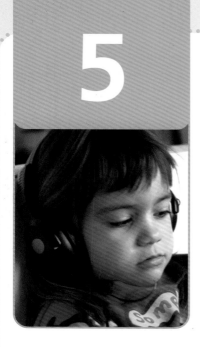

✓ *equable*
✓ *calm*
✓ *anxious to please*
✓ *serious*

A preschooler of this age understands the world better and more accurately judges what he can and cannot do, but is determined that everything he does, he does just right. While your child will not be particularly adventurous, the pleasure he takes in learning will be immense and he will enjoy practicing skills and abilities. He is eager to please and wants things to go smoothly. This makes him a much easier playmate—though best with a child his own age—and more independent in terms of personal care skills. So, for parents, a five-year-old is a joy to be around and for many, it will be one of the most rewarding periods in their entire relationship with their child.

A five-year-old enjoys being at home, around his mother, having his own room, and living in a familiar neighborhood. (If attending nursery school, he'll be very fond of any playgroup leader or teacher, be generally obedient when he's with him or her, and often will tell you what he or she says.) He tends to concentrate on the present (not past or future), liking life the way it is, feeling good about himself and his parents and any

siblings and grandparents. For a five-year-old, parents are the ultimate authorities. That being said, your child will also be adaptable to change, so will be good with unfamiliar people, places, food, and activities. He tends to love life and everything that is a part of it. It's not surprising then that five-year-olds are strong believers: God, Santa Claus, and even the Easter Bunny figure large in their world. If asked where one of the above lives, your child will come up with a concrete destination and when he writes his Christmas wishlist, your child expects to receive what he asks for. A birthday party, too, is very important at this age.

Intellectually, your preschooler will demonstrate great competence in learning languages. He shows interest in new words and has an extensive vocabulary. He now asks questions—how, when, what, and why—to seek information and unlike his four-year-old self, will be content with longer answers. He'll enjoy spelling out signs and words in books. He's starting to figure out things for himself and thus begins to make generalizations

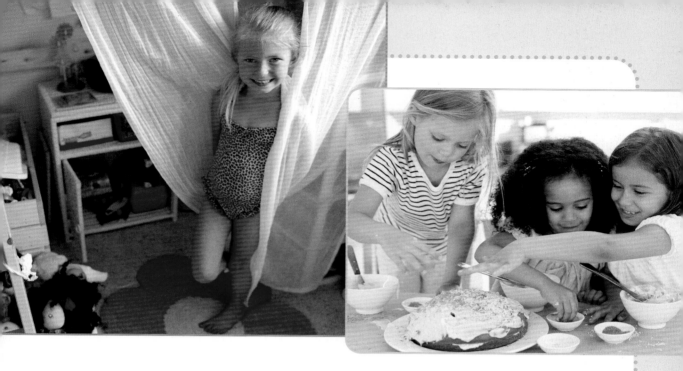

(even if based on inadequate evidence). More and more, he exhibits creative and constructive abilities and enjoys hands-on learning. All these factors are important in determining his readiness for school. Parents can nurture creativity in a five-year-old, not only by providing artistic materials, musical instruments, and puppets, but through games like "20 Questions" and activities that require a child to figure out common problems—for example, new uses for everyday items such as paperclips, a way to group disparate items, or how to share out an uneven amount of money or candy.

Physical play will be an important part of your child's life. Having greater control of his movements and well developed gross motor skills, such as skipping, jumping, and climbing, he's able to confidently enjoy playground equipment without a lot of parental guidance. His improved manipulative skills in cutting, tracing, pasting, and stringing are evident in many of the creative activities he most enjoys. However, he is more interested in solving problems at this stage than engaging in imaginative play, though playing

house is an activity enjoyed by both boys and girls. Books and reading are one of your child's great pleasures, particularly stories that can add to his learning or contain puzzles he can work out.

Five-year-olds can appear more accomplished (compared to their younger selves). They can carry out a great many commands, do simple errands, and are more aware of time and when certain activities, such as eating, watching TV, or going to bed occur. Many can count and some can even read and/or print their name. If taught, your child should know his name, age, address, and birthday. These, moreover, are some of the things that are vital in considering readiness for school.

Though gentle, compliant, and eager to please, your five-year-old won't find it easy to admit the occasional wrongdoing. Because of his desire to be good and to do the right thing, you may be surprised if he occasionally lies or to can't resist taking another's belongings.

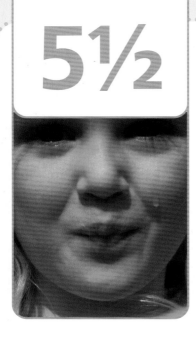

5½ YEARS OLD

✓ *hesitant*
✓ *dawdling*
✓ *combative*
✓ *disobedient*

Going on six can appear to be in a constant state of tension with behavior characterized by opposite extremes such as happy/sad, quiet/loud, or agreeable/defiant. Your child will be more restless and less composed than previously, finding sitting still increasingly difficult. She will have problems making decisions and transitions, will play well one moment but argue the next and will feel torn between choices (she'll often try to choose both play or activity options). She may be shy one minute and bold the next or turn from very affectionate to antagonistic without warning. She will complain readily and disobey often. If she lacks the courage to outwardly defy you, she will dawdle, which amounts to the same thing in that whatever you want her to do will very often not get done. It's important, however, to understand that your child is processing a lot of information and new expectations, and what may look like defiance may actually be her simply being focused on an activity, and lacking the self-regulation to pull herself away and move on to something else. In other words, she may simply be too engrossed in an activity to hear you. On the other hand, particularly if she's started school, her growing involvement with a peer group, and the support she feels in being part of one, can cause her to be challenging.

Your child is still young, and while she may resort to tantrums and meltdowns, she's working on her self-control and self-discipline. Make sure that you

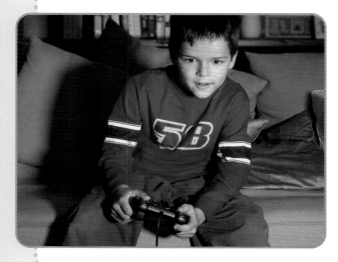

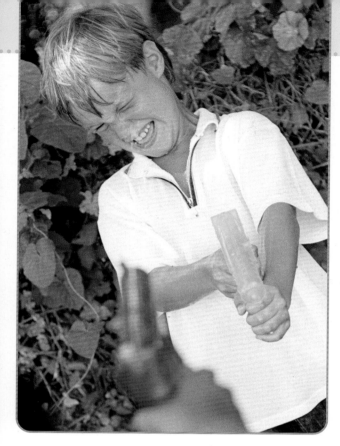

She also will test limits to see how far she can go. In addition to talking back, she may assert food preferences suddenly deciding that she will no longer eat "red" vegetables or only raw tomatoes cut into slices not cooked ones or will have peanut butter sandwiches at every meal. Strong likes or dislikes can also extend to other categories, such as particular garments or activities.

Your child will use more diverse and complex language but if verbalizing freely, her stories or songs may contain hints of hidden violence or dark thoughts—aggression or accidents. Over the past six months, her reading ability is likely to have improved markedly and she should know all the letters of the alphabet and read simple signs and books. She should be able to print her name and count to 20 with few mistakes.

She is now able to express her thoughts and feelings and to understand what you may be feeling and take that into account, even trying to give comfort and express sympathy when she encounters someone who has been hurt. But she also knows that she can hide her thoughts and feelings from you so starts to have secrets. Thanks to an emerging sense of right and wrong, she will be prone to tattle on others.

Your child's sense of independence is developing and she should be able to amuse herself for extended periods. She can look through a book by herself, play a game with her dolls, or watch TV alone. Increasingly she may disappear to her room. She has mastered a great many self-help actions, like being able to dress and feed herself, but may only extend herself if encouraged; otherwise she may passively wait for you to do up her buttons or brush her hair. If she's in a good mood, she may be willing to perform some simple household tasks like putting her laundry away or setting the table.

understand the cause of her being defiant, disrespectful, or acting out in anger. There may be an understandable reason or mitigating factors, such as a change in her routines or in the household. If she is starting "real" school, for example, she may be suffering from separation anxiety, or worried about interacting with new and unfamiliar peers and teachers. She may have trouble adapting to a classroom environment where she has to pay attention, follow directions, and sit still for long periods of time.

There will be physical manifestations of her lack of equilibrium. She may suffer from aches and pains, won't be able to sit still for long periods, may lack fluidity in movements, and reverse numbers and letters. She may start to show an increase in tensional outlets, such as nail biting, pencil chewing, or hair pulling, which also may be because of starting school and finding it difficult.

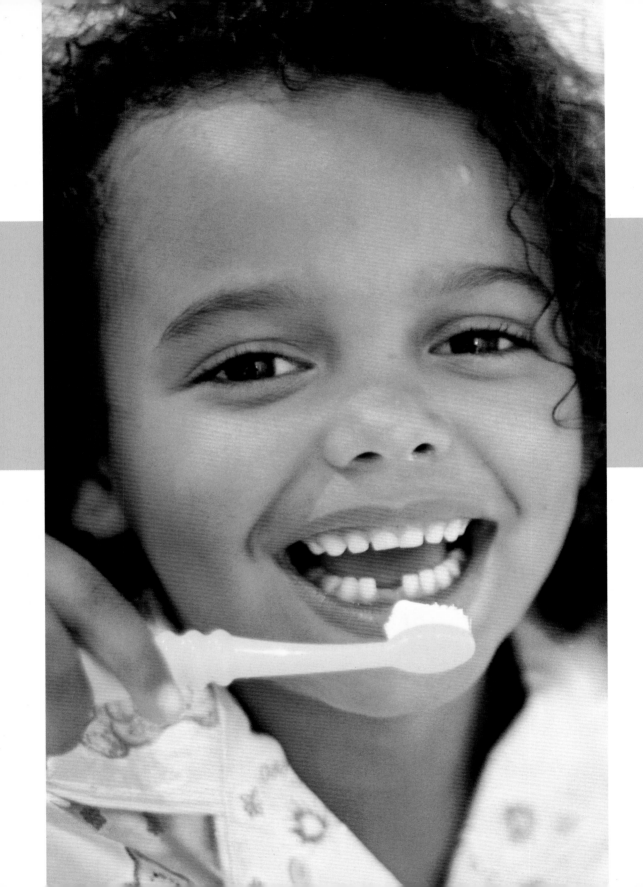

CHAPTER 2
DAILY CARE

Though your preschooler will begin to manage many of the tasks himself, you still have to devote time to making sure he eats well, is appropriately dressed, pays attention to hygiene matters including brushing his teeth and hair, keeps active, and goes to bed happily. You'll also want to ensure that he has lots of time to play—by himself and with others—as well as opportunities to learn about the outside world.

Nutritional needs

Good nutrition combined with healthy eating habits developed during the preschool years will lay the building blocks for future good health. A balanced diet ensures that your child's nutritional needs for energy and growth are met. A good diet also helps protect your child against illness and infection, and aids his mental development and ability to learn.

Your preschooler needs to eat easily digestible and nutrient-rich foods from the four food groups shown below. In addition to his three regular meals, foods from the different groups can be given as his two-to-three daily snacks. Refined sugars should be avoided. If your child regularly eats something from each of the main food groups, he is likely to get all the nutrients (protein, carbohydrate, fat, vitamins, and minerals) he requires for good health.

Calories

Preschool is a time of growth and change for your child; he is developing mentally and physically and needs sufficient calories to grow while not eating so many that he becomes overweight. How many calories he needs depends on his age, activity level and gender. Three-year-olds of both genders need between 1,000 and 1,400 calories per day, with sedentary children requiring 1,000 to 1,200 calories, and active children needing 1,000 to 1,400 calories. From the age of four, sedentary girls and boys need

THE FOUR MAIN FOOD GROUPS

PROTEIN FOODS
Aim for three daily servings of meat, poultry, fish, or egg or plant sources such as nuts, legumes, or beans.

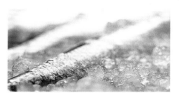

DAIRY PRODUCTS
Aim for at least 1½ cups fat-free or low-fat milk daily or two servings of reduced-fat cheese or fat-free yogurt.

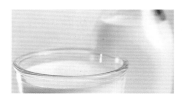

VEGETABLES AND FRUIT
Aim for at least two servings of vegetables and three of fruit daily—fresh, canned, or frozen. (Fruit will provide your child with more energy than vegetables.) Fruit juice should count as only one serving even if given more than once.

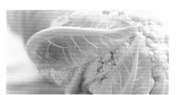

GRAIN PRODUCTS AND STARCHY FOODS
Aim for at least one serving (and preferably two) each mealtime of bread, corn, rice, cereal grains, or starchy vegetables. Make several of the servings whole-grain products, but avoid very coarse ones.

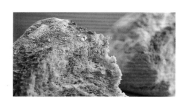

1,200 to 1,400 calories daily. Active girls need from 1,400 to 1,800 calories per day while active boys require 1,600 to 2,000 calories daily.

Portion size

A young child's serving is usually one-quarter to one-third of an adult's. With fruit and vegetables, an easy way to judge a portion is to think of it in relation to your child's hand. A portion at any age is what will fit inside. But if you are looking for a general guideline, ¼ to ½ cup will do for most foods. For protein foods, one ounce of meat, fish, or poultry; two tablespoons peanut butter or ½ egg are each a serving.

Snacks

Preschoolers need to have snacks in addition to their regular meals in order to get the nutrients and calories they need (see also page 47). Snack time may be a good time to introduce new foods. Many times children will refuse food at mealtime, but accept them at snack time.

How much fiber?

Some fiber is necessary in your child's diet to prevent constipation, but too much may fill him up so that he does not want other foods. A high-fiber diet may also lead to diarrhea and can interfere with the absorption of minerals such as iron.

If your child eats a variety of whole grains and fruits and vegetables daily, or a combination of refined and whole-grain types of bread and breakfast cereals, he is likely to be getting enough fiber.

Should he eat fats?

Fat is a concentrated source of energy and vitamins for young children and also provides essential fatty acids. It is best that your child obtains most of his fat from foods such as low-fat milk, oily fish, eggs, nuts, and seeds, which also contain other essential nutrients. Foods like potato chips and cookies may be high in fat but they are poor in other nutrients, so should be limited. Meat should be lean. Children over age two should drink fat-free or low-fat milk. If in doubt, ask your doctor or pediatrician for advice.

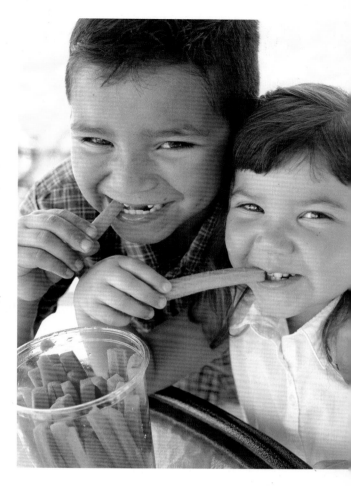

Vitamin and mineral supplements

The American Academy of Pediatrics recommends that some children receive a daily vitamin and mineral supplement up to the age of five. Over-the-counter supplements are generally safe, but only give the dose recommended by the manufacturer—too much can be as dangerous as too little. Chewable tablets or drops are available for children who have difficulty swallowing pills. Seek advice from your healthcare provider.

Iron and zinc requirements

An iron deficiency can slow down your child's growth and development. Try to give him some foods containing iron every day. Good sources of iron include red meat, oily fish (such as canned sardines), shellfish, fortified breakfast cereals, bread, eggs, dried fruits (such as raisins, apricots, and dates), beans and legumes (such as canned baked beans, pinto beans, chickpeas, and lentils), oranges, apricots, green peas, and dark leafy greens (such as cabbage and broccoli). Liver, including paté, although a rich source of iron should only be given to children once a week because it is very rich in vitamin A, too much of which can be harmful. To increase iron absorption give a small glass of fruit juice or some food containing vitamin C at every meal.

Zinc is necessary for a healthy immune system and for growth. Good sources include meat and poultry, whole-grain cereals, zinc-fortified cereals, hard cheese, eggs, legumes, and beans.

Water and other fluids

Most children don't drink enough fluids, but decent hydration is just as important as a good balanced diet. A 2 percent loss in body fluids, for example, can cause a 20 percent reduction in both physical and mental performance. Choose from tapwater, diluted fresh fruit juice, or skim milk. Avoid carbonated sugary drinks.

The amount of fluid a child needs depends on age and weight but, as a rough guide, the average three- to six-year-old should drink around five 8-ounce glasses a day. A child who does not drink enough may experience headaches, lethargy, poor concentration, and constipation. Dehydration also

SPOILED FOR CHOICE

The greater the variety of fruit and vegetables your child eats, the wider range of nutrients he will get. Choose fruit and vegetables from the various color groups and try to offer them in different guises: raw, steamed, or stir-fried, or in stews, sauces, or soups.

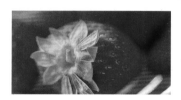

RED
Tomatoes, strawberries, sweet bell peppers, raspberries, red currants, apples, grapes, watermelon, cherries, radishes, rhubarb

ORANGE
Carrots, sweet bell peppers, pumpkin, turnips, squash, sweet potato, oranges, clementines, melon, nectarines, apricots

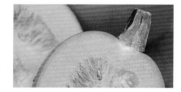

YELLOW
Bananas, zucchini, sweet bell peppers, summer squash, bean sprouts, corn, pineapple, plums

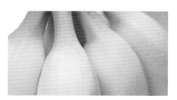

GREEN
Broccoli, Brussels sprouts, cabbage, green snap beans, avocado, apples, pears, salad greens, spinach, peas, kiwifruit

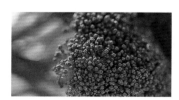

PURPLE
Berries, eggplant, figs, plums, beets, red cabbage

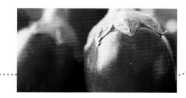

affects the body's ability to transport essential nutrients throughout the body and brain.

What to avoid

While it can be hard to be a food "policeman," it's important that you monitor your child's diet and make sure that you cut out or reduce the following.

Refined sugar

Processed foods such as candies, cakes, cookies, pastries, and sweetened breakfast cereals are high in refined sugar, which has little or no nutritional value and can result in tooth decay and weight gain. Eating sugary food leads to a temporary surge in blood-glucose levels, resulting in a rush of energy (think of kids at a birthday party), which is promptly followed by a slump or sugar-low (tears and tantrums as guests go home). This fluctuation produces an inconsistent supply of energy to the brain, leading to poor concentration and attention span, irritability, and fatigue. Sugary foods, such as doughnuts, cookies, pastries, and candy bars, often also include a fair amount of fat, which increases the risk of disease (see below).

Consuming large amounts of sugar may inhibit the assimilation of certain nutrients, suppress the immune system, and lead to glucose intolerance, which means the body has problems regulating blood-sugar levels.

Junk food

Highly processed and usually full of salt, sugar, sweeteners, additives (artificial colors, preservatives, and flavorings), and fat, these manufactured foods lack nutritional value. They also tend to be high in saturated and hydrogenated fats, or "trans" fats, which slow down digestive, circulatory, and mental processes and clog the arteries, increasing the risk of disease.

Caffeine and carbonated drinks

As well as being found in coffee and tea, caffeine is present in chocolate—a single bar can contain up to 50 mg—and in some carbonated drinks, like cola. Caffeine is a stimulant and diuretic and can cause mood swings since it affects the body's ability to

control blood-sugar levels. It also depletes the body of some B vitamins and such minerals as zinc, potassium, calcium, and iron.

Sweet, fizzy drinks contain added sugar, artificial coloring, artificial sweeteners, caffeine, and preservatives. They also are high in the mineral phosphorus, which inhibits calcium absorption.

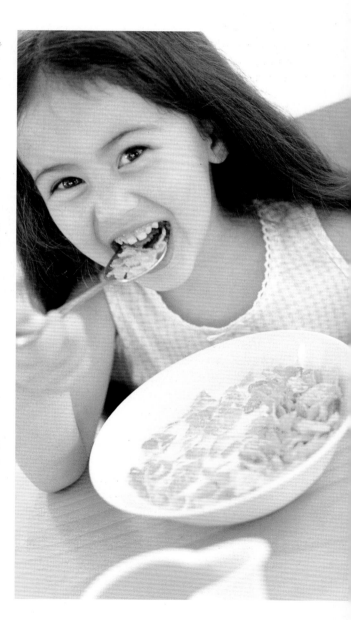

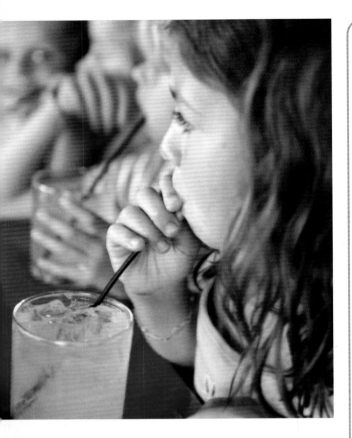

Additives and preservatives

A number of substances are routinely added to manufactured food. ("E" stands for "Europe" but some have also been approved for use in the USA):

◆ Antioxidants (E300–321) prevent food from turning rancid;
◆ Colorings (E100–180) add or intensify color;
◆ Emulsifiers, stabilizers, thickeners, and gelling agents (E322–495) affect the texture of food and bind ingredients together;
◆ Flavor enhancers (E620–635) enhance the taste or smell of a food;
◆ Preservatives (E200–283) prevent and slow down deterioration in food. Any processed food with a long shelf-life is likely to include preservatives.

According to research, additives may adversely affect one in seven children. Young children are especially vulnerable since their systems are immature and they are more exposed to them. While not all additives are potentially harmful, some, such as the orange food coloring tartrazine [E102], have been linked to hyperactivity in sensitive children as well as being the potential cause of allergies, poor memory, depression, and mood swings. The US government requires tartrazine to be declared on food and drug products, so check the label. In fact, most additives and preservatives are listed on labels, enabling you to avoid flavor enhancers, colorings, and preservatives (see box). If you are concerned your child reacts adversely to additives (he has temper tantrums or otherwise behaves disruptively), keep a food diary and monitor his behavior over a period of time before contacting your healthcare provider.

Managing mealtimes

It's not just what children eat that matters but when. Young children are particularly vulnerable to dips in blood-sugar levels, which can lead to mood swings, irritability, and poor attention. Regular healthy meals, supplemented by nutritious snacks and sufficient fluids, are crucial throughout the day to maintain steady blood-sugar levels, ensuring mental clarity, sustained energy levels, and concentration.

Children have very high daily requirements for energy (calories) and other nutrients, but their stomach is still small. This means they cannot eat large amounts all at one sitting. Preschoolers, therefore, need three main meals a day with nourishing snacks in between.

Appetites and tastes

Young children also have different appetites; some eat like birds, picking at everything that's put in front of them; some eat moderate amounts of foods without too much fuss and others wolf down everything on their plate, providing it is of their choosing.

Like adults, children also have their own likes and dislikes when it comes to food, so it is quite possible that there are some foods your child will refuse just because he doesn't like them.

Research shows that children acquire a taste for foods over time, and it takes an average of 10 "tastes" for a child to accept new foods. The theory is that if you can persuade your child to eat just a single mouthful of spinach on 10 occasions, he will learn to like it.

You can also try combining foods you know your child likes with ones previously untried or rejected; you may find that new combinations are enough to encourage your child to try new things. If, however, your child refuses to eat something, and you are unable to persuade him otherwise, take the food away but don't offer an alternative. This may be difficult, but it's important that your child gets used to eating what he is given and not to expect endless alternatives if he doesn't like the first option.

It's also worth remembering that flavors and textures can affect your child—even changing brands can turn him off a certain food. But don't fall into the trap of believing your child prefers bland or so-called "children's food"; many children like strong flavors and will happily try curries, stir-fries, chiles, and similar foods.

To make your child more enthusiastic about mealtimes, it can be effective to give him a sense of control over what he eats. Try to include him in your meal planning, for example, starting with the trip around the supermarket and maybe involving him in the preparation of a meal.

Expect your child's appetite to fluctuate or almost disappear at times. He will go through phases that are affected by things such as growth spurts, moods, even

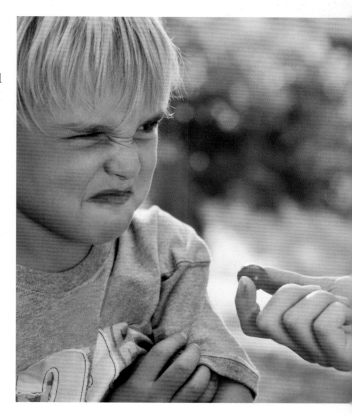

changes in the weather. He may get "stuck" on a certain food, refusing to eat anything else, and then without apparent reason reject it. It is easy to worry about this type of pickiness, but it doesn't necessarily mean your child is not getting the proper nutrition. As long as your child eats a well balanced diet over a period of time, is healthy, and is growing well, the fact that he may only pick at certain foods on a given day, should not be a cause for concern.

Persuading your child to eat

Don't overwhelm your child with large portions or too many choices—he may find them frightening. Instead, offer small amounts of a few different foods in a child-sized bowl or plate. Serving a variety of foods will help keep your child interested. Food needs to look appealing too, so spend a little time on presentation and making food look appetizing.

You also need to pay attention to your child's liquid intake since too much may kill his appetite.

Structure mealtimes so that your child knows what is expected of him—that you want him to eat when you eat, for example, or stay at the table until he's finished. But don't force him to eat everything on his plate if he really doesn't want to.

It can be extremely frustrating if your child does not eat a meal that you have lovingly prepared, and trying to force your child to eat will be a no-win situation for you both. Children are remarkably clever at picking up on the anxieties of their parents and your child may well tune in to your own frustrations about his not eating. Conflict and tension will only to make the situation more difficult and may lead to your child using mealtimes as a way of seeking attention. Instead of becoming anxious, gently coax or encourage your child to try just a mouthful; sometimes this is enough for him to be persuaded to eat the rest of the meal. And even if he eats just the one mouthful, make sure you give him lots of praise.

6 ways to encourage good eating habits

1 **Resist the temptation to offer alternatives** and never use food as a reward or a bribe, or refuse to give it as a punishment—this can encourage an unhealthy attitude toward food.

2 **Don't get hung up on good table manners.** Your child will almost certainly continue to make a mess when he eats. While ideally you would always like him to eat with a fork or spoon, don't be upset if he uses his fingers or hands, holds his utensils the wrong way, or spills things.

3 **Try to eat together as a family,** if only on the weekend. This will reinforce the notion that meals are social occasions and a time to discuss things. It's also a time to teach good eating habits, so make sure you finish up your green vegetables, too!

4 **Involve your child in food preparation.** One of the best ways to get your child interested in the food he eats is encourage him to help prepare his meals. He could arrange salad ingredients, portion out the sausages, or pour some cereal into a bowl.

5 **Apply some peer pressure.** Children often learn by example and if your child sees his friends eating up, it may well encourage him to do the same. Invite one or more friends of your child whom you know to be good eaters over for supper.

6 **Use rewards, such as sticker charts.** These are simple and successful ways of encouraging children to try new foods, especially unfamiliar fruit and vegetables.

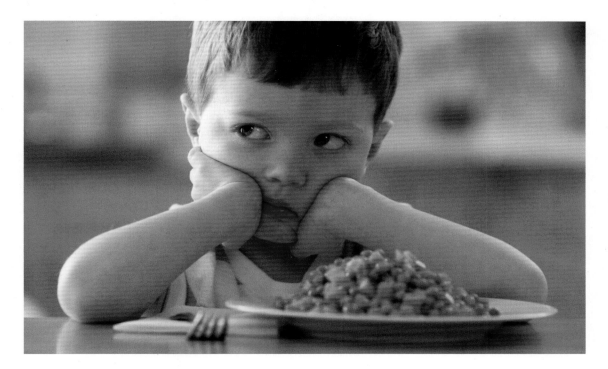

Problems at mealtimes

Feeding your young child may be fraught with problems and mealtimes can easily become a battleground. Parents have a built-in instinct to nourish their child, which can lead to feelings of failure if your attempts are rejected. Of course, your child is only concerned with how he feels that day.

Food refusal

Although there's been a huge increase in overweight children (see page 50), most parents cite food refusal as their biggest problem. Yet although parents will try everything to get a recalcitrant child to eat—persuasion, bribes, distraction, nagging, and threats—they are only encouraging the refusal. Coaxing a child to eat only compounds the problem and makes a preschooler ever more determined to continue to refuse food. He does so because in refusing food all attention is focused on him and he may even persuade his parents to give him just what he wants, even if it is unhealthy or inappropriate. Moreover, if a child is forced to eat foods he doesn't like, this can lead to him avoiding them for the rest of his life. And, if you talk openly about foods you

or your partner dislike or go too deeply into detail about how foods you serve your child are obtained or prepared, this may turn him off of them, especially if he has an active imagination.

If your child is a "poor eater," bear in mind that nothing is really wrong with his appetite nor will he ever starve if you don't make him eat. Instead, you need to desist immediately from all attempts to make him eat (even sidelong glances) and simply ignore his behavior at the table. Treat mealtimes with a casual attitude, neither being grateful if he eats something or angry if he doesn't. However, if he doesn't eat, make sure you don't give him any food between meals. He will learn very quickly, even if he refuses several meals in a row, that he will only get food at mealtimes.

Tantrums

All sorts of things can trigger tantrums during mealtimes. If your child is hungry he will get grumpy, just as adults do. Trying to make him eat food that he doesn't want, or not letting him have a food that he does want, will provoke a similar reaction. If you tell your child off for playing with

DAILY MEALS

Over the course of their preschool years, most children learn to eat what's prepared for the rest of the family—as long as it's not overly seasoned. While there's no harm in continuing with more "child-friendly" options, these tend to be bland and may make it difficult for your child to progress to more sophisticated choices.

BREAKFAST

It is now widely recognized that breakfast is the most important meal of the day; it should provide one-quarter of your child's daily nutrients. A good breakfast replenishes vital brain nutrients and blood-sugar (glucose) levels, which are depleted during sleep and also kick-starts the metabolism, which slows down overnight. Skipping the first meal of the day can lead to children developing an unhealthy pattern of snacking on high-fat, high-sugar foods. The body needs fuel on waking, so when it doesn't get the sustenance it needs, it switches to survival mode and only releases energy for emergencies. This means the body and brain are without the glucose they so badly need. So if your child displays a lack of concentration and poor memory, this indicates that he is struggling because of low "fuel" levels.

A breakfast of carbohydrates (cereal and toast, for example), which are fortified with vitamins and minerals, including the B vitamins and iron, helps with energy production. Carbohydrates also provide glucose, which is the main body fuel, while the milk poured over cereals is a good source of calcium, B-group vitamins, zinc, and magnesium.

A protein-based breakfast (eggs, milk, yogurt, beans, and fish), on the other hand, provides important nutrients and will satisfy your child's appetite more quickly and for longer than a breakfast solely of carbohydrates. The best policy, since the ideal ratio of protein to carbohydrate is unknown, is to make sure you include examples of both at breakfast.

LUNCH

This meal, too, should consist of both carbohydrate and protein foods. Protein will keep your child

---

BREAKFAST SELECTIONS

- Oatmeal with sliced banana
- Boiled or poached egg on wholewheat toast
- Low-sugar breakfast cereal with fruit and skim milk
- Fresh fruit smoothie
- Yogurt with fruit
- Baked beans on wholewheat toast
- Broiled tomato and bacon or sausages with wholewheat toast
- Pancakes made with wholewheat flour, topped with fruit
- Wholewheat muffin or bread with low-sugar jam or low-salt peanut butter

---

LUNCH SELECTIONS

- Lean meat or ground poultry patty
- Cheese omelet
- Mini quiche
- Mixed rice and vegetables
- Home-made sausage rolls
- Falafel in pita
- Poached or broiled fish or fish sticks
- Pasta and tomato sauce
- Tuna fish or sliced chicken sandwich

SUPPER SELECTIONS

- Meat pie or fish pie with a crust of mashed potatoes
- Macaroni and cheese
- Pork and vegetable stir-fry
- Salmon sticks and sweet potato fries
- Chicken and vegetable kebabs on rice
- Baked potato topped with baked beans
- Vegetable fajitas
- Home-made pizza topped with cheese and vegetables

SNACK CHOICES

- Dry cereal with milk
- Meat or peanut butter sandwich
- Vegetable or fruit breads, such as pumpkin or banana
- Fresh, dried, or canned fruit
- Fruit or vegetable juices
- Plain yogurt or yogurt with fruit
- Cheese and reduced-salt soda crackers
- Oatmeal crackers and milk

mentally stimulated and alert and helps prevent the mid-afternoon energy dip that many children experience. However, carbohydrates are the body's most important source of fuel and should play a major part in every meal throughout the day. So a wholesome lunch, whether it is home-cooked, packed, or prepared at nursery school, is vital.

PACKED LUNCH

If your child goes to nursery school, then providing him with a packed lunch is a good way of monitoring his diet. It's very easy to get stuck in the "sandwich, chips, apple, and candy bar" rut, so offer different types of fruit and various breads for sandwiches (see box overleaf for more ideas) or rice, potato, or pasta salads. A thermos is perfect for holding soup for a warming winter lunch.

SUPPER

For many children, this is the main meal of the day and it can be an opportunity to encourage your child to reach the daily recommended intake of 1½ cups of vegetables. As the USDA states, "Make half your plate fruit and vegetables."

There are other reasons, too, to include a higher proportion of carbohydrate to protein. Complex carbohydrates, such as pasta, rice, couscous, and

potatoes, trigger the release of the brain chemical serotonin, which is said to induce feelings of calm and encourage sleep. So, If your child is particularly active or "hyper" at the end of the day, it could be a good idea to increase the amount of complex carbohydrates he eats at this time. However, don't forget the importance of protein, too. It's vital that your child eats a variety of protein foods to get a balance of the essential amino acids that can only be provided through diet.

SNACKS

Preschoolers need to eat little and often, since their stores of glucose are used up more quickly than those of adults. In fact, it's good for children to have a couple of snacks—albeit healthy ones—during the day to keep blood-sugar levels steady. Snacks should provide more than just calories, though. High-fat, high-sugar snacks and drinks will produce a sugar high followed by a sugar slump, often leading to mood swings and irritability.

It also may be beneficial to offer a carbohydrate-based snack, such as a slice of toast or a muffin, an hour or two before bedtime to encourage the production of brain-calming serotonin and to keep hunger at bay. Dips in blood-sugar levels may be a reason for your child waking up during the night.

9 tips for a "successful" lunch box

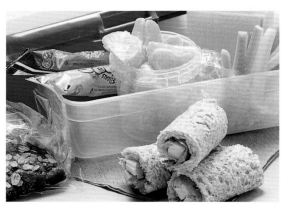

1 **Include the right amount of nutrients** such as a protein food, carbohydrates to provide energy, and essential vitamins and minerals (such as calcium).

2 **Vary the contents as much as possible** but don't include food that you know your child does not like.

3 **Choose an attractive (age-appropriate) container**. Make sure it is rigid but doesn't contain freezer pads or partitions that can limit space.

4 **Freeze yogurt cartons and diluted juice** to act as "coolers." They are healthier choices than so-called low-fat (but high-sugar) fruit dessert in cartons or carbonated drinks.

5 **Store cut-up fruit and vegetables in small plastic containers;** the containers will keep the items crisp for longer.

6 **Use whole-wheat bread instead of white** because it is higher in fiber and is more filling. Alternatively, introduce variety by offering

tortillas, mini buns, bagels, ciabatta, or English muffins occasionally.

7 **To prevent a filling from drying out,** use lettuce or mayonnaise instead of butter.

8 **Wrap a slice of bread (crust removed) around a filling,** or cut a sandwich into quarters to make it easier to handle.

9 **Choose small or sectionable fruit, like grapes or tangerines over a banana;** the latter is hard to store and discolors easily. Vary your choices frequently; try half an avocado, a kiwifruit, cubes of melon, or dried fruit for a change.

his food, or try to make him stay at the table when he wants to leave, a tantrum can result.

In addition, certain rituals, which often only your child understands, can cause a tantrum and food refusal. He might be upset that a piece of meat is touching his potatoes, that his sandwiches are cut into squares and not triangles, or that the meal is not on his favorite plate. Or maybe he doesn't like "red" food. This type of ritual may seem ridiculous to you, but it can be very important to your child.

It's so easy to get it wrong with your child at mealtimes, so it's probably best to go along with as many of his whims as you can. If he doesn't like orange juice with pulp in it, for example, offer him smooth orange juice instead. It is just as good and

certainly not worth having a battle over. It's also important to continue offering a "rejected" food (usually a vegetable) on consecutive days, since your child should remember it and it will become more and more familiar. Preschoolers have fairly short memories, but if you reintroduce an item soon, you are likely to be back at square one when you do.

Of course, you need to stand firm over the important things, such as deliberately dumping his food onto the floor, or spitting it out.

You also need to act when safety becomes an issue; if your child runs around while eating, for example, he might make himself choke. When faced with a tantrum over food refusal, try to remember that your child won't starve himself. Even if he only eats potato chips and cookies for a period of time, these do have some nutritional value.

Modeling good eating behavior

Your child will eat better if he sees you, siblings, or peers, eating the same food. Sadly, the opposite is also true. If you are picky and avoid trying a food before offering it to your child, you will fuel his dislike.

It's also true that snacking parents produce snacking children. If you frequently eat poato chips, candy bars, or cookies, your child will want to eat them, too. Likewise, if you choose healthier snacks, your child will opt for healthier ones as well. Simply by eating healthily yourself, you may not need to employ any other strategies in getting your child to eat well. However, if you are dissatisfied with an aspect of your body image, for example your weight, your dissatisfaction can be transferred to your child. This is particularly true for mothers and their daughters. If you have a tendency to eat for reasons unrelated to hunger, it's more likely that your child will eat food because he feels angry or upset.

Food allergies and intolerances

Allergies and intolerances tend to run in families so if you or your partner suffer from an allergy or intolerance, then the chances are fairly likely that your child will develop one, too. Children are also more susceptible to food intolerance because of their immature digestive and immune systems.

A food allergy occurs when the immune system overreacts to a normally harmless substance in a food by producing antibodies. This can cause a wide range of symptoms from a runny nose, upset stomach, and diarrhea to more serious problems such as asthma, eczema, and breathing difficulties and potentially to a life-threatening reaction, such as when a child allergic to nuts finds his throat swelling or suffers anaphylactic shock (see page 246).

Somewhat confusingly, a child can test negatively for an allergy but may still react to certain foods. This is known as a food intolerance, which is often caused by a digestive problem.

Food intolerances generally develop over time and are characterized by adverse reactions, such as fuzzy-headedness, poor concentration, headaches,

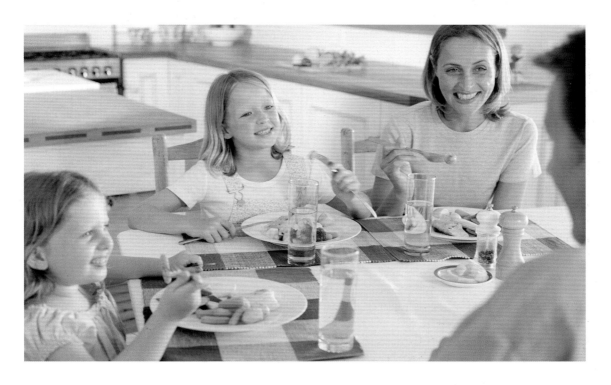

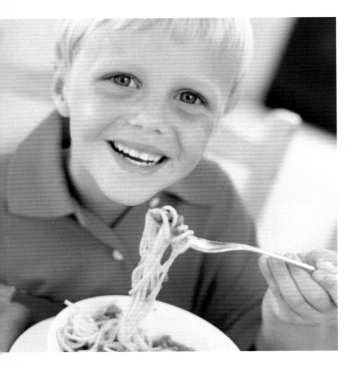

rashes and behavioral problems. Reassuringly, while the number of cases of food intolerance appears to be increasing, the number of people with severe food allergies is still rare. That being said, nut allergy has increased threefold over the last 20 years. The most common food allergens outside of nuts include dairy products, eggs, tomatoes, citrus fruit, wheat, soy, and shellfish. Always consult your healthcare provider about allergy testing and before eliminating any food from your child's diet.

Obesity

Today, obesity is a serious problem, even in young children. Some health professionals believe it has reached epidemic proportions because one in three four- to five-year-olds is obese. Although overweight children suffer few weight-related health and medical problems when young, they are at high risk of developing chronic illnesses, such as heart disease and diabetes later in life. They are also more prone to develop stress, sadness, and low self-esteem as adults. While there may be a genetic basis in certain cases, today's large number of obese children is more likely to be due to a lack of activity (see page 55), eating too many sugary and fatty foods, unhealthy eating patterns, overprotectedness on the part of parents, and possibly, certain chemicals and hormones in food and over-the-counter care products. Children whose parents are obese are more likely to be overweight since they usually share the same dietary tastes and lifestyles.

What you can do

If you are worried about your child's weight, your most important task will be to monitor his food and meals. Don't put your child on a weight-loss diet without getting advice, since this can affect his growth. Talk to your healthcare provider if you have any concerns about your child's weight. Also:

- Make certain that he eats foods low in fat and sugar and avoids junk food whenever possible (see page 41). Serve broiled, roasted, or pan-fried foods instead of deep-fried ones.
- Include some starchy foods in meals, such as potatoes, bread, rice, and pasta, choosing whole-

4 signs your child may be overweight

1 **Babyfat still present.** "Bracelets" of fat around your child's wrists and ankles and "love handles" around his midriff mean he has a weight problem.

2 **Tired much of the time.** Listlessness and lethargy accompany inactivity. Continous lethargy should be investigated because there may be an underlying medical cause, or your child may be depressed.

3 **Breathlessness.** If your child is not asthmatic, getting out of breath when walking or running, or an inability to keep up with other children generally is a sign of being overweight.

4 **Victim of teasing.** Has your child been nicknamed "Chubby," "Chunky," or "Fatso," or given other size-related nicknames by relatives or peers?

MEASURING OBESITY

Body mass index (BMI) is one way healthcare providers assess weight and health. Weight in pounds (or kilograms) is divided by height in feet and inches (or meters) squared. Age-adjusted charts take into account growth changes, and are used to determine if a child is over-weight or obese. Seek advice from your healthcare provider.

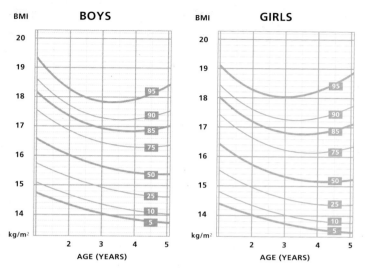

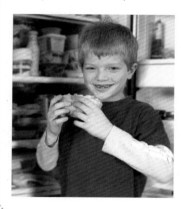

WEIGHT STATUS CATEGORY/PERCENTILE RANGE	
Underweight	Less than the 5th percentile
Healthy weight	5th percentile to less than the 85th percentile
Overweight	85th to less than the 95th percentile
Obese	Equal to or greater than the 95th percentile

wheat varieties of the latter three.

- Serve some fiber-rich foods, such as oats, legumes, grains, fruit, and vegetables, whole-wheat bread, brown rice, and whole-wheat pasta.
- Ensure your child eats at least five portions of a variety of fruit and vegetables each day.
- Encourage him to drink water instead of fruit juice (it is high in sugar), fizzy, or milky drinks.
- Keep an eye on the portion size of meals and snacks, and how frequently he eats. Using a slightly smaller plate can make it easier to adjust portion size downward.
- Make sure that you set a good example both in what you eat and the way you eat. If you constantly snack or eat junk food, eat between normal mealtimes, or eat while watching television, your child will do so too.

That being said, it's vital that you do not set your child apart because of his weight nor tell him he needs to be on a diet. Instead, you should focus on gradually changing your entire family's eating habits and physical activity levels (see page 57). By involving all your family, everyone learns healthy habits and your overweight child will not feel singled out. Children raised in families that are accepting of body shapes at any weight are more likely to have a positive body image and greater self-esteen that is unrelated to weight. On the other hand, derogatory comments and a negative view of obesity in childhood lead to a poorer self-image in later life. Never discuss your child's weight or his overeating with others in front of him.

Dressing and clothes

Putting on and taking off clothes is one of those skills that are mastered in stages though, generally, the latter is achieved much earlier than the former.

While your two-year-old was able to remove her hat, gloves, and socks easily but not dress herself, for example, by the time she's three, she should be able to put on her underpants, pants, or skirt with elasticized waist, socks, and self-stick fastening or slip-on shoes. Shirts and blouses with buttons and lace-up or buckled shoes, however, will probably still be beyond her.

By four, your child will be able to put on most of her clothes on her own although help may still be needed with tricky zippers, buttons, buckles, and laces. Any garments, particularly nightwear that goes over the head, are best avoided.

At five, your child will have almost all of the necessary skills to dress herself but can lack the interest to do it well or completely. Few, if any, children take care of their clothes at this age.

As with the other elements of daily care (feeding, hygiene, sleeping) dressing is an area in which preschoolers frequently oppose their parent's wishes, often as a way of asserting their independence.

Battling over clothes

Problems can arise with your child's choice of clothes and you're likely to find that what your child wants to wear clashes with your own taste and ideas. You may want your child to look tidy and to dress appropriately for the weather, but she wants to wear a favorite scruffy sweater that's two sizes too

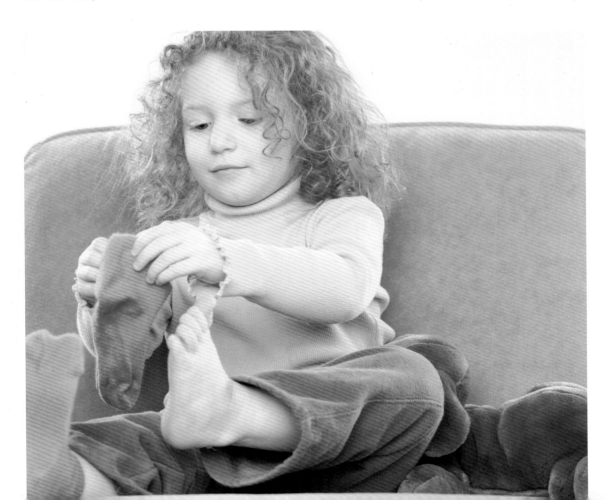

small and old jeans with a giant rip in the seat. Or she may be desperate to be decked in head-to-toe pink. If you object, you're faced with a choice between triggering a tantrum and having a child who looks like a neglected ragbag or a feminist's nightmare.

Protracted dressing

Another problem area can be the length of time it takes for your preschooler to get herself dressed. If your child is slow or easily distracted, the time it takes for her to get ready can be a source of irritation for you both, especially first thing in the morning when you are in a hurry to get out of the house. The more you cajole your child to hurry up, the slower she will become. If you try to intervene, she may have a tantrum because she doesn't want your help; if you get angry with her or lose your temper she'll just get even more upset.

If this is a problem for you, try to find a compromise and, as with much preschooler parenting, pick your battles carefully. Does it really matter if your daughter chooses a skirt that clashes with her top or your son wants to wear odd socks occasionally? At this age, if your child has a little involvement with her wardrobe each day, it will help temper any tantrums and encourage individuality to develop. It will also limit the chances of your child refusing to wear something.

If there are clothes you really don't want your child to wear, either pack them away, "lose" them temporarily, or pick out a few different garment options so that she has a choice about what to put on. However, do remember that she is a child and you are in charge; if you think an outfit is truly inappropriate, for example, for the weather or the occasion, you still get to make the decisions—at least for a few more years!

6 tips for easier dressing

1 **Pack away unsuitable clothes.** If the weather where you live is very seasonal, put all the previous season's clothes into storage when the weather starts to change.

2 **Limit the choice.** Offer your child a choice of clothes, but make it limited.

3 **Lay out clothes correctly oriented.** It can help if garments are laid out on the bed with the fronts facing upward and the top above the pants.

4 **Allow more time for your child to get dressed.** Get up ten minutes earlier, if necessary.

5 **Encourage your child to dress herself** but don't laugh at or criticize her efforts.

6 **Be ready to help.** Bear in mind that some garments, as well as socks and shoes, can be difficult for a child to put on, so be available if she gets stuck.

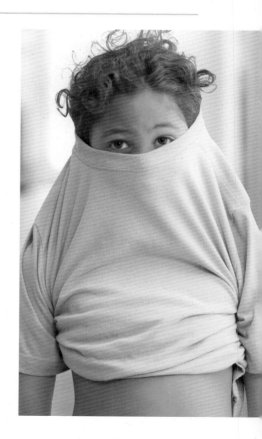

If you sense a battle over getting dressed coming on, you could try sitting down with your child and explaining why she needs to hurry up or why she can't wear shorts and a t-shirt when it's snowing outside. If this doesn't work, and your child refuses to hurry up or has a full-blown tantrum, there is nothing else for it but to pick her and her clothes up and take her to the front door. Finish getting her dressed there so that she understands that going out is the next step.

If your child wants to wear unsuitable clothing or refuses to put on certain items, such as a coat or gloves when it's cold, let her learn from experience how wearing the wrong clothes or going out without these items will affect her (although make sure you have the necessary items handy).

Clothing needn't cost a fortune

Even if your preschooler would be happy wearing that ragged sweater mentioned above, you no doubt want her to look at least presentable. Whether you go as far as fashion-plate mode is personal preference but bear in mind that lively young children rarely respect costly designer outfits. One rule of thumb, at least for day-to-day wear, is to stick with items you won't feel the need to worry about if your child is being a typical preschooler—running through muddy puddles, spilling juice down her front, or crawling around with her toys on the floor, slowly but surely wearing holes in the knees!

That's not to say your child can't look well dressed, just that there's no point spending a fortune, especially when there are stylish junior ranges in department stores, supermarkets, and online. For example, you could also check out eBay for discounted new or lightly used items, or encourage friends with older children to send their hand-me-downs your way. Yard sales and Goodwill Stores are also good places to check out.

It's unusual for a child under six to be particularly brand conscious herself or to face peer pressure to have the latest shoes or the like, but if this does happen, listen to your child and try to understand why she desperately wants that particular item. Bear in mind, however, that it is your decision and saying

OVERLY GROWN-UP CLOTHING

There has been much press coverage in recent times of sexualized clothing for young children, from child-size heels to t-shirts with adult slogans on them, and padded bras for girls still in elementary school. While you might consider such items "amusing" or not dissimilar to tottering around in mothers' high heels and (usually badly applied) lipstick, which toddlers regularly engage in, it's worth bearing in mind that, generally speaking, toddler "dressing up" is occasional, uses items that are clearly the mother's not the child's, and is done in the privacy of the home. Psychologists believe that dressing young children in overly sexualized clothing can lead to issues with self-esteem and body image. So, if over the next few years, you face occasions when you're out shopping together and your child grabs something you'd prefer she didn't wear, remember it's your call. It's might be better to deal with a short-lived outburst of temper now than the long-term consequences of an eating disorder.

"no" does not make you a bad parent (even if there's a tantrum for a few minutes after you do so!).

Sometimes, it's not children themselves hankering after costly designer clothing, but parents. If you are drawn to brands you can't easily afford, reflect upon why this might be. Is it for you or your child? If it's the latter, she really isn't going to know or care whether her outfit is from Dolce & Gabbana or if it's from Walmart. If you believe that other people will judge you for not dressing your child in the trendiest gear, consider if their opinion is really worth worrying about.

Keeping your child active

A healthy lifestyle depends on physical activity. Being active will help your child use up her excess energy, burn calories, sleep better, and enjoy an improved mood. It will also:

- Enable her to maintain a healthy weight, now and in the future;
- Improve her concentration and ability to learn, at playgroup, nursery school, or in kindergarten;
- Reduce the risk of health problems, such as diabetes, joint problems, stroke, heart disease, and some cancers later in life;
- Allow her to lead a happy and healthy life;
- Improve her ability to handle stress;
- Elevate her mood and improve her general well-being.

For your child to be a healthy weight, having her eat a healthy diet—one with the appropriate amount of calories (see page 38)—is one part of the equation; making sure she has sufficient physical activity is the other. There are two main approaches you need to adopt. The first is to minimize sedentary activities while the other is to encourage active play.

Minimizing sedentary activities

It is vitally important to prevent your child from sitting for long periods watching television or DVDs, using a computer, or playing sedentary video games. Not only does watching television discourage your child from active play, but it exposes her to junk food advertisements, which can impact negatively on her eating a healthy diet. Total screen time for television watching and computer and console use should be limited (see page 146).

That being said, active video games like the Wii, can be useful in preventing child obesity. According to a recent research, children burned three times as

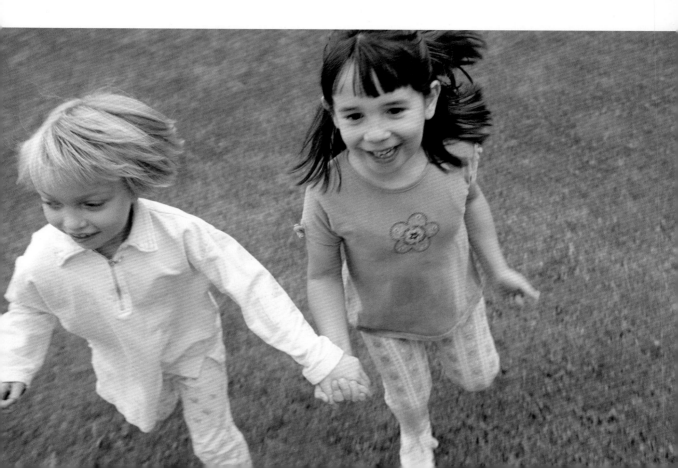

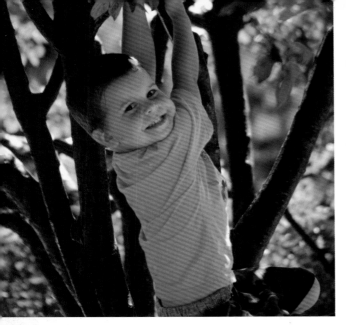

many calories playing "active" video games versus playing traditional hand-held ones.

Encouraging energetic play

The other side of the coin with healthy weight is to get your child engaged in active play. Children need to play and you should offer the time, environment, and equipment to allow your preschooler to do so every single day. Bear in mind that for a small child all play is learning, so there's added benefit.

According to the Centers for Disease Control and Prevention, your preschooler should be encouraged to play actively for at least one hour every day, even if that is just playing tag or climbing on a jungle gym with her friends.

Some ways to play

You should consider taking your child to a gym class, local swimming pool, or to a sports center, but there are simpler and less expensive activities (see also movement games, page 58).

Make walking a positive option. If possible, don't jump in the car whenever you want to go anywhere but try and fit in a weekly (if not daily) walk to the playground, corner store, or just out and about.

Another good alternative is to cycle to activities. By age four, your child will be able to ride a tricycle with ease, turning around sharp bends, and she may even be able to handle a bike with or without training wheels. Scooters, too, provide lots of opportunity for your child to get active, but make sure she wears a protective helmet when doing both (see also page 210). You too, should wear a helmet when bike riding (or using a scooter) so that you serve as a model of safe behavior.

Kick a soccerball around together in your backyard or at the local park. You can practice catching and throwing a baseball or football, or dribble and bounce a basketball and even shoot hoops. When at the playground, encourage your toddler to use all the equipment so that she builds up her climbing and balancing skills.

Put on some music and encourage your child to move to it. Dancing develops balance and coordination and is a great way to do something active together.

Your child may be able to manage roller skates, but again, protective gear is needed. Make sure that she wears all the necessary protection—in particular a helmet as well as knee and elbow pads. Flat paths in parks are the ideal place to learn to roller skate.

Home gym

There is some fairly inexpensive equipment that can help to keep your child active at home. Balls of all types (see abvoe) have a great deal of play potential particularly as they can be used in new and different ways as your child's handling and kicking skills develop. A small exercise ball also offers lots of fun-filled opportunities for your child. She can bounce and roll over on it but supervise her at all times.

A mini trampoline, too, is ideal for working off excess energy and can be used indoors and out. This also has to be used under supervision.

Your child may be able to spin a hula hoop around her middle or if not, several hoops can be laid flat on the ground and your child encouraged to jump or hop in and out of them.

Jump ropes involve play that will develop your child's arm and leg skills, improve her coordination, and encourage healthy bone growth. Skipping is a high-impact activity, so make sure your child wears running shoes when using a jump rope.

Story-telling and role-playing go naturally together, so even reading can be an opportunity for active play. Your child will enjoy acting out a simple tale and burn off some energy in the process.

Children are fascinated by animals, so you could talk about a walk in the park or a day at the zoo, and as you introduce each animal, ask your child to imitate what she thinks the animal is doing. For example, for a frog, she should crouch down and try jumping across the floor or, when you mention a snake, have your child lie on her stomach and stretch her arms out in front. She can raise her head and "hiss" and then try to slither across the floor. And for a monkey, she can somersault, look between her knees, or even put her foot into her mouth. Accuracy is less important than the actions.

ways you can encourage activity

1 **Set an example.** You are your child's most important role model—if you are a couch potato, don't expect your kid to be active! Get yourself moving so the habit rubs off on your child. Walk or cycle to work so that right from the start, your child sees these modes of transportation as "normal." If, however, your child sees you come in from work and then settle in front of the television for the night, she will see no reason not to do the same.

2 **Take an interest.** Encourage your child if she wants to engage in a sport or exercise activity. If she is interested in swimming, take her a couple of times to the local pool to see if lessons might be a good idea or to some local sports events to fire her interests and enthusiasms. If she engages in anything, make sure you're an enthusiastic supporter or join in (don't just drop her off and leave).

3 **Plan family activities** that provide everyone with exercise, like walking, bike riding, or swimming. Make an effort to reduce the amount of time you and your family spend in sedentary activities, such as watching television or playing video games.

4 **Be sensitive to your child's needs.** If your child is overweight, she may feel uneasy about participating in certain activities. It is important to help her find physical activities she will enjoy that aren't embarrassing or too difficult.

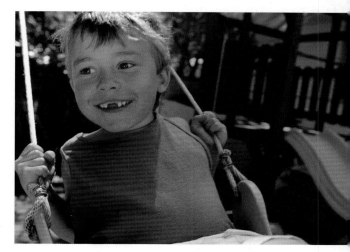

5 **Make sure her environment is safe.** Being active often involves some degree of risk, whether your child is at home or outdoors. You should childproof your home, too, because your child will need somewhere to work off excess energy on days when it's rainy outside. Teach your child about safe practices when outdoors, such as not picking up or eating plants, not getting too close to animals, not talking to strangers, etc., and ensure she always wears sufficient protective gear (when riding a bike, using a scooter, or roller skating) and teach her about safe behavior in the playground, for example, not walking behind other children while they are using the swings, waiting to go down the slide until the last child gets off, and then getting off quickly herself, and holding onto ladders and climbing frames with both hands.

MOVEMENT GAMES

There are a number of games that can be played with one or more children and, depending on the numbers and ages of the participants, may not need to have a "winner"; young children enjoy following instructions and running around. If the children are older, you have the option of penalizing anyone doing the wrong action. Musical games offer an extra dimension.

HOPSCOTCH

By the age of four, your child will probably enjoy playing a simple version of this outdoor game. Don't worry about the numbers too much; focus on her jumping around and having fun. Draw out the squares and let her practice jumping and hopping from one to another. You can play, too! As your child learns her numbers and her agility improves, she will enjoy playing the traditional game alone or along with her friends.

TWISTER®

Your child also might like to try Twister or a home-made variation. Cut out large circles of differently colored paper and place them in rows on the floor. Then call out "right hand, left hand, right foot, left foot" followed by the color for each. A simpler game would involve limiting the game to having your child jump on the colors you call out.

TRAFFIC LIGHTS

Also known as "Stop and Go," you need to stand in front of your child (and any friends) and give instructions: "Green light"—run around; "Yellow light"—slow down; "Red light"—stop; "Traffic jam"—walk slowly.

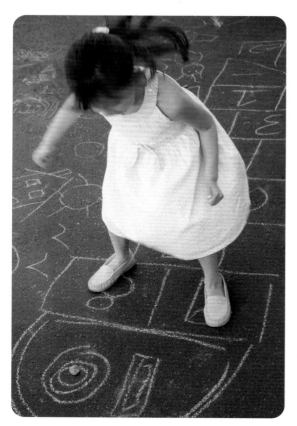

FOLLOW THE LEADER

Have your child (and any friends) stand behind you in a line and then make various movements—walk, jump, hop, skip, turn around, walk backward, and so on—that she (or they) must copy. Make sure you swing your arms vigorously as well.

SIMON SAYS

Stand in front of your child and make up things for her to do prefaced by "Simon says…". For example, "Simon says, hop on one foot." If you just say, "Hop on one foot" without saying "Simon says…", and your child does so, you must point out that she's lost a point or must pay a forfeit for getting it wrong. Try to be as inventive as possible.

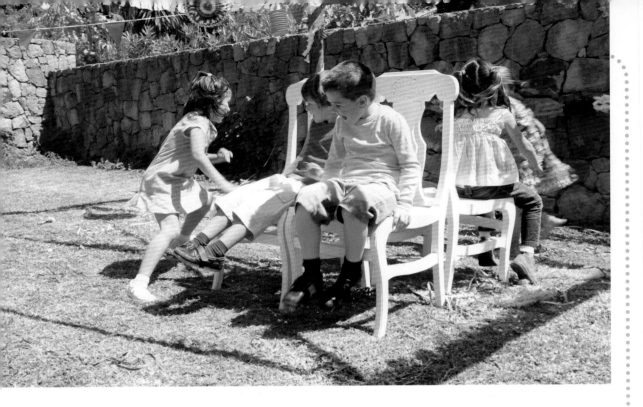

MUSICAL CHAIRS AND FREEZE DANCE

Both games depend on letting your child run around or dance until the music stops. In the simplest version of "Musical Chairs," you ask your child to walk around the chair(s) until you stop the music when she must sit down. The more children, the more chairs, though usually there's one less than the number of children playing. With "Freeze Dance," children have the option to dance around until the music stops and then either sit down or freeze. Strictly speaking the last to sit down or the one who moves is out, but you may decide to let everyone keep playing.

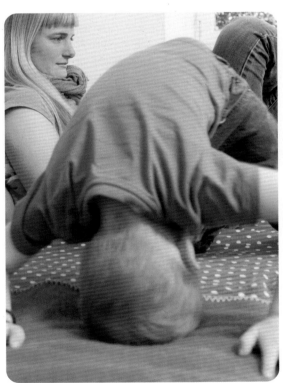

Hygiene matters

Young children are particularly vulnerable to illness and infection (although they will build up immunity in the long run), but it is important to keep a balance between under- and over-protection while imparting personal hygiene rules to last your child through life. It's particularly vital that your child learns the various bathroom skills—toilet flushing, wiping, hand washing, tooth brushing, and bathing.

Hand washing

Germs can be easily transferred to your child's mouth from a pet, the ground, or the toilet, so you need to explain to your child that even if his hands look clean, germs (because they are so tiny) may still be present on his skin. Get him into the habit of washing his hands before eating or touching food and teach him not to eat any fruit or raw vegetables before these have been washed. He must also learn

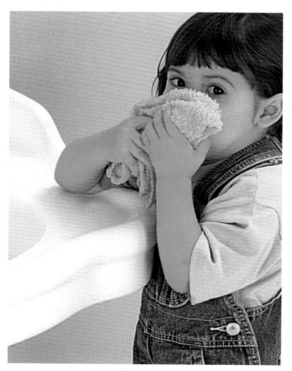

to wash his hands after going to the bathroom, playing outside, or with pets.

Supervise your child's hand washing until you are satisfied he is doing it properly. One of the easiest ways to teach your child to wash his hands properly is to wash yours at the same time. Use soap and pay particular attention to drying your hands afterward. Try teaching him a rhyme or to count up to 10 each time he washes his hands, so that he gets an idea of how long he needs to wash them. Your child may enjoy having his own special soap to wash his hands with—you can get him one in the shape of his favorite animal. If soap and water aren't available, an antibacterial gel or antiseptic wipes are good alternatives.

Wiping

Getting clean after using the toilet may still be something of a challenge for your child; parents usually need to help their children with wiping until they are about five years old. Encourage gentle wiping; if your child wipes sensitive skin too roughly, it may become irritated. You'll also need to show your child how much toilet paper to use—left to their own devices, children tend to use too much of a roll and clog up the toilet. Your daughter should be taught to wipe from front to back to prevent germs from being transferred to her urinary tract.

You can help encourage your child's bathroom independence with products that are gentle on sensitive skin, but also are strong and absorbent. Pre-moistened, flushable wipes are gentle on the skin, easy for your child to use, and may be more effective than regular toilet paper when cleaning after a bowel movement. (Check the wipes are suitable for flusing down the toilet; they may not be in a property with older drains.)

Flushing

You should encourage your child to flush the toilet himself. Once he feels confident enough to do this, you can help him to empty his potty (if still in use, see below) into the toilet and then allow him to flush it. Encourage your child to close the toilet lid before flushing so that he avoids contact with germs that may spray up.

Some children are much more enthusiastic about flushing and may be fascinated by the noise it makes. You may even find it difficult to stop your child from flushing the toilet again and again. If this is the case, don't allow him to use the flush whenever he wants—try to keep it as an incentive to encourage him to use the toilet properly. If he really can't be dissuaded from overusing the flush, consider fitting a childproof attachment to your toilet.

Teaching your son to stand

Your son will probably want to stand up to urinate when he reaches preschool age since he'll probably try to copy his dad or other boys from his play group. Often, children learn best by imitation, so someone, preferably his dad or an older male, will have to show him how to stand up in front of the toilet and aim into the bowl before urinating. However, if he's happy sitting down to urinate, don't rush into having him stand up. Wait until he has developed sufficient control. If you can't involve a male adult, your son will still learn to stand, but it may take a little longer. Once he understands the process, it's just a matter of practicing until this new skill becomes a habit. Make sure, of course, that you teach your son to lift the toilet seat before urinating and, once up, that it remains in place securely (falling seats can cause injuries) until he puts it back down again, closes the lid, and flushes. He'll also need to be taught to "shake dry" afterward without getting drips all over the floor and on his pants.

Standing up and peeing on target, however, is a tricky maneuver for a little boy to perfect. Get your son to direct his penis toward the drain hole before he starts to pass water. Getting it right can take up to a year or more before the floor and walls remain completely free of splashes. Keep a sturdy stepstool nearby; this not only makes it easier for your boy to access the toilet by himself, but will also help him aim more effectively into the bowl.

TOILET TRAINING

As one of the prerequisites for entering nursery school or kindergarten, it's vital that your child is able to go to the bathroom by himself. Most children are physically capable of being potty trained at around two years of age, but some children, particularly boys, don't achieve bladder and bowel control until three or older. You should, however, consult your healthcare provider if your child is not dry during the day by age four; he may have a physical problem. Even if your child is able to use the potty, you'll need to make sure he can use a toilet. A child-size toilet seat, a stepstool, and clothes that are easy to pull up or down can all help.

An older toddler who has perhaps rejected the idea of potty training at an earlier age may respond better to intensive training now. The idea is to create a situation in which your child is able to recognize and respond to the need to urinate within a very short time. This requires dedication on your part (you'll need to give him a few days of undivided attention) but it can be a good way to get everything out of the way at once. You'll need to give your child plenty to drink, encourage him to use the potty on his own, and give him lots of rewards for dry underpants. Try to make the whole thing like a fun game, but don't let him get overexcited; remain firm but encouraging throughout. Once he has got the hang of urinating in the potty, learning to use it for a bowel motion should soon follow.

Privacy issues

Your child may want toilet training to remain something that you do together privately, away from the rest of the family. Even if your child has started off being happy about the attention he's received—particularly if successful—he may without any warning, develop a desire for privacy. He may hide in his bedroom every time he changes his underwear and may be offended if anyone tries to watch or help him. Try to respect these new feelings; this newfound modesty is a sign of his growing independence and self-awareness. He certainly won't want anyone with him in the bathroom if he's going through this phase.

All children have a right to privacy, and this needs to be respected. There are times when it may not be possible to allow your child complete privacy while using the toilet, however. Childcare centers, for example, don't usually allow total privacy in the bathroom. The same applies to public restrooms, where your child will always need to be chaperoned.

You need to explain to your child that different situations may require different behavior. Once he

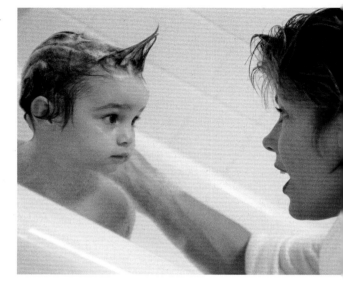

6 things that will keep your bathroom safe

1 **Never leave your preschooler** in the bathtub on his own, or leave any water standing in the tub.

2 **Make your bathtub slip-proof** by using rubber strips or a rubber mat; use a nonskid bath mat to cover most of the bathroom floor.

3 **Ensure that bath water is a moderate temperature**—no higher than 120°F; test the water with your own foot before putting your child in.

4 **Store all medications** including over-the-counter preparations, all electrical equipment, clippers, razors, and scissors out of reach or in a locked cabinet.

5 **Lock toilet bowl cleaner** and other cleansers away.

6 **When not in use, keep the toilet lid closed** with suction cups or a latch, if necessary.

understands, he will be starting to learn about boundaries and acceptable social behavior. For example, he will have to learn that although it is all right to be proud of his private parts, and nakedness is fine at home, it is not acceptable to go out without clothes or to touch his genitals in public (or for someone else to touch his [see page 205]).

Bathing

Your child will probably need—and look forward to—a daily bath to wash off any dirt acquired during play. Make sure he knows which face cloth and towel are his; it is better for hygiene and it may encourage him to use them. In any event, until he is old enough to wash himself thoroughly, you will have to go over what he has done. By now your child should know his body parts, and if given a small sponge or cloth he can wash these himself.

A preschooler's skin can be sensitive, so use mild soaps and shampoos. Try different brands to see which one suits him skin best. Liquid soap may be easier for your child to handle.

Care of the hair and nails

Hair care

Shampooing your child's hair may still be difficult if he, like most young children, hates getting water splashed near his face or fears shampoo getting into his eyes. It's easiest to wash hair in the bathtub and to use a shower attachment for rinsing. Allowing your child some control over hairwashing may also help; let him wet his hair himself with a cloth, by dipping it into the tub water, or using the shower attachment. He may even enjoy wearing his swim goggles. Of course, keeping the hair shorter will make your job easier.

Hair can be rinsed everyday with water or washed two to three times a week with a mild shampoo. If your child's hair is long or curly, use leave-in conditioner after shampooing to prevent tangles. Don't towel dry the hair roughly but pat it dry. If it is still tangled, use a conditioning spray while combing it with a wide-toothed comb. If your child's hair is long, brush it regularly to keep it free from tangles. Be careful not to pull the hair too tightly if you are braiding it or putting it into a pony tail because this could cause thinning or permanent bald patches.

Hair problems

Eating a diet full of vitamins and minerals will ensure that your child's hair grows healthily but dandruff can be a problem. Use a medicated shampoo suitable for children to keep this in check. If in contact with other children, he is at risk of catching head lice.

Head lice

These tiny insects live on hair near the scalp and can be difficult to see. They are caught through close head-to-head contact. Suspect your child may have them if he has a rash on his scalp, is scratching his head, or you can see black and powdery droppings on his scalp or pillows. Nits are the empty white eggshells found further down the scalp.

If you think your child has lice, wet his hair and part it into sections. Comb each section thoroughly with a nit comb with fine, precision-made stainless steel teeth (the comb's teeth should be tight-grooved, otherwise lice can be slip between the teeth and remain unseen) over a sheet of white paper, or when your child is in the bath. Lice, usually gray or brown in color, may be seen on the scalp or comb, or may fall on the paper or in the water. If present, your whole family and close contacts should be treated.

Remove the lice by combing through the hair while it is very wet, starting from the roots, using the nit comb. Use lots of conditioner and wipe the comb between each stroke; rinse out the conditioner and repeat the comb-through. Perform the procedure again five, nine, and thirteen days later to catch any unhatched lice.

You can also use medicated lotion or over-the-counter spray from the pharmacy but not if you are pregnant or if you or your child suffer from asthma or other allergies. However, no medicated treatment is 100% effective and because all contain strong chemicals, they should only be used if a living (moving) head louse is found.

Follow instructions that come with the product when applying it but use enough to coat the scalp and the length of the hair during each application. Depending on the product you are using, it will need to be left on the head from 10 minutes to 8 hours and the treatment needs repeating after a week. Traditional insecticides must not be used more than once a week for three weeks in a row. Some products also carry a fire warning.

Some medicated products may kill eggs as well as lice, although there is no certainty of this. Check for baby lice hatching from eggs three to five days after you use a product, and again at 10 to 12 days later.

If your child has tightly curled or Afro hair, keep his hair short or try braiding it because this can make it difficult for head lice to attach themselves to the bottom of the hair strand. Use a medicated lotion, such as dimeticone, and methodically comb small sections of hair at a time with a lice comb.

Care of the nails

Children's nails usually are pretty healthy, but because there may be the occasional health problem it's important to take good care of them. If something about your child's nails doesn't look right, take your child to your doctor or healthcare adviser.

It's important to teach your child how to keep his nails clean and healthy to make sure germs don't creep in and cause infections. Keep his nails short, using a nail clipper or small nail scissors to cut them. Cut nails after a bath or shower, when they're softer, and to keep them strong, cut them in the shape of the fingertip: almost straight across, but rounded a little at the tips. Cut toenails straight

across to reduce the chance of ingrown nails. Use a file or emery board to help get rid of sharp edges, so the nails don't tear. Don't cut or push back the cuticles, because these protect the nail root.

Wet nails can breed infection so your child should dry his hands really well after washing them or getting them wet. To keep nails from splitting, especially when the air is dry, rub lotion on the fingernails regularly. To prevent toenail infections, make sure your child changes his socks daily. If he's at the pool or using a public shower, he should wear flip flops; fungal infections spread easily in moist environments.

Limit your child's use of nail polish remover to twice a month, because it can dry out or damage the nails. Use an acetone-free remover.

Hangnails

These are pieces of skin at the edge of the nails that tear and sometimes even bleed. They can hurt and if your child chews at or tears one, it can get infected.

If your child is suffering from one, wash his hands with soap and water then cut the hangnail cleanly with a nail clipper or small nail scissors. Don't tear it off. Dab on a little antiseptic cream if the skin is red or sore and cover it with a protective bandage for a day or two. If the hangnail becomes infected, see your healthcare provider.

Thumb Sucking

About 15% of children under five years of age continue to suck their thumbs (up to age three, professionals discourage parents from preventing it). By the age of five years, most children are able to overcome their desire to suck their thumb in face of oncoming social, behavioral, and developmental demands. Older children, who continue to suck their thumb, do it just as a habit.

There are a number of things you can do to help your child quit the habit but using noxious agents isn't one of them; they rarely work. Neither will negative practices such as scolding, teasing, or punishment; in traumatizing your child's self-esteem, they may even perpetuate the habit instead of getting rid of it.

4 things to try to eliminate thumb sucking

1 **Pretend to ignore the action;** in time your child may stop.

2 **Educate your child on its ill effects:** fingers carry germs; repeated sore throats are likely; he may be teased by his peers and others; his jaw may ache and his permanent teeth may be affected; he may develop a chronic infection of the nail folds.

3 **Look out for a precipitating factor** and try to resolve it. This may be boredom, loneliness, or anxiety from scary television shows or a disturbing family routine or situation.

4 **Apply some behavior therapy:** help your child to relax; divert his attention toward something more interesting than his thumb, give him praise when he doesn't suck it, and reinforce good behavior with small gifts such as a star or sticker on a calendar.

Care of the teeth

By the age of two most children have all but the last set of upper and lower molars, which normally erupt any time from 25 months. The average child has a full set of 20 primary teeth by the age of three.

It's important that these teeth are well looked after. They may fall out in time but they will affect your child's permanent teeth; proper attention can mean that more painful procedures can be avoided. Some children (even siblings) are more susceptible to decay and those who have decayed primary (milk) teeth are much more likely to have more problems with their permanent teeth.

Limiting the effects of harmful drinks and foods

Only milk (drunk from a cup) or water are totally safe. Fruit drinks contain naturally occurring fructose, which can cause decay in just the same way as added sugar. Fizzy drinks, including diet drinks and flavored and sparkling waters, are harmful to teeth, not only because of their sugar content, but also because they are highly acidic. They contain carbonic acid which will erode teeth. "Real" fruit juices, too, such as orange, apple, pineapple, and grapefruit, are also extremely acidic.

The best way to avoid such decay is to keep track of how often your child drinks and for how long. If you are going to give your child juice or fizzy drinks, make sure these are only offered with his main meals (when the mouth produces plenty of alkaline saliva, which helps to protect the teeth from acidity) and that he drinks them with a straw. Make sure he consumes them as quickly as possible, rather than sipping them over a long period.

Don't brush his teeth for 30 minutes after drinking juice or a fizzy drink; doing so before will increase the acid erosion on his teeth.

Only offer sweets and candies immediately after meals, when the extra saliva created by chewing will help protect the teeth.

Fluoride supplements and fissure sealants can help a child whose teeth are already decayed.

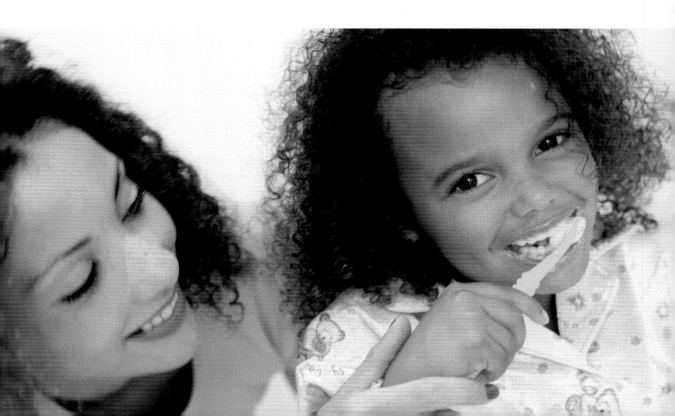

Tooth brushing

It is important to encourage good tooth care from an early age—good habits established now can last a lifetime. A preschooler does not have the manual dexterity or the mental application to brush effectively, so you either need to brush your child's teeth or supervise him as he brushes. If he wants to do it himself, let him, but still do a final brush when he has finished. Technique is less important than the end result; what matters is that all areas of the mouth are reached.

At least twice a day, preferably after a meal, brush your child's teeth with a small-headed brush with soft bristles. The shape and angle of the head are not important. Use a pea-sized amount of low-fluoride toothpaste (around 500 parts per million). You can check the fluoride content of toothpaste in the list of ingredients—it's listed as ppmF. Fluoride is a naturally occurring mineral that strengthens tooth enamel and protects against tooth decay. Some water supplies contain fluoride, in which case your child may need a low-fluoride toothpaste. Too much fluoride causes yellowing of the teeth or fluorosis. Once he's six, your child can use an adult-strength formula. Teach your child to spit out (and not swallow) the toothpaste. He should not rinse after brushing. The more often a child rinses and the more water he uses, the quicker the fluoride exits his mouth. Not rinsing means fluoride is retained in the mouth longer, giving better benefit.

Fissure sealing

This may be recommended for children whose teeth are "at risk." It involves painting a plastic coating on the permanent molars. It is particularly useful for teeth with deep groves, the bottoms of which cannot be reached with a toothbrush.

A new vaccine is being developed, which could help make problems of tooth decay a thing of the past. The vaccine uses antibodies like those in our immune system, which are grown in genetically engineered plants. It is painted onto the teeth.

Fluoride

Fluoride can reduce a child's susceptibility to decay by about half but most dentists today recommend that only children at high risk of decay—for example those with decay in their primary teeth—should take a supplement. Children who are not at particular risk should get all the fluoride they need from toothpaste.

If a child has too much fluoride, it can lead to fluorosis (see Tooth brushing, left). But working out how much your child is getting can be difficult. It is the total intake—from supplements, toothpaste, and the water you drink—that matters. All water contains some fluoride (including some bottled waters), but, unless you call your local authority to ask, you cannot tell how much. If you live in an area with more than 0.7 parts per million of fluoride in the drinking water, you do not need to give your child extra fluoride.

Young children often swallow toothpaste—up to half the paste on a brush—and swallowing fluoride toothpaste can also result in fluorosis.

Pacifiers

If your child uses a pacifier beyond the age of two, it can result in misaligned teeth, which can cause problems with both eating and speech. Moreover, if your child falls while sucking on a pacifier, he is more likely to injure his mouth and displace a tooth. Make sure your preschooler doesn't use one.

Care of the skin

The skin is the largest and one of the most important body organs and performs a wide range of essential functions. It forms a tight waterproof and leakproof layer that helps protect your child's internal organs, and is the body's first line of defense against the penetration of harmful environmental substances, such as micro-organisms (bacteria, viruses, and fungi), allergens, chemical pollutants, and ultraviolet radiation from the sun.

Two main layers combine to form your child's skin. The epidermis forms the thin, uppermost layer of the skin, while the thicker dermis forms a deeper, inner layer. The top layer of the epidermis, called the stratum corneum, is made up of flat, dead cells containing a hard protein called keratin. These cells, known as keratinocytes, are constantly shed and replaced, and are cemented together by a fatty film (the lipid layer) that forms a protective waterproof coating for your child's skin.

It is the stratum corneum that helps protect the body against light and heat waves, bacteria, and environmental pollutants but this is not fully developed until your child is aged four, and although the skin increases in thickness as your child grows, it does not reach maturity until puberty.

The lower or basal cell layer of the epidermis contains the melanocyte cells, which produce the pigment melanin that gives your child's skin its color and protects it against harmful ultraviolet rays. Children also have fewer pigment cells than adults, making them particularly vulnerable to sunburn and the effects of environmental "insults" on the skin.

The dermis contains collagen cells and elastin fibers that give your child's skin its firmness and elasticity. It also contains:

◆ Capillaries (tiny blood vessels) that nourish your child's skin and help combat infection by bringing in white blood cells. They can also expand or contract to help control heat loss;

◆ Sweat glands to produce sweat, which evaporates off the skin, helping cool your child's body;

◆ Hair follicles are the tiny pits in your child's skin that hold the hair roots (the hair shaft projects above the surface of the skin). The tiny hairs on the skin stand up, trapping a layer of air that acts as insulation. Each follicle is attached to a sebaceous gland;

◆ Sebaceous (oil) glands produce an oily substance called sebum, which lubricates the hair and forms a protective moisture film over your child's skin, preventing it from drying out;

◆ Nerve endings enable your child to respond to sensations such as touch.

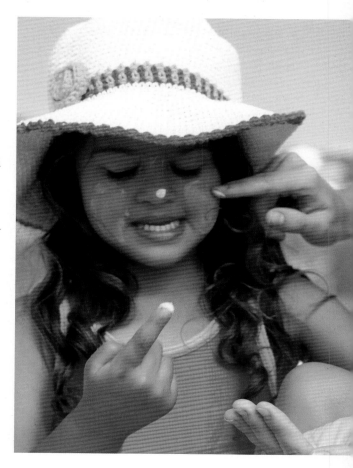

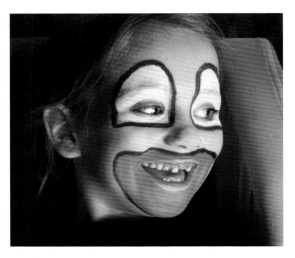

Makeup and face paints

Children like to put on makeup as part of dressing up and also because they see their moms doing so. But bearing in mind that children's skin is more sensitive than an adult's, it's best that these sessions are restricted to an occasional treat.

Whether your child is applying the makeup himself or if face paints are being used, check the ingredients. Make sure the product is nontoxic with just a few (preferably natural or organic) ingredients, nonstaining, and water-based so it is easy to remove. If in doubt, don't use it.

If applying makeup, take a minimal approach. Instead of attempting an entire "look," see if your

General skin care

Always use gentle, fragrance-free cleansers and soaps and apply liberal amounts of moisturizer after bathing to keep the skin moisturized. If the atmosphere is very dry, especially in winter when the heating is on, your child's skin can become dehydrated. If it is dry, it will feel rough to the touch and, if you look closely, you may see little flakes or bumps on the surface.

If this is a problem with your child's skin, apply a hypoallergenic cream formulated for children to his skin—ask your pharmacist for advice if you are not sure which to choose. You also can put aqueous cream or emollient bath oil in the bathwater but take care because this can also make the bathtub extra slippery. Don't use soap since it can dry the skin even more. If the problem does not clear up within a couple of weeks seek advice. It is possible that he has eczema (see page 257).

Your child's lips, too, can dry out or become chapped in dry air as well as when they are exposed to the sun, wind, and cold. The skin covering his lips will feel tight and unless they are sufficiently moisturized, they can start to split. If you notice that your child's lips are dry, apply petroleum jelly to them—the type that contains aloe vera is best. Repeat every few hours.

Many childhood illnesses manifest themselves initially by skin changes so be alert to any unexpected rashes (see also page 260).

SUN CREAMS

There are a range of products formulated especially for children, including sprays, lotions, and foams that cover the skin readily and conveniently without causing any stinging or other discomfort. Sunscreens are preparations containing chemicals that absorb ultraviolet radiation from the sun reducing their effect on the skin. Sunblocks contain physical or inorganic ingredients (such as titanium dioxide or zinc oxide) that physically block the sun's rays (both UVA and UVB). They are usually a much thicker lotion than a sunscreen.

Sunscreens carry a sun protection factor (SPF) rating, which appears as a number on the pack. The SPF rating is a measure of the time it would take you to get a sunburn if you were not wearing sunscreen as opposed to the time it would take with sunscreen on. An SPF 15 product blocks about 94% of UVB rays; an SPF 30 product blocks 97% of UVB rays; and an SPF 45 product blocks about 98% of rays. Even when your child is wearing sunscreen, it is best to limit the amount of time he is exposed to the sun.

3 ways to protect your child from the sun

1 Cover up. Make sure your child always wears a hat that shades his face and good-quality sunglasses with an ultraviolet filter. Keep the back of his neck, shoulders, arms, and legs covered with sunproof clothing.

2 Stay in the shade. Encourage your child to play out of the sun and in the shade as much as possible, but especially when the sun is at its highest—between 11 A.M. and 3 P.M.

3 Use a sun cream. Make sure any exposed skin is always covered with suncream—ideally use SPF (sun protection factor) 30 or above, and make sure it gives UVA (long-wavelength) and UVB (medium-wavelength) protection. Reapply the cream every two hours, and immediately after your child has been in water—even if the label says the cream is waterproof.

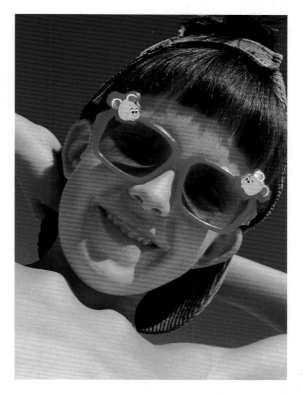

child will be happy with a simple swipe of organic lip balm or a dab of mineral blush on her cheeks or give her her own clean set of makeup brushes and let her pretend to do her makeup as you do yours.

Sun care

Your child's skin uses sunlight to make vitamin D, which is vital for strong bones, so a certain amount of sunshine is important for your child. Sunshine can also help conditions such as psoriasis and eczema (see page 257). Too much sunlight, however, can be harmful. The sun emits two types of ultraviolet radiation (UVA and UVB), both of which can damage the skin. UVB are powerful short-wave rays and are potentially the most dangerous, thickening the skin and triggering production of the pigment melanin. This attempts to protect the skin by producing a tan, but even a tan may be a sign of skin damage. If the skin burns instead of tanning, the damage to the skin is even

greater. UVA rays are weaker than UVB, but are longer rays and can penetrate the skin causing premature aging. They also increase your child's risk of skin cancer.

Because children tend to spend more time outdoors, the average child is exposed to three times more sun than adults. Children's skin is thinner, and may not be able to produce enough melanin to give protection from burning. The paler the skin, the less melanin is produced, and if your child has fair or red hair, blue eyes, and freckles, he is particularly susceptible to burning. Skin cancer has become much more common in the last 20 to 30 years, and too much exposure while young may increase the risk of skin cancer in later life.

Black skin contains more melanin than white skin and is tougher and stronger. However it is still possible for black skin to burn. It also contains more sweat glands, which help regulate temperature control, and more sebaceous glands than white skin.

Despite this, black skin can still be prone to dryness, particularly in cooler climates. Changes in skin pigmentation—such as may be caused by conditions like eczema—are more noticeable on black skin. It is also particularly susceptible to the overgrowths of fibrous scar tissue called keloids.

See the box page 69 for tips on keeping your child protected from the sun and use extra caution near water, snow, and sand because they reflect the damaging rays of the sun, which can increase your chance of sunburn.

Pierced ears

Ideally it's best to wait until your child is older (about 10), so she can take care of keeping her ears and studs cleaned. However, you may do so earlier. If your pediatrician or dermatologist won't do the procedure, ask trusted friends or relatives for recommendations. Make sure that before piercing your child's ears the technician has washed his or her hands or used antibacterial hand gel, put on new gloves, cleaned your child's earlobes with an alcohol pad, and taken an individual sterile ear piercer out of its previously unopened packaging in front of you for each ear.

The procedure will be painful so make sure you talk it through with your child in advance so she is prepared. Advise her to breathe deeply during the procedure. It can also help to cover your child's ear with protective plastic wrap and then apply ice for 15 to 30 minutes before the piercing. The piercer should use a topical numbing cream to help anesthetize the earlobes.

Make sure the earring posts are of surgical stainless steel because this sustance doesn't contain nickel or any alloys that might cause an allergic reaction. Other good choices include platinum, titanium, and 14K gold although some children may be sensitive to white gold, which can contain nickel.

Once the ears are pierced, avoid infection by always keeping your child's earrings clean. Wash your hands with a mild soap and then clean the front and back of the earrings twice a day by using a cotton ball or pad that's been soaked with a little rubbing alcohol, hydrogen peroxide, or cleaning solution provided by the piercing establishment. Gently rotate the earrings and slide them back and forth a few times to help maintain the shape of the pierced hole. Make sure they are not too tight. Do not remove the first pair of earrings until at least six weeks have passed; if you do, the hole will immediately start to close. You can, after six weeks, remove the initial pair and replace them with other earrings, but your child should wear earrings continuously for six months in order for the holes to become permanent.

Make sure your child doesn't irritate her newly pierced ears when changing her clothes or brushing her hair. Giving her clothes that button up and do not fit over the head is a good idea as is putting her hair back with a hair band or up in a ponytail. Try to keep hair products like shampoo and conditioner away from the earrings.

For at least two weeks, its recommended to put small protective bandages over the ears to prevent irritation from rubbing when she puts on a helmet (for bike riding or other sports) and some doctors advise avoiding swimming in a lake or ocean (since it might contain unknown bacteria), for two weeks.

If you notice any redness, swelling, or drainage, or your child complains of pain, itching, or tenderness, contact your healthcare provider to determine if it's an infection or a possible allergy, If it's an allergy to the metal, new posts will likely solve the problem. If it's an infection, antibiotics will be needed. If there is a reaction, remove the earrings immediately and wait at least six months before getting the ears repierced. Keloid tissue (thick scar tissue) is more likely following an infection or allergic reaction.

Play

Play has a very important role in your young child's life. Before he starts school, it's the way he will learn most things as well as helping him develop and practice his skills. Play provides mental, physical, and social stimulation and increases your child's powers of observation and concentration. It also helps to divert aggression, encourages independence, and enables your child to act out stressful situations through role play.

Play is not something that only happens at home; the more play-filled environments you introduce your child to, the more he will benefit. It is important, however, that you oversee play, and join in as much as possible to ensure it promotes your child's physical and intellectual development. Try to strike a balance between structured and self-directed play; the latter will help him develop independence and a sense of his own identity.

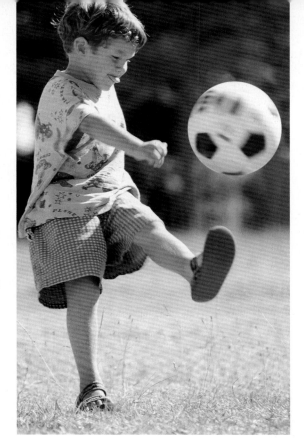

Planning activities

Your child's age, attention span, and stage of development should determine your choice of activities but each day try to include both active and passive play, both indoors and out. If you can, either at a playground or at one of the many preschool activity classes available (see below), try to get together with other parents and children to give both yourself and your child the chance to socialize.

Different types of play are important to avoid boredom and to challenge your child. His physical development will benefit from running, climbing, jumping, throwing a ball, riding a bike, or dancing; his creativity, imagination, and expression will be stimulated through modelmaking, drawing and painting, dressing up, pretend tea parties, and fantasy play; his hand-eye coordination will be strengthened with building blocks, construction toys, and puzzles and his social skills perfected by playing with other children.

As well as the stimulation he'll get from various toys and activities, your child sometimes will also need to do nothing at all and just be allowed to sit and day dream, act out a fantasy in his mind or talk to imaginary friends, unwind, and think about the day, or simply have a quiet moment with you.

Your being involved in his play and activities is a very important factor in your child's mental, physical, and social development. A young child finds it hard to play alone for long and if left to his own devices, will probably get into some mischief. You also need to help guide his play to some extent, to demonstrate how things work, if necessary, and to encourage his efforts at activities such as drawing and making things. When you cannot be available to play with your child, try to involve him in your daily activities. For example, let him help you do the dishes or the dusting, or do some baking together; not only will it be fun for him but he will have an opportunity to learn new skills and actions.

However, as your child gets older, you will need to strike a balance between helping him and leaving him free to play in the way he chooses. If you constantly play with him he will not learn to entertain himself and will become bored or miserable when he is on his own. And if you constantly interfere with, or take over, his play, he will not learn how to do things for himself and thereby gain self-confidence.

The learning home

Primary to your child achieving his developmental potential is whether your home is a supportive environment. The kitchen, for example, is the ideal "science lab" with access to heat, water, a freezer, and food materials. Here your child can not only learn about healthy eating but also about changing states such as freezing and melting and how solids, liquids, and gases are different. Weighing and measuring ingredients for cooking will be ideal introductions to mathematics, while different foods can be the basis for geography lessons, because you can talk about the different parts of the world the food comes from and what the climate is like there. Learning to follow a recipe will teach your child about instructional writing and the importance of chronology (if you don't follow the recipe in the right order, you can end up with some odd results!). And baking or cooking together provides a great bonding experience.

The bathroom is the perfect place for exploring floating and sinking, using soap to make bubbles or make things slippery, and understanding volume and the way liquids change shape to fill a vessel. Using a plastic measuring jug, bathtime can be a way to make use of math.

Bathing also is a good time to work on language development. While washing, your child can make up bubble poems; tell stories about shipwrecks, mermaids, and pirates and even think of musical sea shanties with an orchestra of water-filled containers to bash, rattle, and blow.

The living room is a good place for a cozy book corner (if there isn't space in your child's bedroom). All you need are a few cushions and a plastic crate full of a changing selection of books. Rotating books from your child's bookshelves (or from the library) will encourage your child to take pleasure in reading

(see also page 73). This room, too, often contains the television and DVD player. These aren't necessarily bad for children; what is bad is the lack of conversation and the encouragement of passivity. Limit the time your child spends watching and make sure you watch programs together (see also page 146).

The average dining table topped by a wipeable mat can be transformed into an arts and crafts station. Even if your table is a valuable antique, it can still serve as a den with the help of cloths flung across the top, cushions underneath, and dressing-up accessories. It can become a cave, an igloo, the basement of a haunted mansion, or wherever your child's interests lie. The dining or kitchen table also is, of course, the best place to learn the art of conversation. Make sure, even with differing schedules, that you eat together several times a week, setting the table properly with your child's help.

Everybody—children included—needs a calm, contemplative space to be himself and to collect his thoughts. A bedroom can provide this. Adequate storage makes toys easier to get out and then put away, and giving your child open access to toys and art equipment helps to spark off ideas for activities, avoiding the dreaded "I'm bored!"

The backyard can be a priceless resource for learning. Apart from active play on swings, slides, frames, and so on, to boost fitness and health, it is a great place for open-ended, discovery-based learning. Even the youngest child will enjoy playing with sand, water, twigs, and dry leaves.

A vegetable patch or a flower bed can be a wonderful place for the safe exploration of the natural world and its biology. Here a child can watch plants grow, enjoy bug and bird behavior, look at rocks and soils, and study weather and clouds. Wonderful dens can be constructed cheaply and easily from bought tents, sheets, and chairs or from natural materials. Try to do some gardening with your child. Talk to him about what you are doing, and why. If possible, give your child his own patch to cultivate. Children love to consume what they grow, so plant fruit and vegetables as well as flowers. Talk about the way a plant grows from a tiny seed—even a huge tree. Ask your child if he knows what a green plant needs to grow healthily, such as light and water.

Essential art materials

In addition to the basic equipment (see box) many found, discarded, or reused materials can feed the imagination.

Coloring materials should include pens, pencils, markers, crayons, and paint. Wax crayons (both chunky and finer tipped), pencil crayons for shading, and a variety of felt-tip markers will give your child the opportunity to create many different effects. Metallic or gel pens, chalks, and pastels are also great additions to an art kit. You can buy powder paints that you mix yourself, or ready-mixed ones. Look online or in discount bookstores for inexpensive boxes of oils, watercolors, and acrylics. Solid blocks of paint are also a good option. Ensure you have a variety of brushes, including fine ones.

Clay and other moldable materials—Play-Doh®, putty, and so on—can be a great way for your child to explore different media and techniques, and he can use these materials to make long-lasting artifacts.

Paper—plain white, lined, and colored construction paper—can be as inexpensive or costly as you like. Computer printouts, wallpaper remnants, and so on, can all be reused as well as more expensive "art" paper. You should also have a store of some poster board or thicker card stock.

Sticking materials such as clear adhesive tape, masking tape, and a variety of glues may be needed for attaching different things. Keep glue sticks, white glue, and a glue pot and spreader handy.

Pictures cut from magazines as well as scraps kept from packaging are useful for making collages. So too are beads, sequins, glitter, ribbon scraps, colored wool, and fabric remnants, dried pasta shapes, and natural materials such as leaves, flowers, pine cones, acorns, seed pods, grasses, shells, and feathers.

Household items such as egg cartons, cardboard tubes, bubble wrap, ice cream, and yogurt cartons, netting from fruit packaging, and empty boxes can be used for making models and other art activities. Once you have collected all of these useful items,

BASIC ART EQUIPMENT

- ◆ Apron
- ◆ Scissors (age-appropriate)
- ◆ Ruler
- ◆ Tape
- ◆ Glue
- ◆ Pencil
- ◆ Coloring materials
- ◆ Molding materials
- ◆ Eraser
- ◆ Paper and card stock

store them in plastic crates (available very cheaply from bargain stores), or in large cardboard cartons. Paper files can be made from empty cereal boxes while plastic tool boxes or shoe holders (the type with pockets that hangs on the wall) are cheap to buy and great for holding crayons, erasers, and smaller "found objects." Cutlery trays can be used to store paintbrushes and pens, and small plastic indoor trash cans can be used to store bulkier items such as wool, fabrics, and so on.

Make sure, too, that you have plenty of newspaper handy to cover surfaces. Oilcloth makes a very useful protective table cover.

Reading

As your child gets older, you will find his interest in books becomes more specific as to content. Boys tend to enjoy action and adventure tales, and girls prefer magical tales with a happy ending, but often this is because parents do the discriminating early on. You should make an effort to choose and read a general selection of tales with a mixture of different genres. As your child begins to socialize with other children, he will start to prefer the different types of stories enjoyed by his peer group. If you give him a good grounding, however, he will always be able to appreciate reading in general.

Preschoolers enjoy group story-telling, which allows them to participate, learn, and connect with

3 Party time
4
5
6

3 years old

Your child is likely to enjoy a party, much as she would a play date, but isn't really aware that it is something special and exciting. Keep the party and guest list short (1½ hours) and 4 guests (some recommend same number of guests as age of birthday boy or girl), and go with the flow, which should be very slow and unregimented.

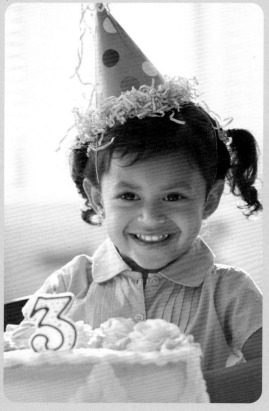

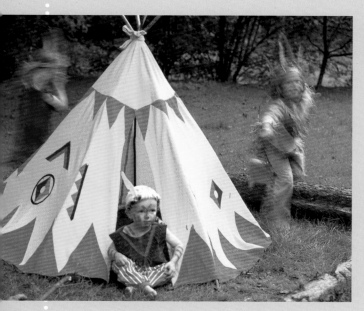

4 years old

Uncritically excited about the food, party bags, gifts, and activities or entertainment (all of which he now expects because he knows a party is "special,") your preschooler will still tire easily and/or become over-excited. Plan on 1½ hours and no more than 6 guests. Play should be informal but don't be surprised if it all ends in tears.

5 years old

Be prepared; fives are filled with excess energy so a party with plenty to do is key, though don't be surprised if children behave in a solitary way rather than share. Now's the time to introduce simple games and/or activities in which the guests (best if same sex) can let off steam. Plan on 2 hours and about 6 guests (fives find it hard to wait for attention or to take turns). Themes and decorations will add to the excitement.

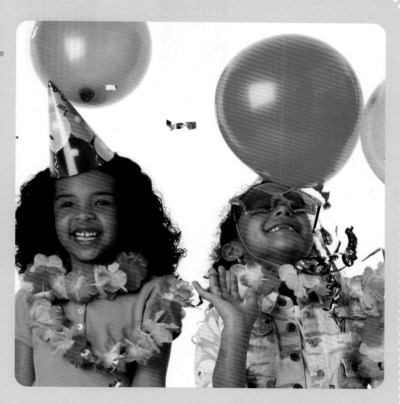

6 years old

Friends are very important and while you may be able to get away with 6 guests, you may also have to invite his entire class! Work around your child's interest (boys will tend to want more action than girls) for activities or games, cake theme, and so on, and 2½ hours will be plenty.

others. Libraries and some children's bookstores offer events but it's easy to set up a small group with other moms and children. It's a good idea to keep sessions short and to choose stories with lots of action, repetition, and noise, and for which you can use facial expressions while reading. Teller and listeners alike will have lots of fun with a story that has a silly "magic word" that the children will enjoy shouting out. It also gives the children something to look for. They will listen intently for the magic word, so that they can repeat it back to you. This, in turn, makes them pay attention to what you are saying, and it makes the experience fun.

Alternatively, you could make some sort of sign or perform an action that the group has to watch for. In any event, choose stories that lend themselves to actions. The more actions and movements you can put in to illustrate what is happening, the more the group will respond and become involved. Pick simple actions like clapping hands or jumping up and down. You could even use soft toys or puppets to help illustrate what is happening in the tale, if appropriate.

As a reader, you should try and make the story more interesting to your child (or children). Exaggerate your facial expressions and movements, and get into the spirit of the tale.

Reading for a purpose

Reading can do more than be entertaining. It's a great way to get your child ready for bed and can help him accept and adjust to problems that he will encounter at home or when she's at school.

A book at bedtime

Reading as part of your child's normal bedtime routine can encourage a restful night's sleep. The perfect bedtime story has to have a strong element of satisfaction and just enough action and adventure to keep your child interested without over-stimulating him. You want to soothe your little one into sleep and leave him feeling that all is well with the world.

Choose short stories, fables, or abridged classic tales that take about 15 minutes to read through. Read the story beforehand so you know whether the words and images conjure up happy things. If you think there is something in the tale that might alarm your child, keep the book for daytime sessions.

Use your voice to soothe and ease your child into sleep. Linger over words that present soft, happy images, and wind down your tale by slowing the pace and lowering the pitch of your voice. You may find that your child drifts into sleep halfway through the story. If so, just let the words dwindle gently and bookmark the page for next time.

Learning about life

Story-telling is great entertainment but it can also be used to educate your child about the way the world

PERSONALIZED FAIRY TALE

All children enjoy being the center of a story and an easy way to make it happen is to take a well-known classic story and insert your child's name into it as the hero or heroine. The main character should be a child of similar age and with good qualities. If the story permits, you can use the names of your child's friends as well as mommy and daddy and the grandparents. Even though the story is based on a familiar tale that you may have read before, you can change the name to make it unique. If you feel confident enough, you can introduce elements to the story to make it your own. So, for example, Sleeping Beauty (your daughter) might be lost in a dream world in which she has her own adventure. The prince could be daddy or mommy, coming to save her and giving her a big kiss. Or if you chose Aladdin, your son would need to think very carefully about his three wishes, and you could discuss the ramifications together. Bear in mind that King Midas wished that everything he touched would turn to gold.

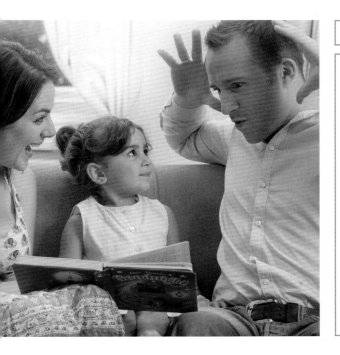

- **3-year-olds**
  Stories about everyday life, not only domestically but at the seashore or a farm; various modes of transportation and the different seasons; animals, both domestic and wild, and alphabet books.
- **4-year-olds**
  Humorous or "silly" books, whimsical or imaginative stories and classic fairy tales.
- **5-year-olds**
  Humorous, "silly," or ridiculous books; books about animals that act like people and books that can "explain" concepts like colors, sizes, and opposites.

"works" as well as help him cope with the new or difficult. Sharing appropriate stories can help your child experience situations in a positive way. For example, reading can be a wonderful opportunity to learn about other cultures. Sharing stories from or about people around the world can give your child an understanding of other societies and how the people in them relate to one another. There's a great tradition of story-telling in other cultures and this should be explored and celebrated. It's never too early to do this.

What's known as "healing" tales—books that teach a specific lesson, or offer help and advice on such things as learning to play nicely, keeping toys neat and tidy, learning to make friends, and not being selfish—enable your child to learn important life lessons in a comfortable and fun environment.

There are many books available that deal with "difficult" situations; these can help your child prepare for a variety of events or situations that he may experience—the arrival of a new sibling, moving to a new home, going to the hospital, the illness or death of a close relative, separating or divorcing parents, or starting school. Using stories in this way means that your child will be able to think through the process in a safe environment, thus

making things familiar for him and taking away the fear of the unknown. Starting kindergarten or nursery school, for example, will be a big event in your child's world, linked to a whole host of exciting and frightening changes. Repeatedly telling stories that include this scenario and putting him in the tales will help him identify with the changes. In this way you will be able to allay his fears as he learns about what to expect.

Toys

Giving your child different types of toys and objects to play with helps develop his self-expression, his hand-eye coordination, and stimulates his creativity and imagination; toys will also help him learn to distinguish different shapes, colors, sizes, textures, sounds, and weights.

There are so many toys and games available it can be hard to decide what to buy. The best toys are those that are right for your child's age and abilities, but that can also be used in more than one way; these are the most likely to retain his interest. Construction toys including bricks that can be joined together and incorporate a variety of other linkable pieces, such as motors, switches, and lights will continue to be used by your child for many years. If a toy is too advanced for your child's age or developmental stage, he will quickly become frustrated and abandon it. If too simple, he will soon get bored with it.

Outdoor activity toys such as scooters, roller skates, and bicycles are fun and give your child an opportunity to get physically fit and let off steam.

If you have a backyard, construct a sandbox and water tray, together with "super soaker" water guns. These are useful for children because, not only are they fun, they can teach your child about such things as floating and sinking and hydraulics. If you do not have a backyard, offer your child a bowl full of play sand or water on a plastic sheet.

Dressing-up clothes including hats, scarves, costume jewelry, and purses can be begged from friends and relatives or bought from Goodwill stores to supplement a dressing-up trunk of commercially bought outfits. Young toddlers enjoy role play and dressing up; older children will enjoy dressing up that is tied in with a historical topic such as pirates, cowboys, explorers, and so on.

Every home should have a collection of puppets and even a small puppet theater (or a cardboard box made into a theater). These toys help to develop language skills, imagination, and story-telling, and can be used to help your child to explore issues that he is having trouble articulating, such as problems with friendship, loss, etc. Using a puppet to "speak" removes a child a degree away from the things he needs to say, and can make him feel safer about voicing his issues.

Electronic and digital games

It's important that toddlers are able to grab hold of the gadgets they see all around them, and to start to discover the digital world in which they'll be growing up. There are many great apps out there that our children can learn from and have fun with—partly because they're such a demanding audience—so the quality has to be high to maintain their interest.

But it's yet another challenge for parents to deal with: how often and for how long should you allow your toddler to play with this stuff?

Generally, "screen time" shouldn't be allowed to replace real-life human interaction and active physical play. This means, that except for rare occasions, not leaving your child alone with a gadget while you do something else; technology should not be a replacement for you. Apps and electronic games should just be other ways to interact with your child, as if you were helping with building blocks or reading him or her a book. Even if an app or

ways to get on top of toys

1 **Only let your child play with a limited number of toys at a time.** If he has too many to choose from he may run from one to another and keep changing his mind about which one to play with.

2 **If your child is given several toys for an occasion** such as Christmas or his birthday, save a few for later and present one as a new toy on a rainy day, or when he is bored or feeling unwell or under the weather.

3 **Check the toys regularly.** Are they still safe? If broken, discard a toy immediately. Has your child out-grown them? If your child has become bored with a toy, but it's still within his age range, put it away for a week or two and then bring it out again. He will probably welcome it as a new toy.

4 **Keep a supply of differently sized batteries handy** (but don't let your child change batteries), and ensure that battery compartments on toys are inaccessible.

electronic toy can be used by your child on his own, it's best to sit next to him, helping him when he isn't sure what to do or encouraging him when he gets things right. You also should make conversation during the game or activity, discussing what's happening and what your child thinks about it.

Excursions

Your child experiences things everywhere he goes. He's like a sponge, soaking up the sights, sounds, smells, feelings, and tastes he encounters. You may think you just are going for a simple day out, but to your child, all outings are rich in incidental learning.

Even a visit to the grocery store can be an opportunity for you to talk together about what you are buying and about the places the food came from. The colors of food will be interesting to your child. Ask him if strawberry red is the same as cherry red. Which is more orange colored—an orange or a tangerine? How many "green" vegetables can your child name? Can you find any food you have not tried before? Talk about the item and try to guess what it will taste like, then go home and see who was right! You can look for "Fairtrade" brands or organic labels on food. Does your child know what they mean? How is such food different?

Science and the natural world are everywhere you look. Use a walk in a wooded area to identify trees, leaves, plants, and bugs using simple guidebooks. Make a collection of items such as leaves, nuts, feathers, and stones for your child to "show and tell" to others. The materials can also be made into collages or dreamcatchers. A walk around a pond can turn into a science trip. Bring a small net and a white dish and look closely at the plants and creatures you find before returning the creatures to the water. Or, take a sketchpad and crayons so your child can make pictures of what he sees in or near the water.

The beach, like many other outdoor environments, is rich in opportunities for hands-on, experiential learning. For example, you are using math (estimating volume, measuring, and looking at shapes) when you construct a sandcastle together. Even history can be introduced as you discuss fortification and dig a moat. Look at plants and

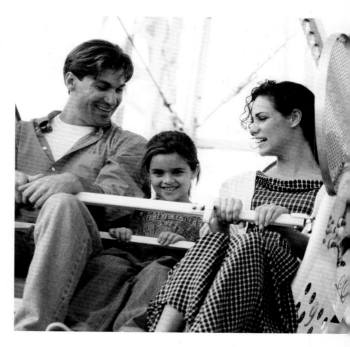

creatures on the shore, and then investigate rock pools. You also can encourage language play by making up lists of sea-related things. Create a game: "In my treasure chest I found …" and make up poetic and outrageous things such as "a mermaid's song" or "a pirate's stinky sock" as well as South Sea pearls and jewel-encrusted daggers. It's not just a memory game; it's about stretching the imagination, something that only expands with regular use.

Make up silly poems and songs encouraged by practicing alliteration (like "salty sea" or "rough rocks"). Give your child examples such as "sticky starfish" and "wild waves." You don't have to say you are using alliteration—just tell your child you are looking for descriptions that start with the same sounds. Encourage your child to find an alliterative description for seaweed, sand, fish, or whatever you can see or imagine.

A visit to any public botanical garden with a greenhouse offers the opportunity to experience different habitats from around the world, such as a tropical rainforest or desert. Heritage sites can often bring history to life for a child. Encourage your child to think about how life was different in the past, compared to today. What sort of jobs did

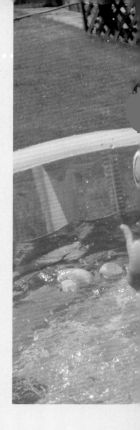

Your child at play

3
4
5

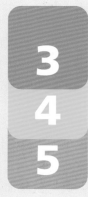

3 years old

Your child still prefers playing with large objects such as wooden blocks or Duplo®, which she can combine into basic structures, or threading large beads on spools of thread. Her delight in large-scale play continues with artistic activities: she will prefer fingerpaints to paint and brushes, for example, and her paintings won't have much shape or structure—whole pages may be covered with a single color. Messy play with sand, clay, and water can keep her occupied for long periods at a time. She will be better at producing lifelike objects with clay while her water play will extend to blowing soap bubbles and sailing boats.

Your child's imaginative abilities will be more apparent with dolls and soft-toy play. Instead of just putting dolly or teddy bear to bed, she may now feed and cook for dolly and organize tea parties.

Outdoors, she should enjoy playing on a slide, swings, and climbing frames.

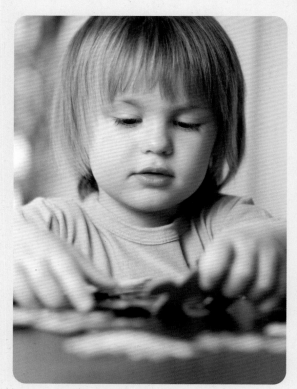

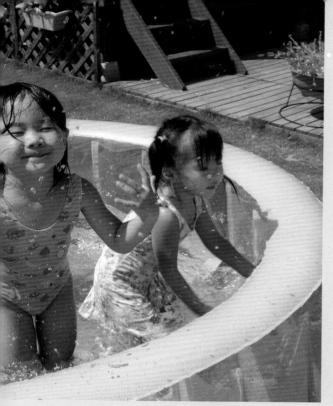

construction toys. Amateur dramatics can involve a wide range of scenarios including the fantastic as well as the domestic. Books continue to be great favorites, particularly those with more detailed pictures.

5 years old

Whether or not your child attends play group, goes to kindergarten, or is still at home, she will enjoy the usual group artistic activities of cutting, tracing, drawing, pasting, stringing beads, and making collages. Now too is the time for enjoying tent houses (indoors and out) and role play with dolls and puppets. Outdoor play can include roller skating, trampolining, skipping, and bicycling, and more organized games with peers. Scientific exploration may be undertaken using magnets, binoculars, magnifying glasses, and flashlights. Drawings may now include letters and numbers and within her capabilities are games that require imagination and the ability to think ("I Spy" or "20 Questions") as well as checkers.

4 years old

Your child will be particularly fond of outdoor play on tricycles, bikes, and scooters and will enjoy climbing frames and jungle gyms, which he uses with increased agility. Give him blunt-ended scissors to cut out pictures in magazines to encourage his manual dexterity and he will enjoy making collages. He will engage in make-believe and may have imaginary companions and objects while pretend play—doctors and nurses, for example—with or without dolls, and dressing up are great favorites. He may enjoy simple card or board games and large, relatively uncomplicated picture puzzles. Using large building blocks, he'll be able to construct impressive stuctures such as houses and forts and may play in them or use other toys such as trucks and wagons alongside. However, he may also start to build with Lego® and other

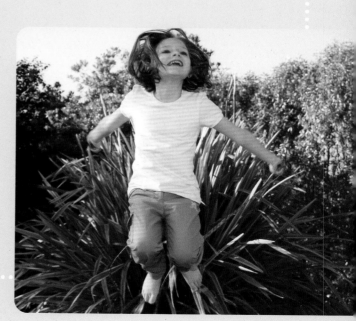

people have, what did they wear? Farms can provide opportunities for your child to get up close to see animals and crops. Many establishments offer activities like feeding the animals, riding on farm vehicles, or picking your own fruit.

Apart from the excellent exercise swimming provides, a day at the pool can be an opportunity to talk about floating and sinking, using swimming floats and rings for demonstrating.

Use a museum trip to find out more about a subject that really grips your child—be that bugs, dinosaurs, or space travel. When you visit an art gallery, take a sketchbook.

Wherever you are, get into the habit of talking about what you see. Ask your child open-ended questions about what he sees: "What if …", "Why do you think …", and stand by for the many questions your child asks you! Never be afraid to say you don't know the answer; if you encourage him to help you "explore" by sitting next to you while you use books and the internet to find out answers, you will be teaching him a vital lesson: how to research.

Group activities

Today, in addition to playgroups that offer your child independent childcare and the opportunity to engage with his peers, there is an enormous range of activities on offer depending on your available time and budget. Most communities have preschooler courses for arts and crafts; drama, music, and dance; athletics from swimming to gymnastics, yoga, soccer, and baseball, and language learning. Some preschoolers have such busy social lives that their parents begin to feel like diary secretaries!

Attending a preschool or activity class will expose your child to his peers and may have the social and developmental benefits claimed, but research has found that the more time children under five spend away from their parents, the more behavior problems (rudeness, defiance, or aggression) they exhibit. In addition, children who spent more time in childcare are rated as less socially competent by their mothers and primary teachers. Researchers have also uncovered elevated stress levels in certain preschoolers when away from the home.

Historically, most children remained at home with their parents and extended family until much older than they do now. They were not segregated with other children. Unlike children their own age, parents and other family members are able to teach preschoolers self-control, empathy, compassion, patience, social etiquette, and an upbeat, constructive attitude for dealing with peer problems. That's why it's vital that you carefully choose and monitor groups your child joins, and that you provide his primary caregiving. Using the internet and other resources, it's very possible to provide your child with lots of varied activities while he remains at home.

4 things you can do to ensure positive group experiences

1 **Keep the number and length of time of each activity short.**

2 **Choose classes that are small and intimate.** No more than 15 students and 4 teachers is ideal as long as the venue has room to play.

3 **Look for teachers who expect friendly, polite behavior.** Avoid classes or groups where children are allowed to get away with angry, antisocial, or disobedient behavior. Ask about the teachers' strategies for coping with undesirable behavior.

4 **Communicate regularly with the teacher.** If you are not present at each class, find out how your child is doing, especially if he is being rejected by his peers or is involved in rejecting another child (for which you need to take corrective action). Make sure your child isn't hanging out with a "bad crowd." If your child plays in peer groups that are characterized by negative emotions or antisocial behavior, his social development will suffer.

Sleep and bedtime

Sleep will help your child grow strong and healthy. Most preschoolers need between 11 and 13 hours of sleep over a 24-hour period and younger children usually have one daytime nap. Naps should not take place too late in the day or go on for too long since either situation will result in the lack of a good night's sleep. As your child gets older, napping will tail off, although some children still benefit from taking one. You should establish a set routine time for napping or expect your child to spend some quiet or relaxing time in his own bedroom. Even if your child can't sleep, some "down time" (about an hour) will help him to relax.

Research has shown that regular bedtimes make for well behaved children but problems such as resisting going to sleep and waking frequently at night are common as are night-time fears and nightmares, sleepwalking, and bed-wetting.

Bedtime routine

A preschooler needs a fair amount of time to get ready for bed. Expect to spend at least 30 minutes on calm and enjoyable activities before kissing your child good night and turning out the light. Action-packed TV shows and DVDs should be left for much earlier in the day. To help your child wind down, he may enjoy taking a bath and reading bedtime stories. Always stick to a regular routine made up of a set time and sequence of events (dressing for bed, brushing teeth, picking a book, and so on) so that your child knows what to expect.

Make sure the room is cool and comfortable and is lit by a nightlight or area light on the very lowest dimmer setting. Playing soft, soothing music is fine. Remember to reserve the bed for sleeping only; it should not be used as a platform for playing. The room should not contain a television.

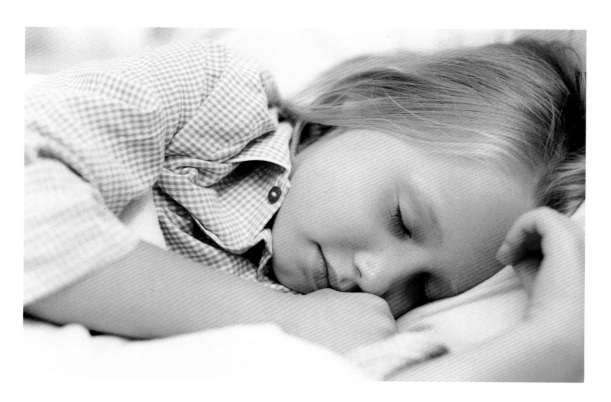

4 vital components of an effective bedtime routine

1 **Create and maintain a consistent routine.** Stick to set going to bed and wake-up times each day.

2 **Make sure the bedroom environment is quiet,** cool, dark, and comfortable for sleeping.

3 **Limit food and drink** (especially any drinks containing caffeine) before bedtime. Bear in mind that many beverages contain caffeine, so check the label.

4 **Tuck your child into bed** in a sleepy but awake state. This will help your child learn to fall asleep on his own and help him return to sleep again if he wakes up in the middle of the night.

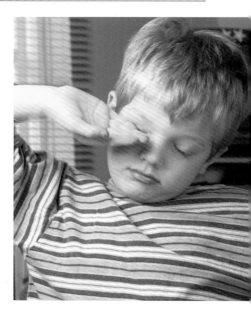

Allow your child to pick out the pajamas he wishes to wear and the stuffed animal to take to bed, etc. His choice of comfort object helps your child feel more relaxed at bedtime and all through the night.

You should also let him pick his bedtime book, but make sure you have set clear limits as to how many books you will read or songs you will sing. Sit close by your child's bed, or get into it with him so that he feels safe and secure. The aim is to make your child as comfortable and relaxed as possible, so take your time and read to him in a soothing voice.

Sleep talking and walking

It's not uncommon for preschool children once fallen asleep to talk or sit up in bed or even to walk around for a short period of time. Talking in one's sleep is quite normal and is not a cause for concern and generally, night- or sleepwalking isn't either. In most cases, a child, within an hour or two of falling asleep, either sits up in bed and makes repetitive motions, such as rubbing his eyes or fussing with his pajamas, or gets out of bed and walks around. In nightwalking, a child is awake but unwilling to stay in bed. A nightlight, some nearby toys, and perhaps a snack or two may keep him in his room.

Sleepwalking involves your child walking around in a dazed and unresponsive way with his eyes open. It can be due to illness or fever, certain medications, a lack of sleep or fatigue, an irregular sleep schedule, or stress (although it is rarely due to an underlying medical, emotional, or psychological problem). If you or your partner are or were sleepwalkers, it's more likely that your child will be one too.

During an episode, it is vital that your child can't access stairs or sharp or breakable objects and that there are no obstacles in his path. Make sure your home is thoroughly childproofed (see page 205) and that he doesn't sleep in the top bunk bed. On discovering your child, gently guide him back to bed but try not to wake him up because this might scare him. Most children usually do not remember sleepwalking and in itself it is not harmful.

However, if the episodes are very regular, cause your child to be sleepy during the day, involve dangerous behaviors, or you suspect there may be an underlying problem, discuss it with your healthcare provider. He or she may recommend scheduled awakening, a treatment that disrupts the sleep cycle enough to help stop sleepwalking. In rare cases, sleep medication may be prescribed.

Bed-wetting

Children vary in when they achieve night-time dryness although by age six, most children are dry at night; see box below for tips on making the process easier. That being said, bed-wetting is extremely common with preschoolers and seems to run in families; if either parent was late in achieving night-time dryness, there is a good chance that your child will be, too. Bed-wetting is also more common with boys, though why this is so is not known.

With a young child, it's important to let nature take its course. A good time to leave off the training pants at night is when he is consistently dry in the morning and, if necessary, gets up in the night to urinate. Continue to use a waterproof mattress cover for some time in case accidents occur.

If your child wets the bed every night, keep the training pants on for a while and try again after a few weeks. There is no point in continuing the "training" if he is not having success because this just will be upsetting for both of you.

If your child is still having problems staying dry at night after the age of five, talk to your healthcare provider, not only to exclude an underlying medical problem but also for some further advice on managing the issue. If your child starts bed-wetting again after having stopped, see box above.

5 ways to help your child stay dry at night

1 **Limit fluids.** Don't let your child drink large amounts of liquid before bedtime.

2 **Bedtime bathroom visit.** Make sure your child urinates just before he goes to bed. Encourage him to go to the bathroom even if he doesn't want to by incorporating it into his bedtime routine.

3 **Lifting.** Try taking your child to the bathroom when you go to bed and possibly if you happen to get up in the night. However, it is not worth doing this if it disrupts your child's sleep and makes him tired during the day.

4 **Keep calm.** Some children take longer than others to achieve night-time dryness. Because you want your child to do this naturally, stay relaxed when accidents happen. Never punish your child for being wet at night! Your doctor will be able to offer help and advice.

5 **Give praise or a reward.** Although you don't want to make a fuss when things go wrong, it is equally important to praise your child when he manages to stay dry. Placing a star on a sticker chart on the calendar days when he is dry in the morning will help your child become involved and feel that he has control over what is happening.

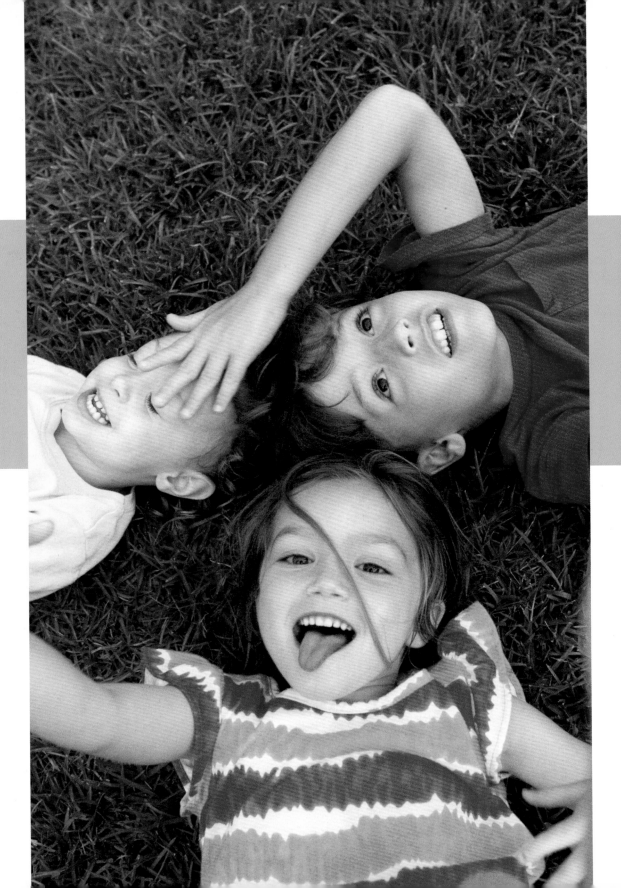

CHAPTER 3
DEVELOPMENTAL CHANGES

Your preschooler's physical, mental, emotional, and social development is at a key stage—and you have a vital role in helping your child reach her potential. Learning to master a wide number of tasks, make sense of her world and communicate her wishes, manage her fears and anger and appropriately display her affections, and become a popular member of her peer group is an enormous task but one that needs to be accomplished before your child is ready for school.

Physical abilities

The preschooler years should be marked by lots of activity; in the previous chapter, you would have learned how important it is to get your child moving and some appropriate activities that she can do on her own or with you. Your child's increasingly sophisticated abilities are a result of both aspects of her physicality—locomotive and fine motor skills—working in concert with each other.

Locomotive skills

By age three, your preschooler is so agile, she's able to make the most of playground visits. Her agility will continue to develop, so that by age four, she should be able to climb trees and longer ladders with skill.

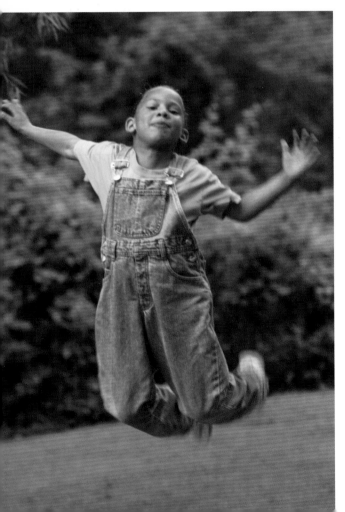

She should have mastered jumping and possibly standing on one leg for a short time. Her balancing skills develop, which are necessary for her to learn to hop, usually around the age of four. When she does so, she'll probably favor one foot.

Most three-year-olds can kick a ball effectively and will start to enjoy trying to kick it back and forth and by four years of age, your child should start to enjoy ball games that include catching, throwing, bouncing, and kicking; she'll be better able to judge direction when throwing. She should be able to catch smaller balls with her hands, and may be able to use a small bat or racket.

By age five, your child should be able to play and enjoy more complex ball games and have honed her motor skills and in particular, her balancing abilities. She should be able to stand on one leg for up to 10 seconds at a time, hop 10 times in a row, skip on alternate feet, and walk along a line with one foot in front of the other. Your preschooler will be able to dance rhythmically to music so may enjoy going to ballet lessons.

If your child started riding her tricycle at age three, she should be proficient by age four, even steering around sharp bends. She then should be ready for a bike, though initially with training wheels. Many four-year-olds can also use skates.

From the latter part of the preschool years, your child is well on the way to mastering all the basic skills involved in movement but she will go on refining them and integrating them into more complex movement sequences. For example, while a five-year-old can both run and kick a ball (although not do both well at the same time), by the time she's six years of age, your child should be ready for organized team sports, such as soccer or softball. Remember to help your child find a sport she enjoys and be a role model by participating in activity as well. And always make sure she wears the necessary protective equipment.

are particularly useful when it comes to dressing and eating. (See box, below, on honing such abilities.)

Most three-year-olds can throw a ball reasonably well over-arm and can catch a large, bounced ball when their arms are held out straight. Your child should also be able to create ever more complex constructions—increasingly taller towers and more elaborate bridges. So, by the age of four, for example, she can build a bridge of three bricks with either hand and build steps with more than six blocks. Imaginative play using large linking blocks will continue to be enjoyed as your child "graduates" to smaller blocks (such as LEGO™) and her scenarios become more sophisticated.

From the age of four, your child will enjoy other types of construction toys, including those with smaller and more realistic pieces, such as cars and planes she can assemble herself and use for imaginative play. Make sure, however, that these are age-appropriate for your child and that she plays with smaller pieces under supervision.

Fine motor skills

As well as locomotive abilities, finger and hand skills continue to be perfected throughout the preschool years. Dexterity, a fine motor skill, greatly improves between ages two and four so that four-year-olds are able to lift and put down objects carefully, even very tiny ones. Being able to coordinate and manipulate increasingly smaller objects are important skills that

6 ways to encourage dexterity

1 **Offer your child increasingly complex jigsaw puzzles;** being able to pick up and fit together smaller pieces will evolve over time.

2 **Let her thread objects.** Start by encouraging your child to place spools or tubes onto a piece of string or yarn, then offer large beads and a shoelace and by four, big buttons with a thread headed with a blunt plastic needle.

3 **Introduce sewing cards.** From the age of four or so, sewing cards are a simple and fun way to learn. You can buy them or make your own by drawing a shape on a piece of card stock and cutting holes (or using a hole punch) in the outline. Offer your child a blunt plastic needle and yarn to sew around the outline.

4 **Let your child "cook."** From age three, your child can help assemble salad ingredients, roll out dough, and use simple cookie cutters with it. She will be able to help you decorate cakes and cookies with a pastry decorating pen.

5 **Provide craft materials.** Being able to use a child's scissors, glue, papers, and pasta or found objects like leaves and shells to create collages; Play-Doh® to make models, and crayons and paints for making pictures not only feeds your child's imagination but helps her perfect many fine motor skills.

6 **Practice different fixings.** Helping your child master zippers, buttons, and buckles will feed her desire for dressing independently.

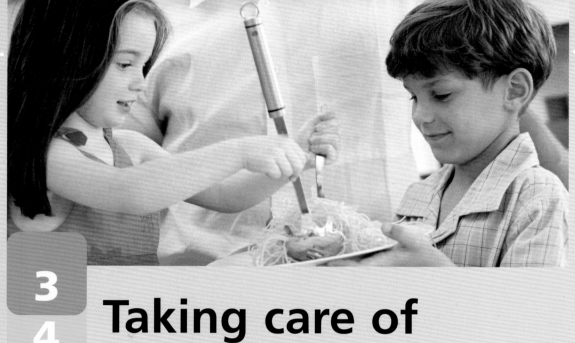

3
4
5

Taking care of herself

3 years old

Routines will be problematical but your child should be able to wash her hands and parts of herself in the bathtub. She will be better at undressing than dressing but can put on socks and shoes (but not fasten them), pull up elasticated pants or skirts, and possibly put on simple dresses and sweaters; she will need help with most fastenings and "complicated" clothes. She can hang her jacket and towel on a low hook, put dirty clothes in a laundry basket, pick up her clothes and toys, eat reasonably skillfully with a spoon, and hold her cup by one handle. Many three-year-olds like to eat with a fork. Overall, table manners are minimal. She may use the potty independently and, like most of her peers, will be dry during the day. She may, like many, not be at night. Even during the day, she may have occasional "accidents" (particularly true for boys).

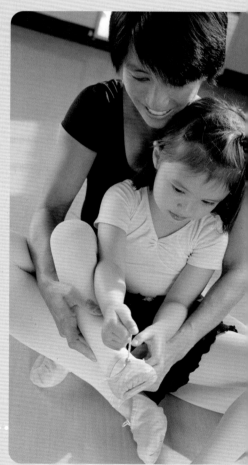

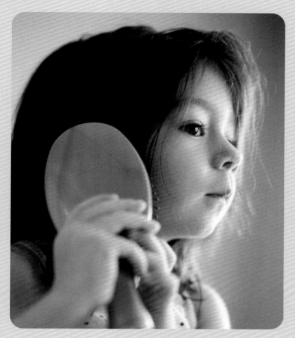

years old

Your child will go to the potty and possibly the toilet by himself (and may demand privacy) and remain dry day and night. He can wash and dry his hands, bathe himself reasonably well except for the hard-to-reach places, and dry himself after bathing. He attempts to brush his teeth and comb his hair. He can blow his nose on his own and get dressed in clothes with large buttons and zippers and can put on shoes on the right feet with self-stick fastenings or slip-ons; some children can do up buckles. He eats well with a spoon and fork and uses a knife to spread jam on bread but cannot cut with one. If he has his own bedroom, may be happy to go to bed and even tell you when he is tired.

5 years old

Your child can perform a number of hygiene tasks competently, like washing her face, brushing her teeth, wiping herself after using the toilet, and washing her hands. She is cooperative and enthusiastic when washing herself in the bath although she may not wash all parts thoroughly. She can select appropriate clothes for the weather and undress herself easily; she can also dress herself competently although her clothes may need to be laid out the right way around. While she can hang up a jacket or dress using a hanger, mainly she doesn't take care of her clothes. If taught, she may remember to cover her mouth or nose with her elbow when she coughs or sneezes. She can pour from a carton and use a knife for cutting soft foods but probably is not able to cut meat well.

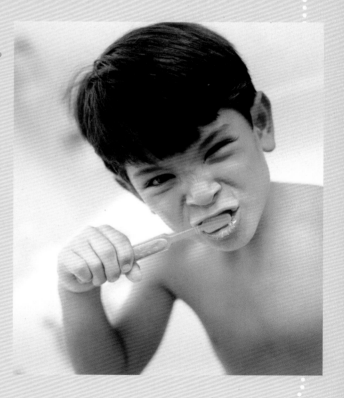

Drawing and writing abilities develop in recognizable stages. At age three, your child will hold her pencil near the point and the positioning of her hand will be more similar to the adult grip, with a pencil being held between her thumb and first two fingers. In addition to drawing circles, your child may also be able to copy a cross. She may draw a figure with a head and probably arms and legs. She will not be able to plan what she is going to draw or to tell you about it before she starts, but is more likely to tell you what she has drawn once she's finished.

HANDEDNESS

Your child's preference for her right or left hand should be clear at about the age of three; more than 90 percent of children are right-handed. But if you or your partner are left-handed, your child is also more likely to be left-handed, and even more so if both of you are left-handed. Interestingly, identical twins will not necessarily have the same hand preference hence the belief that handedness is not just a matter of simple genetic inheritance.

A small number of children are ambidextrous—they can use either hand for all activities or some use one hand for certain activities and the other hand for different ones. However, sometimes a single hand becomes dominant later on.

Handedness develops naturally and there is nothing you should do to help this along or try to reverse it. What you can do, once a preference for the left hand is shown, is to provide special equipment, such as left-handed scissors or utensils, for your child. Otherwise those who are left-handed have no special requirements. Handedness has no influence on the ability to learn.

About this time, too, your child will start pretend "writing." Instead of the many different types of sweeping hand movements she usually makes, she'll begin to lift her pencil off the paper at regular intervals in order to create a series of small marks, some of which may be in a line. She may be able to copy a V shape and a T. She'll have watched your hand actions when you write and begun to imitate the same ones.

By the time she is four, your child will use the adult grip to hold her pencil. She'll be able to copy the letters T, H, V, and O, and when she draws a person, he or she now has a head, body, legs, and often arms and even fingers. She can also draw a simple house. At this time, too, she will probably be able to tell you what she is going to draw before she draws it.

By the time your child is five, she'll be accomplished at drawing and painting with fine brushes. She will color neatly, keeping the color within the outline. She'll be able to draw a person and give him or her facial features and a house with a door, windows, a roof, and a chimney. She will draw many other things and know what she is going to draw. Her ability to copy designs and shapes means she'll be ready to tackle more ambitious arts and crafts like making papier-mâché models.

Printing-wise, she will be able to copy the letters C, Y, and U, among others, and print a few letters spontaneously—with a pen or pencil. This is a good time to teach her to print her name. She'll be able to draw a square and over the next few months, be able to copy a triangle.

Your preschooler's manipulative skills will gradually help her to become more independent in terms of her own daily needs. At age three, she'll be able to hold her cup by its handle with only one hand and put on some of her clothes. At age four she will eat skillfully with a knife and fork and put on most of her clothes herself. By age five, she'll be able to pour juice or milk from a carton without spilling it, and dress herself.

Intellectual and mental abilities

Your child's thinking, reasoning, and speaking abilities have to develop markedly by the time she reaches school age, so that she'll be prepared to digest complex information, make advanced plans, recall strategies she has used in previous learning tasks, think through problems toward a solution, and communicate solutions and ideas.

The components of mind are many, complex, and diverse, and it's a good idea to be aware of what is meant by commonly used terms.

"Understanding" or "thinking" are often referred to as "cognitive" or "intellectual" development and involve reasoning, analysis, and solving problems. It involves first being exposed to something new and then applying this experience to subsequent new and unfamiliar situations. A three-year-old child wanting to coax a treat from her granddad, for example, learns that by looking cute and saying "Pleeeease…" in a certain sort of voice, she has a high chance of achieving the desired result. Over time, her cognition will evolve from the simple and concrete to the almost infinitely complex and abstract.

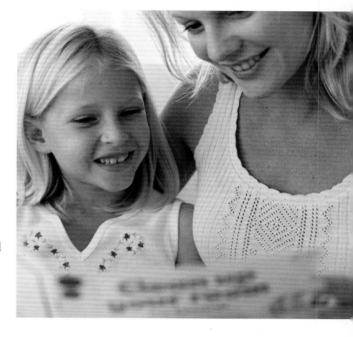

Mental development also involves communication, which consists not only of words but also gestures, facial expressions, cries, and other noises. Sometimes it is about behaviors, such as tantrums. It is about choosing to follow a suggestion (or not), or to obey a command (or not). It is about emotions as well as facts.

"Emotional intelligence" is a term that is used to describe the ability to understand feelings. There are two aspects to this: one is understanding what is said "between the lines," which means both body language and the way tone of voice can convey something more than the words themselves. The other is about the ability to see things from another person's perspective. This latter type of information is very different from the former: it is abstract, yet it is of fundamental importance because children have to learn how to build relationships and friendships. It begins within the first few weeks after birth and continues as children start to imitate others and later to engage in cooperative or collaborative play. Specialists increasingly believe that the development of emotional intelligence comes before the development of reasoning and structured thought.

Perception is a mental function that is fundamental to development. The ability to hear is mature before birth while being able to see is mature by the age of five or six years. But the way in which the information is handled and processed is, in part, culturally and socially determined. Adults are good at filtering out extraneous information, but preschoolers usually attach equal importance to everything that happens within their range of sight or sound. This can manifest as a child being easily distracted or unable to concentrate when, in reality, it's simply that she has different priorities.

Thinking

While the ability to think can be measured as "intelligence," "IQ" (intelligence quotient), and "intellectual ability," a preschooler's thinking can be difficult to measure because the skills required are not yet well developed. Moreover, according to American developmental psychologist, Howard Gardner, there is more than one type of intelligence. According to Gardner, in addition to the commonly measured logical-mathematical and linguistic abilities, we also are gifted, in various degrees, with spatial (artistic), bodily-kinesthetic, musical, and naturalistic skills as well as interpersonal and intrapersonal abilities. In order for a child to realize her full potential, all types of intelligence must be recognized and encouraged.

Building "thinking," cognitive, intellectual, or "mental" skills involves several different dimensions:

- Problem solving. A toddler has limited ideas on how to solve a problem but a five-year-old will consider many possibilities and then test them through trial and error, striving for success.
- Concentration. A toddler's focus is limited; she darts from one thing to another very easily. An older child concentrates on a game until the end point is reached, or until the challenge is tackled effectively.
- Memory. A toddler's recall is limited and is confined to objects or people she sees frequently;

 ways to aid your child's thinking skills

1 Use "scaffolding." Creating temporary "structures" can enable your child to move from one level of understanding to another. If, for instance, your three-year-old cannot solve her jigsaw, and doesn't even know how to begin, you might help her pick out the four corners and then help her find the flat-sided border pieces. That might be all the help she needs to solve the rest of the puzzle. By providing a "scaffold" of learning for your child, you help her reach new learning heights. You'll find that you can gradually reduce the level of assistance until she reaches the point where she learns independently.

2 Build her memories. Whenever possible, remind your child of what she did before (yesterday, on vacation, at the museum)— talking over incidences and experiences—and by playing matching games like "Snap," where she has to recognize common objects.

3 Have fun with numbers. Incorporate numbers into everything you do; count items when you shop, the pieces of a game, the clothing your child puts on, and the houses in your street.

4 Point out patterns. Many kinds of patterns— visual, auditory, and motor—can be found in your child's world. Encourage her to tune in to these patterns by drawing her attention to things that appear in the landscape, things that can be heard in songs and speech, or that can be followed, such as by fitting puzzle pieces together.

5 Play games. These involve communication, solving problems, facts, and emotions, as well as trust, deception, pretence, and competition. Games are probably critically important for certain kinds of learning, and should evolve from the very simple and concrete (like "Peek-A-Boo"), to the complex and abstract (simple charades).

when she's older, your child be able to recall information she learned days, weeks, or months before.

- ♦ Symbolic thought. During her second year, your toddler began to think about matters in her head, without having to actually see things. This is the emergence of symbolic thought, which continues to develop.
- ♦ Inquisitiveness. A toddler has a limited ability to explore and gain information. A five-year-old child, however, is able to ask questions in order to satisfy her thirst for knowledge and to acquire vast amounts of information from others.

Thinking styles

Each child approaches learning differently although psychologists have identified two main styles, with the majority of children falling somewhere along the continuum.

If your child spends a great deal of time thinking and planning before she actually does anything, she has what's known as a reflective learning style. She imagines various different possibilities in her mind and runs through these, carefully weighing up the pros and cons. Only when she feels confident does she try out her ideas in practice.

A reflective learning style involves patience, planning skills, and the ability to wait.

On the other hand, if your child immediately flies at a problem with great enthusiasm, preferring to discover things as she goes along, she's displaying an impulsive approach. She is not particularly troubled by early failures; she learns from these as they occur and quickly moves on. Before a reflective child has lifted a finger, the impulsive learner has tried out several different solutions.

Each style has its own advantages. For instance, a reflective style is useful when there is plenty of time and there can only be one attempt at finding a solution. On the other hand, an impulsive learning approach is useful when time is short and a solution is needed quickly. Like most children, your preschooler probably shows elements of both learning styles at different times.

Thinking processes

The most popular psychological theory of mental development is that a child uses mental "schemes" to represent, organize, and understand her experiences. A toddler starts off with a few basic schemes for making sense of her surroundings but these gradually extend as she grows older and fits any new information she's learned into an existing schemata. For example, a two-year-old already familiar with the concept of "cat" on seeing another animal with four legs, such as a sheep, thinks it also could be a cat. She uses her existing schemata for "cat" and assimilates the image of the sheep into it.

An older child, however, is also able to change an existing schemata on the basis of new information. Suppose she sees the sheep and realizes that although it has four legs like a cat, it is larger, with woolier hair, some horns, and so on. As a result, she accommodates this new learning by increasing her existing schemata so that now she has one idea of cats and another for sheep.

Your growing child has an emotional need for her world to be balanced and to have a settled understanding of the world around her. In order to maintain this equilibrium, she constantly modifies her mental development as she learns. Curiosity is motivated by your child making sense of something she doesn't understand in order to regain her sense of balance.

Learning styles

Your child's thinking can be aided by appreciating how she learns. If, as Howard Gardner posits, there are different intelligences, you may find that your child's learning style also depends on her particular abilities. Your child will be one of four types.

Auditory learner

If she is a language-oriented learner, she will think in words instead of pictures, and verbalize concepts to make sense of ideas. She needs to hear about facts and directions in order to "digest" them. You can tell that she is an auditory learner if she learns easily from listening to instructions, is a good talker, and sounds out words phonetically when spelling.

Visual learner

If your child remembers things she has seen rather than heard, she may be a visual learner. This is likely to be the case if she remembers images and diagrams; can recall movies, talking about different scenes when she describes them; enjoys drawing and likes visual puzzles such as mazes, and is something of a daydreamer. As she learns to read, it is especially important to suggest visual clues to her. She will devour picture books but will also enjoy "chapter books" if she is encouraged to visualize the story like a movie playing in her head. Story writing can be encouraged in the same way.

Kinetic learner

Physical activity is the key for this type of child. She will want her whole body to be involved in learning and you may need to teach her to count by making steps and when reading to her, letting her tap out rhythms or walk about. Your child is likely to be a kinetic learner if she is highly active and finds it hard to sit still, emphasizes her speech with large, whole body movements and gestures, and shows you things rather than explains them. You will need to think outside the box with your child! Kinetic learners enjoy hands-on activities and may be gifted at sports and creative thinking but can find school life difficult. They often are labeled as exhibiting signs of attention deficient disorder.

Logical learner

If your child likes to find patterns and work out relationships between objects and ideas, enjoys finding out about how things work, drives you insane with the amount of why-based questions she asks, and likes mathematics and playing strategy games, she may be a predominantly logical learner. Hold your child's interest by carrying out "science" experiments together and encourage her to explore any hypothesis she has about what she is investigating. Do not provide your child with answers but allow her to test her own ideas.

Communication

No matter your child's age, communication is a two-way process; it involves an exchange of feelings and ideas, passing back and forth between you and your preschooler.

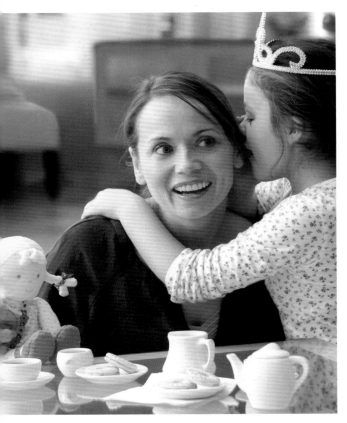

Even though a young child can speak, she conveys her feelings nonverbally as well. Using a broad range of gestures—such as walking away, clenching her fist, staring directly at you, and cuddling—you understand what she means even when she doesn't say a word. However, between the ages of three and five, your child's verbal communication skills will grow rapidly and she will love chatting with her friends as they play cooperatively together, exchanging ideas and comments at the same time. She will, however, still continue to use body language, although this becomes more complex as she combines individual gestures to make a new meaning. For instance, if she pulls at her ear, looks steadfastly at her feet, and her cheeks redden, you should suspect she is hiding something from you.

Between the ages of three and four, your child's vocabulary will increase to more than 1,000 different words, and she will understand many more. Her sentences become longer and contain many verbs and adjectives. She asks questions. At four to five years of age, she will have a spoken vocabulary of approximately 1,500 words. Her speech will start to resemble adult speech in the way she uses it to communicate her feelings and ideas. She will use the past tense and other word endings. Your child should speak clearly enough so that an observer who is listening closely can understand most of what she says.

By the time she is six, your child will be much more effective at giving accounts of incidents, both pleasurable and distressing. She will begin to recognize the emotional benefits of talking things over with others. At this point in her development, your child also may recognize she can use body language deliberately in order to convey her intentions. For example, she smiles at someone whom she wants to play with, or she deliberately frowns and stamps her feet when she wants you to know she is angry.

How to help your child

The acquisition of speech, like other developmental milestones, takes time and there's lots of learning involved, so be supportive. Don't make a big deal when your child makes mistakes. Help your child expand her vocabulary by telling her the names of different objects and the meanings of words and asking her questions about things she is doing—like what is she drawing, for example. Use as much detail as possible. Instead of saying "Put your toys away," say, "Please put your toys in the toy box." Use your normal speaking style, but try to speak more slowly, using less complex sentence structures so that your child can tune in more easily. Always provide a good model of language. For example, if your child says "Mommy's car," you can reply by saying "Yes, that's right, Mommy's car is outside."

Look at your child and make eye contact when you talk to her; this helps her focus attention on your comments. And encourage her to look at you. Remind her, as she gets older, to make eye contact when speaking to another person. The social actions accompanying speech will be increasingly important.

Conversation is partly about taking turns, but it also allows children to experiment not just with new words, but also with ways of saying them, and ways of joining words together to create new meanings. Conversation is also about listening, so you have the opportunity to demonstrate to your child the importance of listening, and to reward that behavior in your child. With both children and parents, some are much better at listening than others. Good listening skills, and plenty of opportunity to practice, are both important in helping your preschooler build up her vocabulary.

Try to listen when your child wants to talk. You may be busy with other things, but set aside time to have a discussion. Young children are often unsure of the exact words to use or maybe can't talk fluidly yet, so it takes them more time to speak. When your child speaks to you, don't rush her, but do help her stay on track. Even a four-year-old can easily lose the point of a discussion if she isn't given a gentle reminder from you. By the time your child is ready for school, conversations with older people—carers, neighbors, or older relatives—take on new dimensions because she has so much more language to use, and more complicated stories to tell.

Commands

From around three years of age, thanks to increases in her thinking skills and memory, your child should be able to understand and perform commands involving at least two pieces of information. She should, for instance, be able to comply if you say, "Please bring me that book, and put your teddy bear in your room".

Most of the commands you give your child will not be open to bargaining, and you will expect her to carry them out. But at times your child won't want to do what you ask, perhaps because she is busy with another activity or because she thinks your instructions are uninteresting or unimportant. That's why it helps to give her an explanation. She won't fully understand the reasons, but doing so will encourage her to think beyond her own immediate wishes. So, for example, if you ask your child to stop making so much noise, point out to her that you want her to stop because you are getting a headache. Explanations help your child realize why you are asking her to behave in a particular way.

In addition, point out the emotional consequences of her following your instructions; you could tell her, for example, that you'll feel good if she puts her toys away neatly, or that Daddy will be sad if she breaks his favorite pen. Linking the instruction to an emotional outcome in this way makes your instruction more significant for your child, and she is therefore more likely to respond positively to it.

Questions

Starting at four years of age, when she will have enough language and sufficient intellectual skill to frame a question, your child will begin asking you things. Although somewhere between four and six years of age is usually the peak time for constantly asking questions, its only at about five years old that she starts to think through both the kind of problem she is trying to solve, and the kinds of question she wants to ask, before putting a question into words. But even before then, children typically think about choices, consider the possibilities, and ask questions about them. For instance, offered the chance to go to the store with Dad, or stay at home with Mom, your child may ask whether Dad might buy a treat or Mom will play a game. The answer to the question might determine whether going shopping or staying home looks like the better choice. Your child is considering the future possibilities for each scenario and imagining how each might feel before deciding whether to go or stay. This requires a fairly high level of abstract thought.

Questions come in all sizes. Big ones might relate to birth and death ("Where do babies come from?" or "Is Grandma in heaven?"). Others may be "What if…?" type questions ("What if the pool is closed?"), and others may start "Why…?", as in connection with behavior ("Why did you turn the TV off?"), or about situations or events ("Why is this apple green?", "Why can't we go there?"). It is important not to deter your child from asking questions and to answer with honesty, even if all you can say is "I don't know." You may find your child's questions irritating, but answering them helps her extend her vocabulary and knowledge. And, for your child, questions are a great way to start a conversation.

Questions also arise from your child's natural curiosity about her environment and the things that go on in it. For a young child, learning about the world is important and, as you'll come to realize, it is a lot easier for your child to ask a question than for you to provide a good answer. Although occasionally you child may ask questions that you are unable to answer or she may not properly understand your answer, you should take your child's questions seriously and answer as best you can. For questions that don't have easy answers (such as, "Why did Grandma die?"), only provide information that is appropriate for your child at her current age ("She was very sick and the doctor couldn't make her better.").

The ability to ask questions comes from being able to make complex sentences, as well as to think in abstract terms. Your child may ask some questions because she has doesn't understand the things happening around her and needs more information to make sense of things. You can help your child to develop both her thinking and style of questioning by asking her "What if…?" and "How does…?" questions. This helps your child develop different styles of interaction as well as explore the world in an abstract way. You should try to encourage your child to ask about the way something works, instead of allowing her to break it open to try to find out.

In terms of expanding your child's thinking, it is better and more challenging to ask open-ended questions that can be expanded on than closed questions, which have yes or no answers (so "Why do you like vanilla ice cream?" is better than "Do you like vanilla ice cream?"). If you are planning an excursion to a museum, for instance, you should say "What shall we do when we get there?", which can lead to many possible answers instead of asking, "Shall we see the dinosaurs first?"—the answer to which is "yes" or "no." Where a question is "closed," your child won't be encouraged to suggest other possibilities that exist.

Concentration

Over time, your child will be able to function in much more complex ways. From around age three, she'll be able to stick with an activity for longer, becoming less distracted by external events and better able to focus on the task in hand, even if it is a little difficult. If she does gets stuck, she will be more able to frame a question that will help her to deal with the problem and to come up with different solutions; if, for

example, she is working on a jigsaw puzzle, she's better able to choose appropriately shaped and sized pieces.

Your child's use of trial and error (as a way of exploring things) becomes increasingly sophisticated and she will use a great deal of persistence in trying to understand objects and make them work. So most activities, even though they may still be quite simple, commonly last much longer than when she was younger. Moreover, left alone, your child will find new ways to stretch and entertain herself. At the same time, her play becomes more imaginative and complicated; she may act out roles, such as being a doctor or fireman, or create complicated scenarios involving model toys or animals.

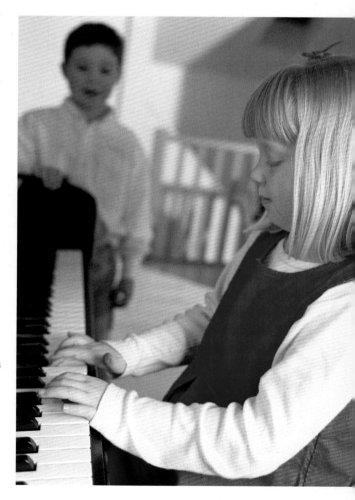

Curiosity

Your child is a natural learner. She instinctively tries to make sense of everything she sees, hears, and touches. This natural curiosity—her desire to discover the undiscovered—drives her to learn more at every opportunity. Everything she sees represents a new and exciting opportunity to explore and learn more. And this intrinsic motivation to reach new heights continues throughout her childhood.

You will need to keep a close eye on your child because she will want to open every box, empty out every container, or search every cupboard. She's not purposely being bad, she just wants to find out how things work. By the time she reaches school age, her curiosity will be channeled and more controlled, and new learning opportunities should be the means to satisfy her eagerness to acquire more knowledge.

A thirst for learning

Even before she starts school, your child may show an interest in reading and numbers. Let her interest and ability guide you. If she seems ready, you can help teach her letters and numbers. A lot of reading and counting occurs naturally throughout your child's daily routine so she will start to recognize the names of stores that you frequently go into and may count items that you put in your cart. Praise her when she demonstrates these early learning skills— she thrives under your approval. The information she acquires through her natural thirst for learning will give her a good start to formal schooling.

Do not, however, be tempted to advance your child too quickly. All children need a normal childhood and your child can become stressed if a lot of pressure is put on her to achieve. By all means, feed her interests but make sure you don't overstimulate her; it's important to just let her express her creativity in play.

Self-perception

Throughout childhood the way your child perceives herself changes. Around three years of age, your child's self-perception is so strong that it usually overshadows consideration of others. Your child may demonstrate through bad behavior that she refuses to accept that what you want is more important than what she wants.

Between three and four years of age, your child will know a lot about herself, for instance, that she is a girl (or a boy), her name and age. She can list these things for you, when asked.

By the time she is five or six years old, your child will be able to describe herself reasonably accurately; she has a sense of who she is and how she relates to the people around her.

As part of self-perception, your child needs to hone her ability to think about and distinguish between feelings, to recognize them as discrete emotions, and then use them to direct her behavior. This is covered further in the next section.

How to help your child

Understanding herself—what's she's good at and what she finds difficult—will be your child's greatest key to success. One way of getting her learn about her abilities is to help her set and meet her goals. Goals can be big ("I want to be rich") or small ("I want an extra cookie"). They can be for things she wants to do today ("I want to go skating") or in the future ("I want to have karate lessons or to go to the beach on vacation"). The key thing is that they are for specific things your child really cares about, and are realistic but challenging.

Where possibile, faciliate your child's goals. You can't make her rich but you can encourage her to save any pocket or birthday money and watch it accumulate, and she could have an extra cookie if she completes a task, for example. Bear in mind her choice for your summer vacation. Have your child set goals and review them regularly.

Bear in mind, too, that your child watches how you react to situations and manage your emotions. You also may be inadvertently teaching your child ideas that can affect her self-image. Do you have "food issues" or express a belief that girls shouldn't be boisterous, or that boys shouldn't be caring?

The emergence of personality and the growth of emotions

The unique individual that is your child—a result of both her genes and environment—will not be fully known until she is much older, but during the preschool years, certain aspects of her temperament will become more constant and more obvious to you. These both impact on and are affected by her emotional responses and will have a lot to do with how she develops socially (see also page 119).

Temperament

By the time she is four compared to two, your child is more likely to be more patient, more articulate, will have started to develop insight into the feelings of others, and has learned the art of reasoning. However, she is also likely to be quarrelsome at times and to fight with her friends as they all try to exert their independence.

By the age of five, individual personality traits will be apparent. You may notice that compared to her peers, your child is more fearful, or more extroverted, or more caring. Personality is not static so these early traits are not completely reliable hints to her mature personality. In fact, as children get older, they begin to change at an accelerated rate. Different surroundings and experiences affect even inherited traits, so that a child can change and accommodate to things as they change around her. You may be surprised if your boisterous and booming toddler becomes a quiet and hardworking school child.

Learning to understand and accept the temperament of your child is an important stage in nurturing her personality and helping her find a way to fit in with her environment. If, for example, your child is reluctant to go to parties or to a friend's house to play, you can develop strategies to prepare her and give her the confidence to cope with the situation. The important thing is to focus on her

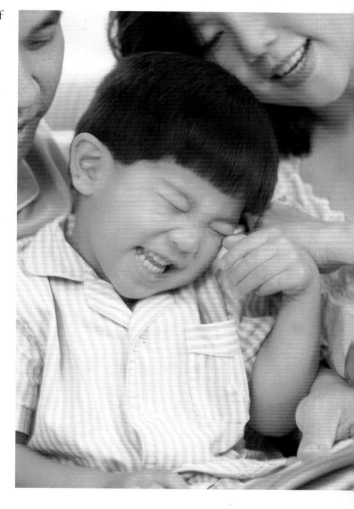

strengths. Take a step back and look at who your child is. If your child is "strong-willed," for example, set her challenging tasks or give her complicated toys. She has perseverance, after all, and is able to manipulate and analyze. If you deal with her temperament in a positive way, she will thrive.

Bear in mind, too, that while it is helpful to acknowledge particular features of your child's temperament, it is not a good idea to label her as having a particular personality trait. Your child's personality is still developing, and hearing herself described in a certain way may upset her and also may make her live up to the description. In addition, if you believe you you've mapped out your child's character, you may become blinkered and be too rigid in how you manage her.

Gender identity

Over the preschool years, your child will develop her sense of "boyness" or "girlness." This psychological phenomenon is distinct from a sexual preference and usually depends on body shape. At age two your child may have told you that she is a girl, but it's not until around age six, that she'll comprehend that she was never a boy and will always be a girl (toddlers believe that a person's gender is changeable and depends on what he or she does or wears).

What causes gender differences is unproven though experts cite "nature" or "nurture" or both. Those in favor of nature, claim there are built-in differences in human infants from almost the time they are conceived. For example, proponents are convinced that boys demonstrate "maleness" due to their higher levels of testosterone, the hormone that

"TYPICAL" BOY AND GIRL PRESCHOOLERS

Though each child is an individual and there are wide differences in behavior among children of the same sex, experts agree that there are some useful generalities.

Boys walk, talk, feed and dress themselves, and toilet train later than girls. At an early age, they are more interested in things and more likely to show and feel frustration. At age four, they are more muscular than girls so they enjoy more active, aggressive and vigorous play. They are keen to be dominant and to have their own way. The right side of the brain develops more quickly in boys, leading to a greater grasp of space. This they explore through movement games such as climbing and chasing, and measuring activities including driving cars through space or shooting darts across it.

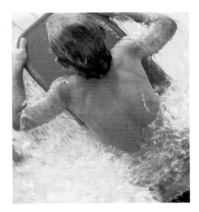

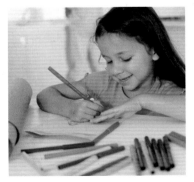

Girls walk and acquire self-help skills early and they talk a lot more than boys of the same age. From a young age, they are more interested in people than boys and more willing to follow the bidding of others. At age four, the left side of the brain, which is associated with language, becomes more active, and girls spend even more time talking—to parents, playmates, and toys. This enables them to build relationships at home and at playgroup. They also are more practiced in using fine muscle skills, such as those for drawing and painting.

is linked to aggression and activity, which starts to affect body cells in pregnancy. Girls are more nurturing and caring because of the physiological processes involved in a woman's ability to bear children. Experts who favor nurture or environment, however, claim that gender differences are more likely the result of parents treating boys and girls differently. For example, it's been proved that parents find aggression in their sons more acceptable than in their daughters and conversely, fear and sadness less acceptable in their sons than their daughters. In one famous experiment, infants dressed in pink were handled more gently and delicately by adults whereas those in blue were bounced around—even though the actual gender of the child was unknown.

Almost certainly, however, both factors contribute to a child's gender identity and while there is little you can do about preexisting genetic factors, it is important that you offer your preschooler, no matter her gender, a wide variety of play opportunities and experiences that support the development of many skills. (Parents generally show more interest in their child's play if it is gender-appropriate [boys playing with soldiers and cars, girls with dolls and tea sets]).

Children learn about their sexual identity by watching and copying adults around them. Your preschooler is susceptible not only to your behavior and attitudes regarding gender but also to those of friends and relations and on television and in other media. Even if you and your partner both work and share household responsibilities equally and make an effort to police any examples of gender identity in your actions or speech, your child may persist in acting out a conventional gender role—your daughter walking around in high-heeled shoes and wearing makeup, your son brandishing a sword.

Preference for one's gender begins early. From the time babies first show interest in other people, girls and boys both prefer others of their own sex and from 18 months of age, they choose different toys and activities. By age four, girls and boys spend three times as many hours playing with either all-girl or all-boy groups, and at age six, eleven times as much with their same gender.

In order to explore what it is to be male and female, and thus to learn more about herself, it's natural that your preschooler engages in gender games. You may try and eschew gender-stereotypical toys and activities like dressing fashion dolls and using light sabers to play at intergalactic war, but your child may prefer such activities above all others. Moreover, in order to differentiate girls from boys, you may often hear your preschooler use gender stereotypes in her speech—(to her mother on rummaging through the toolbox "You can't use a hammer! Only Daddy can!" or "Of course I know how to kick a football. I'm a boy!")

Some children, however, do go against gender type: your son may be shy and gentle or your daughter fierce and adventurous. Don't be concerned, therefore, if your son wants to wear high heels or your daughter plays "shoot-em-up"; there is no evidence that playing with gender-opposing toys or engaging in gender-opposing activities will have any lasting impact whatsoever.

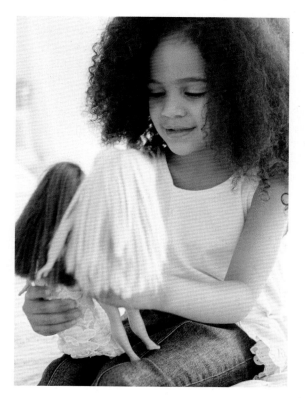

Sex play

Preschoolers are very interested in their bodies and as they get older are also curious about those of others. As a toddler, you may have found your child touching her genitals and, as she gets older, you may catch her engaged in other sex play such as touching another child's genitals; or she may rub up against you in a suggestive way. It's important to recognize that such behavior is commonplace and normal but you may feel uncomfortable about it, particularly if it stirs sexual feelings on your own part. In such instances, rather than a issuing a reprimand or punishment, it's best to try interesting your child in another activity or addressing her interest more directly by answering any particular questions she may have about sex and sexual behavior. Talk to your child about what behavior you find allowable—touching herself but not anyone else—and don't leave her alone for too long with other children without supervision. Make sure, too, she learns to respect your privacy; if you close your door, she should know she must knock first.

Your preschooler will have questions about where babies come from, male and female genitals, and sexual activities—even if she doesn't voice them. If she does, it's best to give simple and succinct answers and provide further information when or if an additional question is asked instead of engaging in extended explanations. While your answers will depend on your comfort level, you may decide that the whole truth isn't necessary at this stage, especially if you think your child isn't able to comprehend what you mean. For example, should your child walk in on you during lovemaking and demand to know what you are doing, you might answer "Just giving daddy a cuddle" or "Something that mummies and daddies do" instead of explaining the mechanics of the situation.

The development of emotions

Recognizing emotions both in herself and others will enable your child to express them and to understand why she and others feel the way they do. This can help her deal with difficult situations and react more appropriately and effectively as she gets older. Instead of falling into a sulk when some treat is refused, she may be able to "negotiate" a more favorable settlement if she learns to keep her emotions in check.

6 questions your child might ask

1 **"Where do babies come from?"** Your child may want to know how a baby gets in and out of the mother's tummy or may refer to what she expects to be the answer—"What supermarket did you buy me in?" or "Do I have seeds for making a baby?"

2 **"What are you doing/what's that noise?"** If you are caught making love, your child will be curious about what's happening.

3 **"What's this?"** Anything she comes across that is related to sex and sexual activity from male and female genitals, to condoms and birth control pills.

4 **"Can I see …?"** Your preschooler may ask to see (or even touch) your or your partner's genitals.

5 **"Why does my penis/vagina …?"** Your child will be curious about how his/her genitals "behave."

6 **"Why don't I…?"** Your child may identify her gender as either male or female but want to know why she doesn't display mature characteristics like pubic hair or breasts.

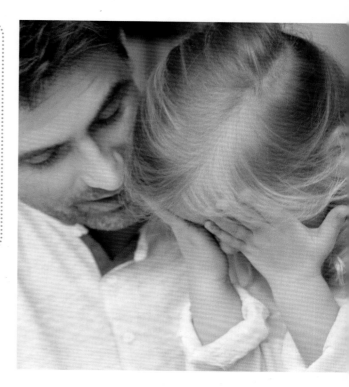

Unfortunately the "terrible twos" don't always cease on your child's third birthday and your young preschooler may still struggle with strong emotions. Some three-year-olds are extremely confident but others are fearful and insecure. Extremes of emotions, though both positive and negative now—loving certain things to excess, greatly disliking others—characterize many a four-year-old but at five years of age, your child should be generally positive in her outlook, calm, and serene, with the maturity to take most troubles in her stride.

Your child's emotional needs

Although every child is different, all have the same fundamental emotional needs; the challenge for you as a parent is to recognize those needs and to find ways of meeting them. Dominating the preschool years is the emotional need to feel loved and valued unconditionally; your child needs to feel that you care deeply for her no matter what she does and that you accept her as a worthwhile individual.

Also vital is her need to feel safe and secure; she needs to feel relaxed and happy when she is at home, in your company, and to feel that you can protect her from all dangers. She also needs to achieve; she thrives on success, has to learn to cope with failure, and seeks your approval when she improves.

Finally, there is also her need to have friends and to be popular, to become independent, and to cope with the ups and downs of everyday life.

Instead of looking at each of these in isolation as if they are items on a list to be checked off one at a time, the best way to understand and meet your preschooler's emotional needs is by asking two questions. Is she happy and settled? Is she making progress? If the answer to both questions is "Yes," then you can be confident you are meeting her emotional needs through your effective parenting, even if you haven't particularly planned it that way. If the answer to both is "No," then it is likely her emotional needs are not being met (although her lack of progress could be due to a developmental problem and not an unfilled emotional need).

How to help your child

A healthy attachment to your preschooler is vital (see also page 119) since it is mainly through this two-way connection that her emotional needs will be met. Therefore, maintaining a strong bond between you should always be your top priority. One way to do so is through communication. If you encourage your preschooler to voice her feelings to you instead of keeping them locked up, her

7 signs your child may be stressed

1 He has poor eating habits and appetite loss.

2 His sleeping patterns are disrupted at night, with an increased frequency of nightmares.

3 He displays increased aggression toward other children and adults.

4 His behavior is withdrawn when previously he was outgoing.

5 His concentration and attention has dropped.

6 He has a lowered ability to tolerate frustration.

7 He exhibits regressive behavior (thumb sucking, toiletting accidents).

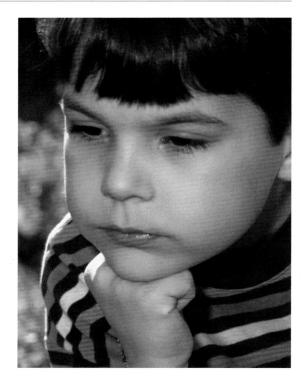

openness will go a long way to stopping emotional problems from building up. When she is troubled by something, she'll tell you, and that will ease her anxieties. Good communication with you also makes her feel loved and valued.

But meeting your preschooler's emotional needs also involves helping her cope when things go wrong, for example, when she isn't successful, or when she has a disagreement with her best friend, or when someone at nursery school laughs at the way she is dressed. Resilience is her ability to recover or bounce back when things don't go her way; it is her ability to cope when the odds are stacked against her. Some children are, by nature, more resilient than others. And some children tend to buckle under stress.

You can help boost your child's resilience by showing empathy and understanding when she is troubled. That will make her emotionally stronger. When she does tell you the difficulty she faces, it's important that you don't make her feel she is at fault

or that she has to struggle to cope. Instead, suggest ways to turn the situation around—inviting her best friend over for a play date may enable both children to put the matter behind them.

Remind your preschooler of incidents in the past that she found challenging and yet managed to cope with and talk to her about what she did then that worked. In other words, help her learn from her past experiences. That way she will discover solutions herself without you having to solve the problem for her. And when she loses her confidence and expresses negative comments about herself, point out her strengths by reminding her of all the things she is good at. Working with your child using these strategies also confirms to her that she is important to you and that you think she is wonderful, which further adds to her resilience.

You also need to take her feelings seriously. She may only be a young child, but her feelings are as important to her as yours are to you. Of course her world is less complex than yours and her worries and concerns are much simpler, but they are very real to her all the same. So don't trivialize her when she tells you she is upset about something, don't be annoyed with her if she appears to cry unnecessarily, and listen to what she tells you when she is unhappy. As well as helping her express herself, that approach also makes her feel special. You know she is special to you because she is your child, and you know she is terrific. Yets she needs you to demonstrate that so that she feels special. Tell her how much you love her and why you think she's such a great child; she has heard you say this many times before but she can never hear it enough.

Give her plenty of attention whenever you can. It's not just about spending time with her. What matters is that when you are with your preschooler, you focus your attention on her, whether playing with her, reading her a story, or chatting together. She feels very contented when you show interest in all aspects of her life. Comforting her when she is upset also helps. In most instances, all you need to do is put your arms around her, give her a gentle hug, and tell her that everything will be all right—that usually will be sufficient to drive her unhappiness away. Once she has calmed down, talk to her to find out what is causing her distress, and then try to find a way to solve the problem.

Do your best to avoid negative comparisons with other children—whether your child's friends or siblings. You may be tempted to encourage her to improve by pointing out how another child behaves better, or achieves more, than she does. You hope that by giving the other child as an example, she'll try to copy him or her. But that strategy rarely works. Comparisons with friends or siblings typically make a young child feel even less secure and can cause a rift between your children, or between your preschooler and her friend. Instead, focus on your child's strengths. Emphasize her good qualities. Your child's confidence is fragile and easily rattled. That's why it is good to tell her why her friends like her, or why you enjoy her company. This will make your child feel more positive about herself.

Taking an interest in her achievements has the same effect. Even though you may find it hard to get excited every time your child completes a jigsaw, particularly if she does so regularly, to her it is an achievement, and she wants evidence of your interest and approval.

Moods

Every preschooler experiences a range of moods—happiness, sadness, anger, jealousy, irritability, sullenness, and aggression—throughout a typical day. Part of growing up involves learning how to manage these different emotions so that your child maintains balance and stability in her life. As your child gets older and has an increasing awareness of those around her and her own feelings, her moods may become more complex. Although most young children are predominantly happy and content, there may be times when your child will feel irritable.

Often, such moods will be short-lasting and may be related to tiredness, boredom, hunger, or thirst but, in some cases, your preschooler's mood of discontentment may have an underlying cause that

REGRESSION

This is a healthy psychological strategy that your child sometimes uses involuntarily to protect himself emotionally during times of stress, but it is also his way of letting you know he's not coping well. Your child may resort to behavior, language, or mannerisms associated with an earlier developmental stage because it can make him feel safer. For instance, if you and your partner have frequent arguments, your fully toilet-trained child may start to have "accidents" if he's around when you do so. Likewise, if a new baby arrives in the family, your preschooler may start to suck his thumb and talk in a baby voice. In this instance, regression enables him to compete with the new baby for attention.

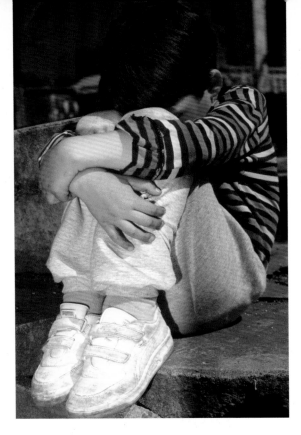

needs to be addressed. It is up to you to recognize these moods, and to provide help and support whenever it is needed.

A moody child, who tends to let negative feelings dominate, can be difficult to live with. Her friends will soon drift away from her because they find her unpredictable, and the child herself will spend more time being miserable than enjoying herself.

In contrast, a child who is aware of her varying moods, who is reasonably capable of controlling them, and who is also sensitive to the varying feelings of those around her, is more likely to have a strong sense of well-being and contentment. Your preschooler's level of emotional management and understanding is a combination of the sensitivity she was born with, the skills that she learns growing up, and the interaction between these abilities.

How to help your child

You can, however teach your child to deal with her moods more effectively. Possibly the most useful strategy is to encourage her to express her feelings through words, rather than behavior. That's not always easy for a preschooler because her language skills are still underdeveloped, and it's a lot easier for her to hit someone than to tell him or her how frustrated or angry she feels. Nevertheless, encourage your child to describe her emotions rather than to act on them. Tell her that you want to know what she feels inside, explain that you will help her put her emotions into words, and be patient as she slowly learns to express herself through spoken language instead of physical actions.

Try to create a listening environment at home, one in which your child is able to say what she's feeling and thinking in the full knowledge that she will be listened to. Have discussions about other people's emotions, too. Ask her to think about the feelings of her friends and her siblings when she plays with them. This will go a long way to helping her gain control over her moods. Psychologists claim that girls and boys have the same potential for managing moods, it's just that their strengths lie in different areas (see box, page 105). You might not be able to change what moods your preschooler goes through but you can influence the impact these moods have on her behavior.

Grumpy phases

When your preschooler contradicts you at every turn, you can sometimes feel as if nothing you can say or do is right. This does not mean that you are doing anything wrong, it's just that your child is going through an irritable phase. Often this will coincide with times of change, when she is feeling unsettled. Tiredness may also be a factor. In some cases, though, children go through such phases for no apparent reason, and the mood will lift as suddenly as it began. Like adults, children can seem to get out of bed on the wrong side for no apparent reason. If your child is in a grumpy mood, keep smiling and be positive, encouraging her to get on with her day.

Irritability in the short term may be related to being hungry. It may also be that your child has had a poor night's sleep and needs to rest for an hour or two. However, irritability may also indicate that she has something on her mind. Asking your child about what she has been doing at day care and maybe asking specific questions about friends at nursery school may uncover an explanation.

Managing anger and aggression

Dealing with anger will be challenging for your preschooler. Having passed through the intense tantrum stage of the toddler years, she is now expected to make more of an effort both to curb her anger and to express her aggression in ways that are neither frightening nor harmful to others. She needs to take more responsibility for managing her rage instead of relying on you to calm her down as she did when she was younger. She's old enough now to realize that extreme outbursts of anger and aggression are unacceptable and avoidable.

strategies for dealing with anger

It's important that you give your child practical techniques to deal with his anger and/or displacement activities when he feels tense and irritable. Suggest that he try the following:

1   Your child could come to you the moment his anger starts to rise.

2   He could walk away from the situation that is fueling his temper.

3   He could watch a DVD until he calms down.

4   He could pound a large lump of modeling clay.

5   He could engage in activities such as running around in the yard, kicking a ball as hard as he can, hitting a ball with a wooden bat, pedaling a toy up and down the sidewalk, or making a swing go back and forth at high speed.

How to help your child

Be open with your child about what you expect; tell her that now she's "a big girl" she must stop behaving like a younger child. Explain that you are very unhappy when she loses her temper and that you expect her to try harder to control it the next time. Let her know that there is nothing wrong with feeling angry, but that it is wrong to express her anger forcefully. As well as that, teach her practical strategies for controlling her temper, techniques that she can use whenever she feels her blood starting to boil (see box).

Make a list of any options; ask her for some suggestions as well, and then let her choose which methods she should use whenever she starts to feel angry. Practice these with your preschooler in role-play so that she knows what to do when the real thing arrives. In addition, suggest that she voices her anger as soon as it arises, instead of bottling up until she explodes. Explain that it is better for her to say "I'm getting angry because I can't finish this jigsaw" than it is for her to say nothing, simmer for several minutes, and then throw the jigsaw on the floor in fury.

You can also help your child gain control over her anger by showing her alternative and acceptable ways of expressing her fury that don't hurt anyone. These displacement activities are not always practical (for instance, running around outside when bedtime is approaching or when it is raining) but there may be times when you can use this approach effectively. Direct her toward this activity when you see her start to become riled.

Anger and aggression-management strategies might not work at first, no matter how often you practice them together. Don't worry, though. Your child will improve with time and experience. When you see her temper ignite, remind her what to do to keep control. Give your preschooler a big hug and lots of praise when you see her control a potential surge of anger. She'll be as delighted as you with her success in anger management.

Jealousy and rivalry

Unlike anger, which usually has an outward expression and generally dissipates quickly, jealousy is typically internalized and lasts for a long time. That makes it an altogether more challenging mood for your child to manage. Jealousy is an unpleasant feeling—a mixture of resentment, fear, insecurity, possessiveness, and suspicion—and it is always very destructive. At best it makes your preschooler unhappy and dissatisfied, and at worst it makes her behave nastily.

Your child can be jealous of others her own age, whether in her family or not, when she thinks she is treated less favorably than they are. She can also be envious of possessions, and she may even be jealous when she sees you giving your attention to her older brother or younger sister. This form is rivalry is natural. But your preschooler has to learn to keep her jealousy under control or she will feel miserable all the time and will be permanently convinced that she always gets a raw deal compared to everyone else.

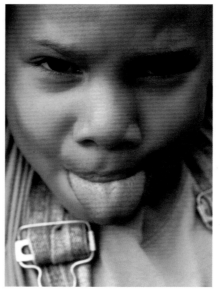

To help her master this powerful emotion, avoid making her feel guilty about being jealous. Remarks such as "You should be ashamed of being jealous of your brother" or "Only horrible children get jealous" simply encourage her to hide her true feelings from you. It also is likely to produce a poor self-image, since she will begin to see herself in negative terms. Instead, let your preschooler know you understand what it is like to be jealous of someone else. There is no harm in admitting to her that you also feel jealous at times, so long as you add that you don't let these feelings upset you or spoil your enjoyment. She'll be relieved to know that she can discuss and share this with you.

Encourage her to talk about her jealousy, instead of acting on it. That's better than suggesting she

pretends these feelings don't exist—denial won't make them go away. Ask her to explain to you why she feels jealous, and try to identify reasons why she shouldn't feel this way, for instance, because she has more toys than she thinks, or because you spend more time with her than she realizes. When your preschooler learns how to manage her moods effectively, she'll find life so much more enjoyable.

Fears and insecurities

Every preschooler is afraid sometimes. While some fears can actually be good for your child—if she's afraid of strangers, for instance, then she won't go off in a car with someone she doesn't know— most fears cause inconvenience. Fears at the preschooler stage are perfectly normal, and fortunately, most disappear spontaneously without requiring any special help.

Many preschooler fears are in response to objects or events. For instance, there is the fear of small animals and insects. Small animals can be more frightening to a young child than large animals, maybe because they move so fast and are so unpredictable. Your young child feels she has no control over them and so she may be very afraid when she realizes that a normally caged gerbil or hamster, for example, has become free.

Then there is a fear of the dark. In darkness, your preschooler's imagination can run riot. In a matter of moments, she can become totally convinced that a wicked person is hiding in the blackness that surrounds her at night and she'll scream out to you in terror.

You may also discover that loud peals of thunder cause your child to hide under the table or bed covers. She will be terrified of the noise, even though thunder cannot physically touch or harm her. Like many other fears, this is totally irrational yet extremely powerful.

Other preschool fears arise in response to emotions and relationships. For example, your preschooler wants to achieve, but if she is afraid of failure—perhaps someone laughs at her when she drops a ball—she might be afraid to try anything new in case the challenge proves too difficult for her. She may flatly refuse to climb up the ladder of the slide because she knows her pals can reach the top rung and she is afraid she won't manage this.

Sometimes a child fears losing her parents' love. If she is regularly made to feel rejected by her parents, she can to start to fear that she will lose their love entirely, and is very anxious in everything she does.

How to help your child

You should try in the first place to prevent your child from developing fears (although bear in mind that she may acquire fears despite all your efforts). Advanced preparation helps. If you know that she has to face a stressful episode in the near future (for example, she has to have a travel vaccination jab),

then let her know in advance. Tell her what to expect about the procedure, and point out that you will be with her at all times. Remind her of the times she had one in the past and coped well. And remain calm yourself. Any fear you have will quickly spread to your child. So if you are anxious about the challenge she faces, don't show it otherwise her fear will intensify. Maintain a calm and relaxed outward manner, and try to avoid suggesting in any way that she should be worried about what lies ahead.

If your child does develop a real fear, do what you can to help her beat it. Most important of all, treat her with respect. Her fear could seem trivial to you, but it is very real to her. She's not behaving this way just for fun, so don't treat her in a way that might suggest you think she is being silly. Give her lots of reassurance. As far as your frightened preschooler is concerned, the object of her fear is insurmountable but she will gain emotional strength from your confidence in her. Certainly, you should make sure that she doesn't arrange her life so that

reasons why a preschooler is more prone to fears

1 **He has a very vivid imagination**. That's why, for example, your preschooler argues vehemently that the shadow cast across his bedroom wall is actually a monster with special powers. His limitless imagination means that he can be extremely frightened about something that you regard as trivial.

2 **Fantasy and reality can merge sometimes in your child's mind during play**. This means, for instance, that an exciting play episode can suddenly become very intense and real for him, and a bad dream can seem as if it is really happening.

3 **He has an imperfect understanding of his environment**. Although he comprehends a lot about the world around him, there is a lot that

he still doesn't fully grasp. He doesn't know that flies do not gobble up people, that he can't be washed down the drain in your bathroom sink, or that a small bird will not carry him off somewhere. Of course he will learn these things in time, but for the present, his limited understanding leads him to believe that anything is possible.

4 **His sense of danger becomes more developed**. He is now more aware of the risk of physical injury and hurt from, say, falling down, a bite from a small animal, and a vaccination from the doctor. His heightened sensitivity to these hazards can become transformed into specific fears.

she avoids the focus of her fear altogether. For instance, she won't ever overcome a fear of dogs if she constantly avoids them altogether. In fact, that will make matters worse because she won't learn new coping skills. She has to face her fear—with your support—and see for herself that she can manage.

Fear generates a physical response in your child. Her muscles will tense, her teeth clench together, and her hands will grip tightly. So encourage her to relax her body muscles when she feels afraid and to breathe more deeply—these physical changes by themselves will have a calming effect on her and she'll feel more confident. When you are afraid, you may use the technique of telling yourself not be afraid, that you will cope and so on. Suggest to your preschooler that she says similar things to herself when she is afraid—this further boosts her coping ability. You can also use her imaginative skills to resist fear; she can visualize herself successfully going through the frightening experience unafraid (this prepares her for the real thing) and she can imagine that you are safely alongside her when she is afraid. Keep supporting your child, until she has beaten her fear. Some fears are harder to change than others but they can all be changed eventually. Your child needs you to persist with your support for her.

Separation anxiety
This form of fear or anxiety emerges when your child realizes she has to temporarily part from you,

for instance, when you try to leave her at playgroup or nursery school or with the babysitter. She clings to you tightly, howls, and won't let go. Her terror at the thought of leaving you seems very strong.

Prepare your preschooler in advance for temporary separations from you. Don't wait until the last minute before telling her that you will leave her there, because that gives her no time to prepare herself for the emotional challenge that lies ahead. And talk positively about the separation. Point out that she will have lots of fun when she is there, and highlight all the things she can look forward to (there will be other children to play with, her temporary carer has lots of activities planned for her). If you plan to leave her at, say, a new playgroup, take her to visit beforehand so that she is familiar with the other children, the building, and the adults there. Similarly, let her meet the babysitter a couple of times before employing her.

Do your best to stay calm at separations. Your child will take her lead from you. Give her lots of reassurance, especially when she starts to appear insecure as the temporary separation approaches. Explain that she has nothing to worry about and that she will enjoy herself. Keep the actual moment of separation brief, no matter how upset she appears. Don't linger too long, even if she cries. Give her a quick kiss and a cuddle, make sure she is with the person who will look after her while you are away and then leave immediately. The more you draw out the separation, the more your child will cling tightly to you, and this will increase her fear of separation even more. When you return to pick up your child, tell her how pleased you are that she managed so well without you beside her. Show an interest in everything she did while you were away from her.

Bad dreams and nightmares
Although your child mostly has pleasant dreams, she may have a nightmare that is so frightening she wakes up crying and distressed.

Occasional nightmares seem to be part of normal development and they can be triggered by a range of different factors, for instance, eating cheese last thing at night, watching an exciting DVD just before bed, the onset of an illness, or concerns about a friendship.

If your preschooler does have a nightmare, don't try to shake her out of it—she may not be fully awake when she cries out. Instead, once you realize she is having a nightmare, speak to her gently in a soothing reassuring voice. Stroke her forehead or cheek softly. Even if she remains asleep, she'll be sensitive to these loving, physical contacts. Tell her quietly—but repeatedly—that she is fine, everything is all right, and you are with her to keep her safe.

Remind yourself that nothing dreadful will happen to your child as a result of this nightmare. At worst, she'll tremble from the effects, and at best she will forget all about it by the time she wakes up the next morning. If she doesn't wake up from the effects of the nightmare, let her stay asleep. It is very common for a preschooler to sleep right through a stressful bad dream, so do what you can to avoid waking her. If she does wake up, listen to what she tells you. She may have trouble distinguishing her dream from reality at that moment and may talk as if she is still in the dream. Instead of trying to make sense of her comments, respond by reassuring her.

Once your child's nightmare is over and she is fully awake, take her out of bed, perhaps to go to the bathroom, or to the kitchen for a glass of milk and a cookie. This change of surroundings will probably make her feel better. Then put her straight back to bed. It is best not to keep her up for too long because she may lose her tiredness altogether. Emphasize that she won't have another bad dream that night (children seldom have more than one nightmare each night).

Comfort objects and comfort habits

The chances are your preschooler has a favorite cuddly toy that she loves snuggling with—and it is probably one that she's had since she was a baby. Or maybe she cuddles a well worn remnant of her receiving blanket. At least half of all children under the age of five years still use an object like this.

Why comfort objects

Psychologists use the term "comfort objects" to describe this sort of cuddly item because cuddling it brings a child a feeling of comfort and well-being. Nobody, however, knows for sure why a young child should feel the need for one. It's not that children who are emotionally insecure crave one more than emotionally secure children, because almost every child uses a comfort object sometimes. In fact,

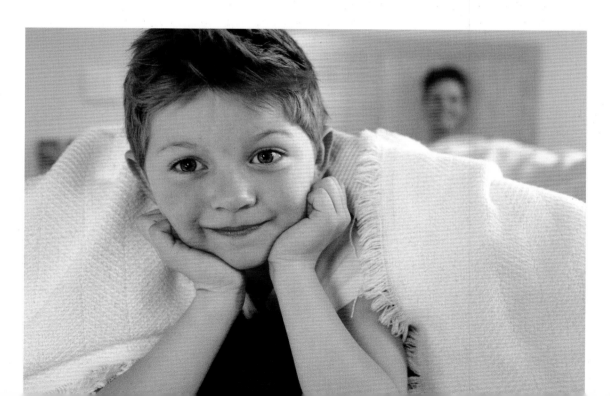

research has shown that a child who uses a comfort object before she reaches school age typically has better relationships with other children once she is in school and is less likely to be shy, lacking in self-confidence, and even to have fewer nightmares. It's as though having a comfort object could actually be good for your child.

Maybe it's the familiarity that appeals to her. Your child likes her object's instantly recognizable feel, smell, and even taste. She knows exactly what it will be like to hold, and this provides her with reassurance and comfort. If she has a comfort object from the time when she was very young, its attraction for her probably lies in that link. A child is likely to have fond memories of her early years and uses an object associated with that period to provide feelings of security and safety when she doesn't have her parents with her. It makes her ready to face the world independently and is similar to being armed with a good-luck charm when you have to deal with a situation that makes you nervous, say, a job interview. This is what your child is doing, though in her case she prefers a comfort object to a lucky charm to help her beat her anxiety.

There is nothing intrinsically wrong with a preschooler using a comfort object, though you may be uncomfortable about seeing your child trail an old cuddly toy around with her wherever she goes. Don't worry; she will probably grow out of it by the time she's five. The main advantage of a comfort object during the preschool years is that it is virtually guaranteed to induce positive feelings in her, and that can only be good for her.

Simply knowing that she has her comfort object clutched firmly in her hand may be sufficient for her to deal competently with any crisis. For instance, allowing her to take her comfort object on vacation means that she will be able to sleep happily in a strange bed in an unfamiliar hotel bedroom. Or allowing her to take her favorite cuddly toy along with her to the doctor or the dentist will ensure that she cooperates during the appointment.

FANTASY PLAY

Young children are blessed with vivid imaginations, which they use to explore and come to terms with a wide range of emotions. An imaginary companion, for example, can help a child to experiment with "forbidden feelings" and experiences, so it's a good idea to encourage these imaginary friends, even supplying a few props for the "friend" to play with.

Sometimes, however, a make-believe world becomes a little too real, and your child will become upset or frightened by some element of the situation or play—a scary jack o' lantern, an overly jolly Santa Claus, or an accident to an imaginary friend. Imaginative play is important to your child's development, so don't belittle or make fun of these incidents. Instead, try to join in and solve the problem—let your child draw a smiling face on a Hallowe'en pumpkin that you carve—but let him continue to manage his fantasy play as he'd like.

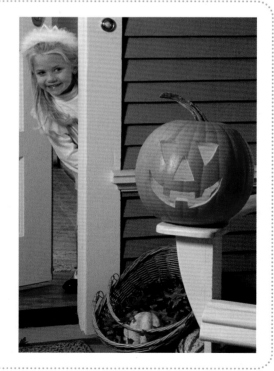

The main disadvantage of a comfort object, though, is that it can be a nuisance, especially if your child becomes too attached to it. You'll already be aware of this if you've ever had to deal with her refusal to go out the front door until she has found the item. It doesn't matter at all to her that you are ready and waiting to go and that everyone else is also ready. If she can't find her comfort object, everybody has to look for it. She'll probably be miserable for the whole outing if it is left behind.

Then there's the image created by a child who has a comfort object with her. A baby with a cuddly toy is cute, while a five-year-old clinging desperately to a grubby old teddy bear gives an entirely different impression. She may look immature and babyish. Although she isn't bothered by this, you might be, especially if you think that her peers will tease her.

Hygiene is also an important issue. Old receiving blankets and stuffed toys get dirty and harbor germs. Part of the attraction for her is the comfort object's well worn texture, so your preschooler won't thank you for cleaning it—she may even be furious because washing gives the comfort object a different feel, scent, and flavor.

6 questions to assess the importance of your child's comfort-object habit

1 **Has the habit just started or has it continued without a break since early childhood?** If he has been biting his nails since he was a toddler and has just continued with the habit until now, then this is a habit, nothing more. However, if he never bit his nails during early childhood then suddenly started at the age of four or five, this could be a sign of an underlying worry.

2 **When does he use his comfort object?** Some children cuddle their old teddy bear in private when they are happy and relaxed, say, while watching television at home in the evening, or reading a book in bed at night. The use of a comfort object is of a concern when a child insists on using it even in public, say, at nursery school, in front of his peers.

3 **Are there any other areas of his development that cause you concern?** If his comfort-object habit is a sign of a deeper anxiety, you may be concerned about other aspects of his development too. For example, he might also be more irritable than usual, or sleep badly during the night. Usually, signs of stress affect more than one area of your child's progress and development.

4 **How resistant to change is his habit?** In many instances, though not all, a comfort-object habit can be a sign of a deep worry when it is highly resistant to change. This is particularly true when the habit starts suddenly. If your preschooler persists despite lots of discouragement and support from you to help him stop, there may be something more to it.

5 **How long has he been doing this?** Preschoolers often drop comfort-object habits as quickly as they pick them up. One day, for instance, he insists on twiddling his hair all the time and yet the next day he doesn't touch it at all. The habit is often more significant psychologically if it lasts for more than a month or so without change.

6 **What effect has this on his life?** A normal comfort-object habit will have little impact on your child's life. Yet, if you find that, for instance, he insists on sucking his thumb while he is walking down the street, getting dressed, or while he is eating, and that he becomes very distressed when you tell him to stop, this is a likely indication that he is worrying about something.

Preschoolers can also have comfort habits instead of comfort objects. Typical comfort habits include: hair-twiddling (while concentrating hard on something or while relaxed when watching the television), which, if it goes on too long, may thin her hair in that area; thumb sucking (this is an extension of sucking a pacifier in earlier years), and if it persists, may make the skin on her thumb rough or broken and damage her teeth; genital rubbing (masturbation in childhood is comforting, not sexual—so don't overreact with embarrassment, shock, or disgust) and nail biting (she nibbles away at her fingernails or at the skin surrounding her fingernails), which if the habit persists can cause unsightly skin blemishes and possibly infection.

Breaking the habit

Almost certainly, your preschooler will grow out of her comfort object or comfort habit spontaneously by the time she starts school, whether or not you do anything about it. Yet there's no harm in helping her drop the habit earlier if you want. Whenever you decide that the moment has arrived for your child to give up her comfort habit, avoid making it a battle of wills. She'll only become more determined to persist if you start fighting with her about it. The more that her comforter gains in importance for you and for her, the more she will hold on to it, determined to resist all attempts at change. So take a positive approach. Tell her "You look like a big girl when you go to nursery school without your blanket" instead of "I'm really angry at you taking that stupid blanket with you everywhere"; or "I'm really proud of you when you watch television without sucking your thumb" instead of "You look silly with your fingers stuck in your mouth all the time"; or "Your sister is very happy with you when play with her without holding your teddy bear" instead of "Your sister doesn't have her teddy bear all the time and I wish you were more like her."

It's not easy for anyone, child or adult, to break a habit, so your approach to discouraging her use of comforters should be supportive, encouraging, and steady. Don't go for the "cold turkey" strategy, which involves the immediate and complete withdrawal of the object or habit. That's far too demanding. She won't be able to break her habit that quickly. Better to suggest that she tries to avoid using the comforter for a specific amount of time (for ten minutes at first), then gradually extend this period. Her ability to survive without the comforter will increase slowly.

Likewise, don't use punitive measures. For instance, resist the temptation to paint her thumb with a commercial foul-tasting-but-harmless liquid to stop her thumb-sucking habit—the chances are she'll just get used to the taste or suck a different finger instead. Instead, say "No" and then gently but firmly remove her thumb from her mouth.

The fact is that she does enjoy the comfort habit and she may not see any reason to change things at the moment. So expect some resistance when you ask her to stop. Persist with your discouragement anyway. Your preschooler will be more willing to give up her comforter or comfort habit when she feels that this change in behavior brings her some benefit. That's why you need to tell her how happy you are with her new behavior. Other ways of rewarding her for not using the comforter include pointing out that she looks like a "big girl" now, reminding her that her friends will not laugh at her any more and maybe giving her a special treat because she has tried so hard. You can do this even when she only stops the comfort habit for a few moments.

When it's extreme

Some preschoolers continue to use their comfort object, or continue with their comfort habit, long after most of their peers have given these up. If yours does this, you may worry this is a sign of a deep emotional problem. The chances are she'll be ready to give it up soon, but in the meantime, you need to establish its importance (see box, page 115).

Daydreaming

If your child is a daydreamer, with her head in the clouds, always thinking about something else other than the task she is supposed to be completing, you'll know how frustrating it is to try to get her focused. No matter how hard you try, she always seems to end up distracted in her own world, deep in thought, dreaming about other things. If, for example, you ask her why she hasn't put away her toys, which you asked her to do ten minutes ago, she'll probably reply. "Sorry, I forgot. I'll do it in a minute." Even when she does make an effort to sort things out, the final result is not as organized as you had hoped for because her mind wandered onto something else soon after she started.

Daydreaming is a harmless activity for your preschooler, and it provides her with a rich fantasy world. When daydreaming, she can invent anybody she likes and have any conversation she wants. One of the marvelous features of this psychological phenomenon is that your child is totally in control of what happens in her daydream; she decides what goes on, who is there, and what they say to each other. She doesn't have that sort of control in most other aspects of her everyday life, so it's hardly surprising she enjoys daydreaming so often. However, you may worry that she could be learning so much more if she was more attentive to the world around her.

A child might even develop daydreaming to the point where she has a daydream friend, such as a character she creates in her mind whom she treats as real. She may, for example, set the table for two, sit in one of the chairs, and then proceed to talk to the empty seat as though she can actually see someone there. She might even pour her imaginary friend a cup of juice and offer her a cookie. Similarly, she might be furious with you if you don't make room for her friend during storytime, or if you close the door to the room before her friend has crossed the threshold. Don't worry; your preschooler knows her imaginary friend does not exist.

4 steps to ensure your child's attention

1 **Reduce distractions where possible.**

2 **Use your child's name** to preface what you are going to say—say nothing more until you are sure he is looking at you.

3 **Keep saying his name** until he turns to face you.

4 **Once you have his full attention,** give him the instruction or information. If he looks away while you talk to him, or appears to slip into a daydream, remind him to continue looking at you. Don't give the instruction until you are absolutely satisfied that you have his full concentration. This ensures that he hasn't allowed his mind to wander onto other things.

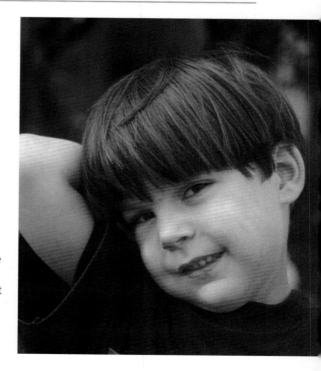

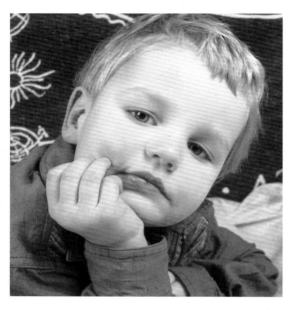

There are many potential psychological benefits from this type of daydreaming. Most obviously, the friend does exactly what she's told to do. Your child doesn't have a problem about deciding what toy to play with next, or what game they should play together; her imaginary friend obliges without argument or challenge and livens up an otherwise dull and boring day.

A daydream friend can also boost your preschooler's confidence. For instance, if she is afraid to climb the ladder that leads to the top of the slide she can turn to her fictitious pal for emotional support. The friend can offer her encouragement and reassurance, giving her that extra push needed to spur her on to greater achievements. In addition, an imaginary friend lets her vent her anger without any repercussions. That's why you might see your preschooler severely reprimanding an empty space for naughty behavior—exactly the way you did to her a few minutes ago. She gets rid of her frustration by taking it out on her imaginary companion.

As with all types of daydreaming, you need to set boundaries around her use of the imaginary friend, particularly if your child makes excessive demands on behalf of her friend (for instance, always wanting to have a seat at the table for her) and this may become tiresome. Be prepared to say to her that her imaginary friend doesn't need to be with her every minute of the day.

Discouraging daydreaming, improving attention

You might worry that your daydreaming preschooler has a serious problem with her attention and concentration, and that her frequent forays into the world of imagination signify an underlying disorder. Or you may worry that she needs to daydream because she is unhappy with her real world. Neither of these possibilities is likely, however (unless the frequency of daydreaming is so extreme that your child appears totally disconnected from the world around her). In most instances, daydreaming is a harmless childhood activity—your child knows the daydream is not real.

Even so, you may want to gently discourage the practice and to help her become more attentive to the world around her There are several strategies you can use for this purpose. For a start, remove distractions when trying to grab your preschooler's attention or when asking her to follow an instruction. For instance, there no point in asking her to tidy her toys when she's already watching television. Even though she'll nod in agreement, she won't have absorbed what you asked her to do. Instead, mute the sound or turn the television off altogether before speaking to her. The same applies when she plays with her friends. Wait for a suitable moment before you say anything, probably when she and her friends are quieter, then break into their conversation. You won't succeed in catching your child's attention simply by trying to talk over their conversation—the louder you talk, the louder they will talk.

If your preschooler seems to daydream so easily that your instructions are rarely followed, make sure that you have her full attention before telling her what to do. Then ask her to repeat the instruction back to you—this is a good way to get her focused on the task in hand, and it also helps her memory. If she can't repeat your instruction accurately, tell her again. Repeat this process until you are sure she has listened accurately.

Social development

Egocentrism, the belief that the world and those around you exist solely for your comfort and entertainment is universal in toddlers and is demonstrated by a refusal to share, take turns, or the refusal to wait for a parent to do something for them. Gradually, the realization comes that the world does not revolve around this one, small person and that the feelings of others need to be taken into consideration. Developing an understanding of the perspective of others may come earlier if a child has siblings or if she spends time with groups of children, perhaps at day care.

By the time she's three, your child should show that she understands another person's situation rather than relating it to her own experience, for example, by seeking out your help if she sees a younger sibling cry.

Around four years of age, she will be able to consider conflicting emotions before responding—pleasure, if her younger brother is reprimanded for taking her toys but sympathy when he bursts into tears. Your child will also be more able to wait for things to happen as she gains more of an understanding of what is going on around her and that not everything that happens relates to her.

At five years of age, your child should be able to appreciate the needs and wishes of others, although this does not necessarily mean she will put the needs of others before her own. A preschooler of this age becomes concerned about her siblings and friends and will take care of a younger brother or sister, perhaps holding hands protectively when they enter a roomful of children or an unfamiliar place.

Ensuring the bonds of attachment

The relationship you have with your preschooler strongly influences all other relationships in her life. Therefore, the strength of attachment she has to you (and your partner)—that is the two-way emotional connection between you and your child—is extremely important. By now, of course, the bond between you

will be solidly formed. Your preschooler feels close to you, is happy and relaxed in your company, shares her thoughts and feelings with you, and likes to cuddle you—these are the hallmarks of a strong parent-child attachment. However, even at this age, there is lots you can do to continue promoting a healthy psychological connection.

Perhaps most important of all is to continue appropriate loving physical contact with her, such as cuddling, hugging and kissing, holding her hands when you are out together, stroking her cheek or hair gently, and even patting her on the back when she has behaved well. Those warm, affectionate gestures make her feel loved, valued, safe, and secure. Some parents mistakenly think this sort of contact with a child is "babyish," and that by the time she is four or five years old, these physical demonstrations of love should stop. That's a pity, because having an appropriate physical dimension to

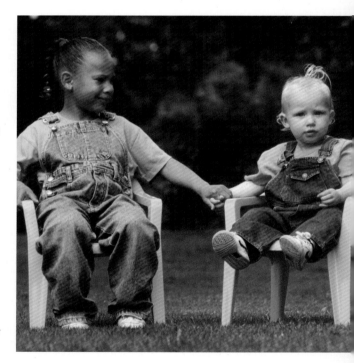

your relationship remains important throughout your child's life, and helps keep a strong attachment.

Continued sensitivity to your child's needs also enhances bonding during the preschool years. She needs you to be available to her, to hear her concerns when she worries, to reassure her when she lacks confidence, to guide her when she is uncertain, to calm her when she is upset, and to encourage her when she faces a challenge. In other words, just continue with what you are already doing anyway. The sensitive interactions you have with your preschooler every single day all contribute to the two of you having a solid emotional connection.

This period in your child's life can be the stage when she starts to assert herself, and you may find yourself spending more time than you would like setting rules and limits on her behavior. There may be confrontations because your preschooler doesn't like to hear you say "No" to her. That's part of parenting. While no child or parent enjoys battles of will or conflicts over what is and isn't allowed, you needn't be afraid that this will impair your attachment with your preschooler. On the contrary, a balanced approach to setting limits and guiding a child's behavior is recognized by psychologists as an important feature of a strong bond. So stand your ground, and be prepared to stick to the rules and standards you have set.

Sharing

Sharing is one of those crucial social skills that enables children to mix happily with others either at home or in nursery school, but yet rarely comes naturally to a preschooler. When you think about it, you won't be surprised that sharing is unpopular and that a preschooler needs time to come to terms with it. Most children start learning to share some time after the age of three.

 ways to encourage sharing

1 **Ask your child's permission.** If you want your child to share possessions, always ask him whether his friend can have something; never presume your child will agree and never hand the item over if he refuses. Making him share his possessions against his wishes will only upset him and make him more resistant to sharing next time.

2 **Be fair.** Don't always make your child give up his toys for a visiting child; the same applies to siblings—don't always expect an older child to be the "sensible one" and give up her toys for her younger sibling. Don't rush in to pass a ruling on which child should have a particular toy; give children an opportunity to come to an agreement on their own first.

3 **Try to avoid confrontation.** If your child has a particular toy that he and his friend always fight over, perhaps a doll or a dressing-up outfit, ask the visitor to bring his own along. This will help to create a happy environment where other toys are more likely to be shared.

4 **Set easily understood limits.** Where items are provided for everyone to share, for example, equipment in a playground or instruments in a music class, explain there's a time limit. After your child has had a reasonable turn on the swings or tambourine, for example, show him that another child is waiting and interest him in doing something else. Set a timer if you have to so that each child gets a turn and has to make way for another when the timer rings.

5 **Praise your child for good behavior.** When your child lets someone else play with one of his toys, praise him enthusiastically. Never become angry with your young child for refusing to share.

For your child to share properly, she has to understand that a sibling or friend with whom she has to share has needs and desires too, just like her, and that this sibling or friend feels the same way about her toys and games as she does. In addition, she must be willing to temporarily part with a toy that she likes very much and wants to play with herself. It's not easy to give like this. Moreover, sharing requires a leap of faith, a trust that the other child will return the toy soon and in the same condition it was given. That's all challenging for a preschooler. By four years of age, your child should have a good, but not infallible, understanding of the concept and arguments with playmates over particular toys should become less frequent.

How to help your child

The best place for your child to learn how to share is probably at home. In that safe environment, under your guidance and supervision, she'll be more willing to take risks with sharing because she trusts you will treat her fairly. You can make a start in teaching her this social skill by giving her a small bag of candies. Once she holds the bag, ask her to give you one of her candies instead of keeping them all to herself, and suggest that she offers one to her brother or sister (or friend). Be ready to give her gentle persuasion because she may refuse to cooperate with your request at first. Persist until she shares, however grudgingly. Then give her lots of praise. Encourage her further by making clear the practical implications of sharing. Tell her "The other children will like you better when you share, and they will share their toys with you as well." The more you encourage sharing at home, the better; you'll find that your child will slowly apply the same principles to social situations outside the home.

Setting a good example yourself is also important. Your child imitates a lot of your behavior because she loves you and wants to be like you. Show her that you enjoy sharing things with her, with your partner, and other children too, and with your own friends. A sharing home atmosphere encourages everybody to be more generous with his or her possessions. If you only have one child, the same

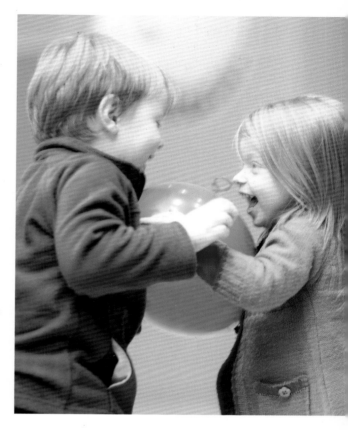

suggestions apply. An only child can be just as good at sharing as a child with siblings, as long as her parents show her how. Whenever cousins or friends come to the house to play, remind your preschooler beforehand about the importance of sharing and, afterward, comment on how well she shared. You can help the learning process along by asking your child's playmates to come and play in your home so that your child is called upon to share her toys sometimes.

Before children are able to share, they learn about owning things. By the age of two, your child will probably have realized that although some things are hers, others belong to other people. (You can help her understand this by pointing at things, saying "Daddy's shoes," "Mommy's nose.") Appreciating this is the first step in coming to grips with sharing. Learning to share things and take turns is a natural progression in child development. However, there are a number of measures you can take to help

Your child and his friends

3 years old

This is the start of cooperative play and very often your child will share a toy—or offer something else in its place—but you will have to intervene from time to time "settle" differences. He will, however, still spend lots of time playing by himself or alongside other children. Your child generally prefers being with one other child, who he will consider a "special" friend but occasionally he will play with more children. Overall, he can spend about three hours a day playing with others. Over the course of this year, your child will play more often as part of a group and there may be lots of cooperation, and often clowning and fooling around. Friendships will become intense and your child may prefer others with a similar temperament and/or energy level. Some children may be excluded from group play. It's not unusual for playtimes to end in tears and bad behavior.

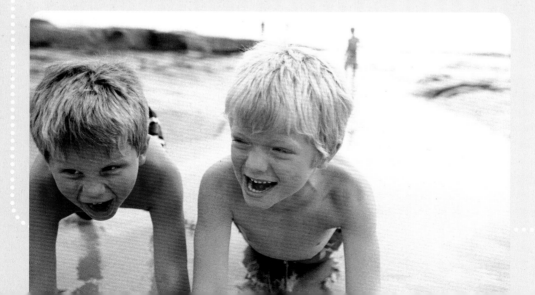

4 years old

Other children are now a source of pleasure and exciting activities; your child prefers other children over adults and can spend hours playing with them. Playtime generally goes smoothly with cooperating, sharing, and taking turns, but you may need to settle disputes and may have to coax your child to accept a new playmate. Your child should enjoy being part of a group and will be better at expressing what she wants to happen and be more tolerant of others' infractions of game rules. She might have a special friend, but in any event, wants to be liked by other children. A leader or a follower? Over the course of the year, some children issue orders and find that others carry them out. Or, your child may become very strongly attached—even for a short while—to another child, possibly of the opposite sex, and take her lead from them.

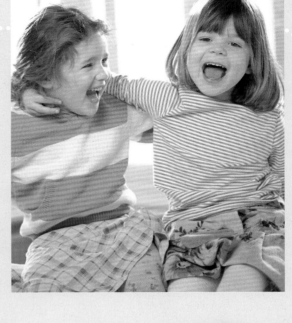

5 years old

Your child now is an accomplished playmate, particularly with one or two children of his own age, and can be left unsupervised for longer periods. This is useful since play with others will take up more of your child's time from now on (though not as much as when he's at school). A five-year-old, however, still enjoys being with his family the most. You can plan on him spending a good part of his day with friends. He also will play with both girls and boys (something that will change as he gets older).

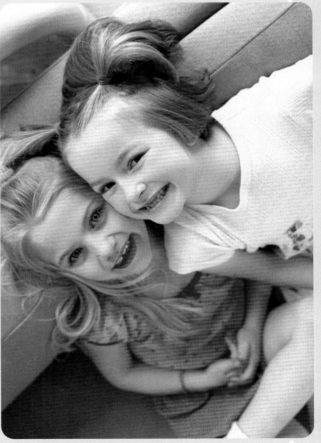

things along and hopefully make for a more harmonious atmosphere (see box, page 120).

Sharing a parent

As well as having to learn to share toys and other possessions, children have to learn to share their parents with others, whether this be other adults or a younger sibling, or even chores that need doing. Your child needs to understand that she cannot always be the focus of attention of her parents, who may want to spend time with others or who have their own activities to fit into the day. Provided she has your company, it is good for your child to learn how to amuse herself. No parent can be a playmate every minute of the day.

A child, particularly a first child, may find it hard to let you visit others or do your everyday tasks instead of playing. If you experience this, try to involve her in your activities. If you are dusting, give her a cloth; if you are doing the laundry, let her help you put the clothes into the machine; if you are writing a shopping list, ask her to make her own list by scribbling, or if she is older, by drawing the things you need. If this isn't feasible, don't stall her repeatedly; explain what you are going to do and when you will be able to play with her. Make sure you keep your promises—if you say you will play with her when you have finished the laundry, try your best to do it. And, when you do play with her, give her quality time. When you do something together, make her the focus of your attention.

Empathy and kindness

You may feel you face an uphill struggle when trying to teach your child to be caring and thoughtful about others, but you'll find this task much easier than you expect; you just need to find ways to harness her instinct for kindness. Empathy develops over time, although it may be apparent early on (a young baby may cry if she sees her mother do so).

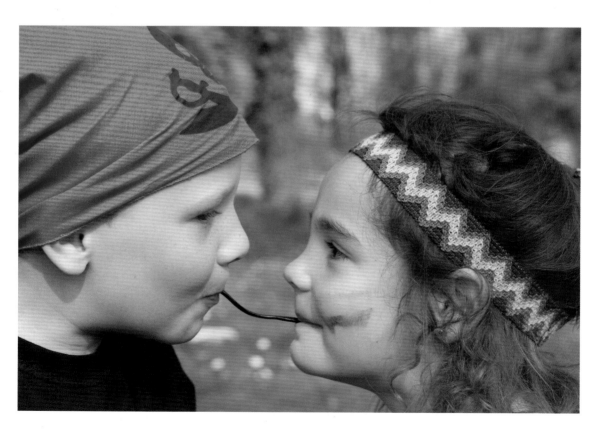

When your preschooler sees other children or adults are upset, her natural reaction is to try to comfort them. She intuitively wants to ease their distress, even when she doesn't understand why they are unhappy or what practical help they might need. That's also why your child is generally very caring toward a younger brother or sister. She will be prepared to stand up for her siblings and won't allow them to come to any harm if she has anything to do with it. These acts of kindness and empathy happen spontaneously. It is as though a young child intuitively knows when to be caring toward others, when to help them, and when best to offer emotional support.

Despite these natural tendencies toward kindness, however, there are lots of incidents of antisocial behavior among preschoolers every day. There are a number of explanations to account for this. First, your child has many basic instincts (as well as the instinct to be kind to others), and these instincts compete with one another. For instance, her need to satisfy her hunger might be more powerful than her instinct to be caring—so she pushes her friend out the way in order to grab the candies.

Second, your preschooler is influenced by the behavior of those around her, especially by you and your partner. If she sees you bicker with each other about loading the dishwasher, or fight over the choice of television programs, the chances are she'll do the same when she is in a similar situation.

Third, your child's natural impulse to be kind and empathic may be suppressed by the influence of television. Most contemporary role models in children's television programs are admired for their strength, physical abilities, and capacity to beat an opponent. Even though these fictional characters show occasional acts of kindness, such actions may go unnoticed in the eyes of your young viewer who may be more interested in adventure than she is in sociable behavior.

How to help your child

As well as setting a good example yourself (after all, you can't reasonably expect your preschooler to behave in a kind way if you behave uncaringly or unkindly in front of her), make a point of praising any kindness that she demonstrates, because there will be many times when your preschooler is considerate to friends or family. When that happens, tell her how pleased you are with what she's done. Make a big fuss of her for being so caring; your positive reaction will encourage her to behave kindly on other occasions.

You could also consider buying her a pet to look after. This needn't be a dog or a cat, just a small pet such as a goldfish or a hamster. The basic responsibility of feeding a small pet teaches your child to think about the needs of others. However, you'll need to supervise while she looks after the pet, but let her know that she is in charge.

Explain to your preschooler that her behavior also has practical consequences. For instance, tell her clearly "When you helped your friend, she felt better" or "If everyone was unkind, nobody would help you." Statements like these help your child understand the wider implication of her empathic, kind behavior. She begins to realize that kindness affects her as much as it affects others.

And give her opportunities to be kind to others. For instance, she can have responsibility for basic household chores, such as putting away the toys each night or helping set the cutlery on the table for the family meal. Giving your preschooler duties like these teaches her to think about others and encourages her to be kind toward them.

You can also involve her in charity. Whatever amount of money she gets to spend, for instance, for birthday presents, suggest that she gives a share of her money to charity. This is a very practical form of kindness that provides her with direct involvement. Make sure that she physically puts the coins into the charity collection—that makes it very real for her.

As well as positive encouragement of empathy and kindness, have zero tolerance for antisocial, uncaring behavior. Don't let incidents of unkindness from your child go by unnoticed, even though they may be relatively minor. A strict nonaccepting attitude at home lets your child understand that you expect kindness and empathy at all times.

Manners

Preschoolers often lack manners. It's highly likely that you have spoken to your child about this on a number of occasions, and yet your pleas for politeness seem to fall on deaf ears. It's as if learning good manners is a hard job for a young child because somehow she has managed to build up a whole repertoire of bad manners, such as sneezing without covering up her nose and mouth, touching other people's things without asking their permission, talking loudly (or even shouting) in public as if nobody can hear what she says, forgetting to say "please" or "thank you," and making unacceptable noises from one body orifice or another.

Her lack of manners can be frustrating whether it's her behaving dreadfully the moment you have a visitor or not showing any interest when given a gift. Worse still, her nose-picking during mealtimes sickens you and can be a very effective appetite-suppressant! Manners matter, as far as you are concerned, and you would like to see her awareness of them improve.

In most instances, though, your preschooler's poor display of manners is totally unintentional. She doesn't deliberately set out to have bad manners, it's just that she simply doesn't think enough about politeness because she's too busy thinking of something else, like what's on television or the latest toy that you bought her earlier that day. Or maybe she isn't fully aware of the impact her behavior has on others around her.

Sometimes, however, her lack of manners may be designed to have an effect. For instance, there was the time she made an insulting comment about the size of another child's nose and then she and her pal howled with delight as they collapsed in a heap of giggles. On that occasion, she intended to be rude because she thought that was funny. Then there was the time she belched loudly while sitting with her friends and then they all rolled around in fits of laughter. Yet these occasions are much less frequent than you probably suspect.

Good manners and politeness have to be learned; they are not inborn and they rarely develop spontaneously. By the time she is a preschooler, your child can begin to understand the idea of "good" and "bad" manners, however, and from then on the slow learning process gets underway. She won't learn good manners overnight.

Barriers to manners

When teaching manners to your child, expect to meet resistance for a number of reasons. First, the reality is that while adults like good manners, children often prefer bad manners, which is why she and her friends laugh when one of them is rude. All it takes is for your child or one of her pals to break wind loudly, and before you know it they all double up with delight. Most children—and if truth be told, many adults—get a good laugh out of those situations. They find them extremely funny.

Second, your preschooler has already discovered that bad manners usually generate a strong reaction from you. While you give mild praise when she behaves politely, or perhaps not even mention it all, she gets your full attention the moment she speaks rudely to a sales assistant. She knows that if you are too busy to spend time with her, she can change all that by making a vulgar comment or rude noise, which is just loud enough for you to hear.

And finally, good manners require effort, and sometimes your preschooler just can't be bothered. It's easier for her to sit and say nothing when you give her a snack than it is to thank you for it; and it's easier to say nothing when she is with her peers and to think only of herself, than it is to make polite conversation.

That's why you need to explain to your preschooler why manners matter. Keep your discussions about good manners very practical, spelling out the positive benefits to her personally. For instance, point out that behaving politely will make her more popular with her peers. Tell her that although a display of bad manners will make her buddies laugh at first, nobody wants to play with a child who constantly picks her nose or makes rude noises and bad smells. In the long run, good manners help your child to make friends more easily. And the same applies with adults. Her mom and dad, aunts and uncles, nursery-school teachers, and other grown-ups in her life always will think more favorably of her when she is polite.

Teaching manners

Use positive language when teaching good manners. No child likes to be told all the time that she is doing this or that wrong, or that people are irritated by her behavior. Think how you would feel if she said to you "I think the way you eat your food is terrible" or "I'm sick and tired of constantly having to remind you to cover your nose and mouth when you sneeze." Your self-esteem would drop and you'd be utterly miserable—it's no different with her. You should say "You are a such neat child, and that's why I am surprised the way you eat isn't as tidy as it could be. Maybe you just need to eat a little more slowly" or "I know you can sneeze politely because I've seen you do it sometimes. Maybe you just need to remind yourself to do that every time." It's amazing how much more responsive your preschooler will be to constructive comments than to negative ones. Embedding your observations about her manners in some form of praise, and offering an alternative course of action to improve her behavior, encourages your child to listen to you.

She also needs to understand the purpose of good manners. It is obvious to you, for example, that she should always say "please" and "thank you," but it may not be obvious to her. Take nothing for granted and give a full explanation each time. Likewise, be patient when she asks questions about manners, for instance, "Why is it good manners to do that?", each time you try to teach her a new aspect of politeness. You'll find that some manners are hard to explain. For instance, can you really provide her with a good reason why she should ask permission to leave the table when she has finished her meal?

Have realistic expectations. Don't try to teach her too many good manners at once—she'll feel totally overwhelmed. Instead, pick one aspect of good manners to start with, perhaps one that is easier to learn, for instance, saying "please" when she asks for something. Talk about that with your preschooler, explaining that you are much more likely to give her what she wants when she asks politely; then shower her with praise when she eventually does what you asked her to do.

Set an example of good manners yourself. After all, it's not fair to expect her to cover her mouth when coughing if she sees you splutter all over the place with your mouth unguarded. Your good manners provide a role model for her to follow. Likewise, never laugh at her bad manners, even though they may be highly amusing. For example, you might struggle to stop yourself from snickering when you hear your child's sweet voice telling her grandmother to, "Get off your lazy butt and get me a cookie." If you do laugh at such behavior, your preschooler may take this as encouragement to do the same again in the future.

Yet it's a matter of balance. You don't need to react every single time your child's manners fall below the standards you have set. Sometimes she just forgets what to do or say; it's as simple as that. Everybody makes mistakes sometimes—even you— so you can safely ignore occasional lapses in politeness. The most effective way to teach your child manners is to praise her when she shows good manners rather than to reprimand her when they are bad. Highlight what she does right, not what she does wrong.

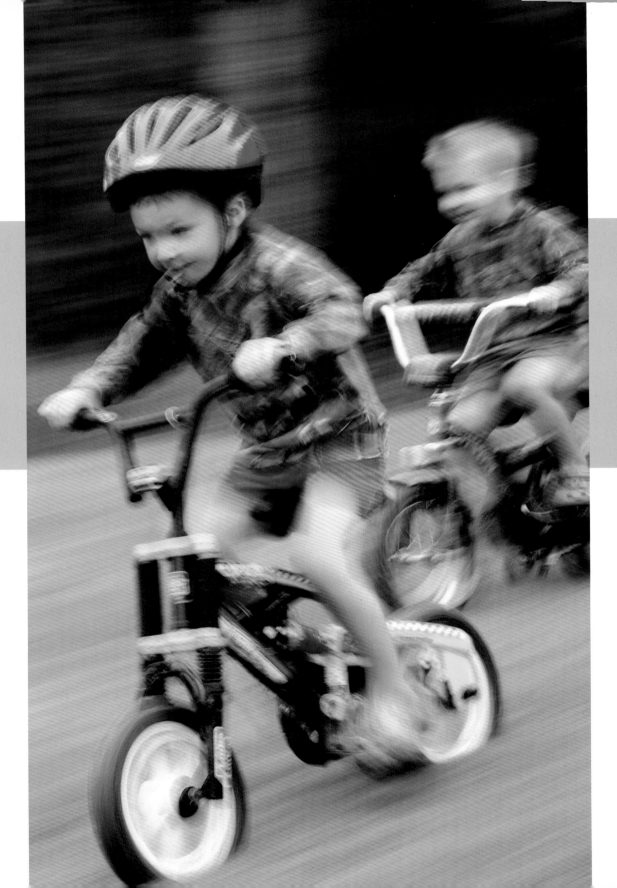

CHAPTER 4
PARENTAL CHALLENGES

In addition to age-old situations like managing bad behavior, including lying, bullying, and tantrums, and encouraging your child to be independent and making sure he is ready for school, today's parents have to deal with the influence of the internet, computer games and cell phones. While it's important that your child benefits from what modernity can contribute, it's also vital that, like all previous children, he be an acceptable member of the community. Your role in ensuring that he knows what good behavior is and is able to act accordingly, is paramount.

Managing bad behavior

Establishing a loving family discipline isn't about controlling your preschooler or forcing him to conform to a set of rules. It's about helping him think of others, about the effect of his behavior on those around him, and to gain self-control over his urges and desires. Discipline is about your child gradually taking more and more responsibility for his own behavior rather than you having responsibility for that on his behalf. In fact, the actual origin of the word "discipline" comes from the Latin word meaning "learning." In other words, your child learns through discipline. That's why you should approach discipline with him as though you are trying to create a system that enables him to learn rules so that he can behave properly, rather than a system that coerces him into behaving properly.

Establishing rules

Parents differ in their approaches to disciplining their preschoolers; some are stricter, some are more flexible, some explain more, and some use punishment more than others. You have to decide which style of discipline is best for your family. At this age, however, your child's understanding and reasoning has developed to the point where you can justifiably expect him to follow rules—for most of the time. He realizes that there are other people in the family who have feelings and ideas, and that living in a family involves thinking about mom and dad, and about his brothers and sisters as well as about himself.

This doesn't mean that he'll willingly follow the standards you have set without ever mounting a challenge. Young children are by nature

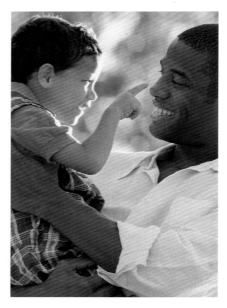

egocentric (in other words, they tend to think of themselves first) and it is only through encouragement and experience that they begin to consider others. Your preschooler's responsiveness toward family discipline (for example "You must put your toys away when you have finished playing with them" or "You must take your turn to put the plates on the table for supper") develops gradually. His natural instinct is to think that a rule applies to everyone else but him, so you'll need to help him accept that rule does indeed apply to him, too.

The first step is to make your preschooler aware of the rules. While they may be obvious to you, they might not be so obvious to him. For instance, you probably have the rule that the living room should be tidied when visitors are due, and this seems self-evident. Yet your child might not see it that way. As far as he is concerned, leaving the room in a mess could be perfectly acceptable. So make your family rules explicit. Your child's willingness to follow the rules can only develop when he knows exactly what they are. Keep repeating the rules until you are sure he understands them.

Consistency is also vital. There will be times when you bend the rules, for example, you might tolerate your child's grumpy behavior more when you know he is unwell, or you might let him stay up later than usual when it's a special occasion. Most times, though, it's best to stick consistently to the family rules that you have laid down because this will help your child adjust to them.

As an adult, you are able to transfer a rule from one situation to another. You know, for example, that the rule about your child not hitting another child means he isn't allowed to hit anyone at all, ever. It is a general rule that should be followed at all times. Yet your young child might not realize that. For instance, he might think the rule means he can't hit his friends in nursery school but that it's still okay for him to hit his big brother. That's why you need to give him very specific and practical explanations. For instance, instead of saying "It's not nice to hit people" he'll understand more easily if you say "Don't hit anyone, not your friends, not your parents, not your brother or sister, and not your cousins. If you do, I'll still love you but I'll be very annoyed with you." A clear and unambiguous description will be easier for him to grasp.

There is no doubt your young child is more likely to adhere to your discipline at home when he sees everyone else in his family do the same. You can hardly expect him to follow the rule "No feet are allowed on the furniture" when he sees you resting your feet on the coffee table.

Rewards and punishments

Make a big fuss of your preschooler when he does follow your rules—he loves praise and approval. This is much more effective than continually reprimanding him for something he has done wrong. Always use more rewards than punishments—positive discipline that gives attention to what your child does appropriately is much more motivating than negative discipline that focuses on what your child does inappropriately. So give him a cuddle or a special treat (see box on rewards, page 132) when, say, he helps his brother without prompting from you. In addition to rewarding your child spontaneously when he regularly demonstrates desired behavior, you can, together with your child, plan a reward in advance in order to achieve a desired behavior ("If you keep your toys tidy for the next few days, you can have ...."). But bear in mind that your preschooler will be unable to wait for too long to receive his reward.

No matter how well your preschooler conforms to the standards set by your loving family discipline, there are likely to be times when he breaks a rule and you decide to punish him. However, be careful to avoid empty threats. If you warn your child that such-and-such will happen if he misbehaves once more, follow that through. If you don't, he will learn quickly that you don't mean what you say and he'll soon start to ignore your threats. That's why you must ensure that any punishment you use is fair (that it's deserved), that it is reasonable (that it's not extreme but proportional to the infraction), and that it's enforceable (that you can actually carry it out).

FAMILY COUNCILS

Many families, and particularly those with older or stepchildren, find that regular meetings are ideal for sharing information and dealing with problems. While some families do this casually—over the dinner table, for example—others favor a more formal regular meeting involving specific topics, such as the weekly schedule, forthcoming outings, or "rule" changes. Four-year-olds and up should be able to enjoy and contribute to such gatherings and may even take a turn as leader.

For such events to be successful, make sure:

- Everyone gets a turn to speak and is listened to;
- Pleasant and positive suggestions are encouraged while negativity and criticism are not;
- Agreement on what needs to be decided on—a sum of pocket money for an allowance, a vacation destination, a new bedtime hour;
- Review suggestions made in the previous week(s) to see how they turned out;
- Limit the amount of time for the meeting; a preschooler may not be able to sit still for more than 15 to 30 minutes.
- A good time is had by all. Use the occasion for praising your child's behavior in the past week and sharing her accomplishments.

Never, ever, threaten to leave your child and walk off. Not only will this be extremely distressing to him but you almost certainly will have to eat your words!

Tell your preschooler what the punishment will be if he doesn't do what he's told. Give him advance warning, for example, "If you do that one more time, I will take that toy away from you for the rest of the day." If he ignores your warning and proceeds to repeat exactly what you asked him not to, say "I told you if you did that again I would take your toy away. You did that again, so I'm going to take it away now. I love you but you have misbehaved." That establishes a clear link between his behavior and the subsequent punishment. Don't change your mind about punishing him just because he bursts into tears once he realizes what trouble he's in—of course you can cuddle and soothe him because he's upset at the thought of being punished—but in most instances you still should do exactly as you warned. Bear in mind too that discipline loses its impact when there is a long time lag between the misbehavior and the punishment because your preschooler might not remember why he is being punished. For instance, reprimanding your child in front of his father when dad comes home in the evening because of his misbehavior just after dad left the house in the morning is too big a time gap—punishment should come as soon as possible after the misbehavior.

Think closely about the way you manage your preschooler during a typical week; if you realize that you give out more punishments than rewards, or

types of rewards

1 **Stickers and stamps**. Gold and other colored stars or appropriate picture or word stickers or stamps ("Well Done") can be their own rewards or collected in a book for yet a further reward.

2 **Items your child likes**. Toys, books, garments, art supplies, athletic equipment, and the occasional edible treat (ice cream or soda).

3 **Special activities**. A trip to the movies, a day out at a fun fair or adventure park, a visit to a toy store or creative activity center, a sleepover at the grandparents, going to a football or baseball game, visiting the zoo, aquarium, museum, or planetarium.

4 **Special privileges**. Choosing a DVD or television program for the family to watch, selecting a restaurant for dining out, having a friend over to play, or deciding what should be served for dinner.

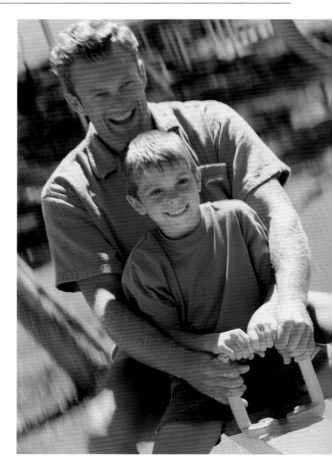

you just feel that you punish your preschooler too often, swing the balance in the other direction. An excess of punishments creates a negative downward spiral that makes both you and him miserable. Use rewards and punishments that are meaningful to your child, not those that are meaningful to you. It comes down to knowing him well and recognizing what he likes and dislikes.

Time-out

This procedure can be used for any young child as part of a strategy to improve his behavior. It involves sending a child to a specified place, such as a chair, with no entertaining distractions (generally not his bedroom) for a period of time—generally one minute for each year of age. Before using time-out, you need to explain to your child what he needs to do or stop doing to avoid the time-out and that you will give him a warning before you institute it so that he has a chance to change his behavior. Time-out needs to be used in conjunction with positive reinforcement of desired behaviors, and should only be used when your child understands the reason; it should not be used for nonspecific "bad behavior."

Spoiling

Saying "No" to your preschooler at times is part of a loving family discipline. Telling him "No, you can't have that/do that/or touch that" or setting limits and sticking to them consistently helps your child learn that he has to follow your expected standards of behavior. In contrast, if you give him everything he asks for, allow him to do whatever he wants, and permit him to think only of himself, he will become spoiled. In the short term, giving in to him will make you happy because you won't have the challenge of setting boundaries (so you can avoid having confrontations with him and can have fun buying him lots of presents) and he will be happy too because he does what he wants and he gets a steady stream of new toys and clothes. But in the long term, spoiling him will make you both unhappy. Your preschooler will become totally uncooperative and demanding, which will make your life more stressful, and he'll feel dissatisfied for

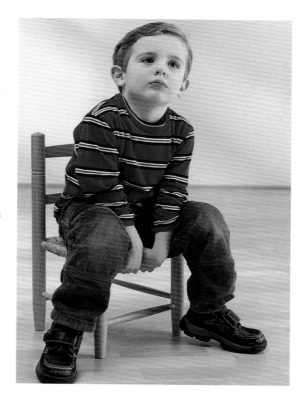

much of the time. Not only that, his peers won't want to play with him because he won't want to share, take turns, or play by the rules of a game.

Parents who spoil their child usually do this out of love but so too do parents who practice an inconsistent discipline without rules and limits. So when you find that your friends or relatives start to tell you that you spoil your child, stop for a moment and think about the way you manage him. Consider the potential negative effects that spoiling could have on him, and remind yourself that spoiling him isn't the only way to express your love for him.

Whether or not you continue to spoil your preschooler is up to you, but if you to decide to move toward a more balanced, consistent discipline, you won't find it too difficult. Remind yourself each day that setting rules and limits is in his best interest, because that helps him gain control over his feelings and think about others. Start to say "No" to him. Expect him to be furious with you (after all, he likes the way things are at the moment) but hold your ground and don't give in even if he rages. Start to ask him to make choices instead of agreeing to all his demands, for example, "I love you but I'm only going to buy you one of these three toys. Which one would you like?" Give him minor responsibilities for others, such as helping his brother put away his clothes or serving his friend a piece of cake. As your preschooler slowly adapts to your new expectations, tell him how pleased you are with his behavior—positive reinforcement is always effective.

Lying

Virtually every child is capable of lying sometimes. It's a normal part of development. A three-year-old might insist that the crayon marks on his bedroom wall were drawn by someone else, even though they weren't there an hour before and he's the only one who's been in the room during that time. Even the most honest child can distort the truth, especially

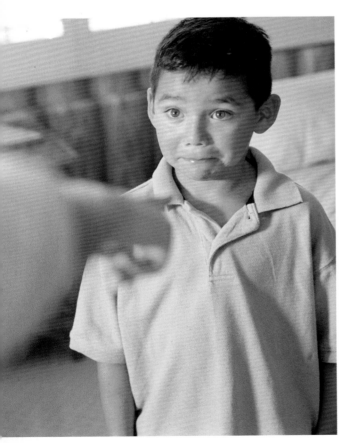

when faced with a furious adult questioner. However, you will want to discourage lying right from the start because honesty is a key part of every relationship. It's very difficult to trust a child who lies regularly. And if lying becomes a habit during the preschool stage, it may become even more frequent as your child grows older.

From the age of three onward, you can be confident that your preschooler knows the difference between right and wrong and that he also knows that lying is unacceptable; so if he lies to you, there is usually an important reason. Whatever the type of lie your child tells you, make sure he understands that it is wrong to lie and that you always want him to tell the truth.

Your reaction on discovering that your child is lying will heavily influence what he says in response to your followup questions. In a classic study, children were led individually into a large room that had a hamster in a cage in one corner, and a pile of enticing toys in the other. The researcher told the children that unless the hamster was watched constantly, it might escape and run away, and she asked them to use a rolled-up newspaper to keep the hamster in the box. The researcher then left the room. As you would expect, the lure of the toys soon became too strong to resist, and each child inevitably moved toward them, turning his back on the hamster. At that precise moment the researcher, who was observing through a one-way mirror, tripped a switch causing the hamster to disappear down a hidden trap door. When the child returned to the cage he was stunned to see that his charge had vanished. He was even more stunned when the researcher stormed back into the room, demanding to know where her precious hamster had gone! The results of the study established three important principles about children's lies. First, every child will tell a lie to avoid discovery if he feels threatened enough; second, a child who is very scared to own up will try to maintain his lie even under severe questioning; third, a child who feels he is not listened to when he tries to explain why he lied will conclude there is no point telling the truth.

Dealing with lies

Prevention is better than cure, when it comes to lying. It is better to raise your child in a way that discourages lying before it happens than to punish him after you've discovered he is lying to you. Have clear rules about lying, for instance, "Don't tell lies to me or to anyone" is easy for your preschooler to understand, whereas "Telling lies isn't a very nice thing to do" is too vague. Another preventative strategy is to explain to him that his behavior has consequences. A young child doesn't always fully grasp that his actions can affect others. Explain to him that "Telling lies makes me sad" or "If you tell lies, none of your friends will like you."

No matter how hard you try to discourage your preschooler from lying to you, however, there may be times when he's not entirely honest. Once you have discovered that he has lied, speak to him openly about what he has done, letting him know that you are sure he has lied to you. Listen to his explanation. His justification for the lie will not be acceptable to you but let him give you his side of the story anyway. Respond calmly and seriously. You may be hurt, troubled, and possibly embarrassed by

your child's lie, but don't overreact. Leave him in no doubt that you are unhappy with what he has done, though do bear in mind that if your reaction is too extreme then he will try even harder to hide the truth from you the next time. It's also important to recognize that your preschooler has probably lied out of his instinct for self-preservation, and not because he wants to upset you. So don't be pessimistic. The fact that he lied to you on this occasion doesn't mean he will grow up to be a persistent liar.

By all means punish your child for lying, but don't make it too severe or he will feel like he is a victim. You could put him to bed early that night, give him a strong reprimand, or stop him from playing with his favorite toy for a short while.

The best time to punish your child for lying is right after you have discovered the lie and have heard his side of the story. Any later and the rebuke will have less impact. Immediate punishment also means that the incident can be brought to an early close. While you want your child to know that you totally disapprove of his behavior when he has lied to you, you also want him to know you are not

reasons why a preschooler might lie

1   **She might lie in order to protect herself.**
    Your child knows when she has broken a rule and she may deliberately lie to you in order to protect herself from your anger or punishment. She is aware this is wrong but she lies to you anyway in the hope of avoiding discovery.

2   **She might lie to protect a friend.**
    Friendships are very important at this age. Your preschooler may try to cover up for her friend's mistake either by giving a distorted account of events or by taking the blame herself. She feels this is sufficient justification for her lie.

3   **She might even lie because she thinks that telling you what you want to hear** (even though it is untrue) will make you happy. That's why she tells you she has tidied her room, even though it's still in a mess, because she knows you would be pleased if her clothes and toys really had been put away.

4   **She might lie as a result of peer pressure.**
    If she and a group of friends are caught doing something they should not be doing, then she may lie along with her peers because she does not want to break ranks. She may be afraid of group rejection if she tells the truth.

rejecting him. He'll learn that you can dislike his lies and yet still love him at the same time. You have to tread a fine line between reprimanding your child for lying and making him afraid to tell you the truth. He needs to understand that you would rather hear the truth, even though it may upset you and cause problems for him, than to have him lie to you. This way, you encourage his honesty.

In addition, praise your child when he does admit his guilt about something he has done. Tell him how pleased you are that he didn't lie even though he might have been strongly tempted.

"White lies"

There is no point is discouraging your preschooler from telling lies if you are dishonest in front of him. Never leave yourself open to the accusation "But I heard you tell a lie." At this age, your child will think it is perfectly acceptable for him to tell a lie if he hears you lying; he won't be convinced by the argument that he should "Do as I say, not as I do."

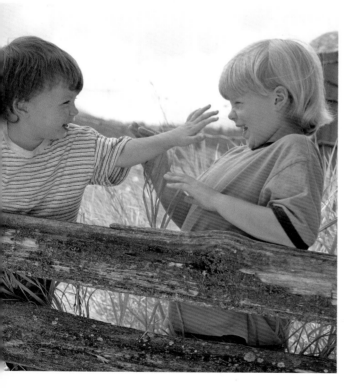

Yet despite all your good intentions, despite all your determined efforts to encourage honesty at all times, you may find yourself telling a "white lie" (that is, a deliberate lie told in order to protect someone's feelings) in front of your child. Like the time your mother-in-law came to visit and she asked you if you liked the sweater she had recently bought you for your birthday. You and your child had laughed together at the atrocious color of the present when you opened it the day before, but you stand with him by your side and tell your mother-in-law, "Yes, I loved it." No wonder your preschooler will be totally confused by your double standards. After all, you have repeatedly discouraged his lies, and now you have to tell him why you broke the very rules that you set.

Explain that sometimes a small lie can be justified when it is designed to protect another person from distress. This does run the risk that your child may then use this as justification for all his own lies in the future, claiming each time that "It's only a white lie." That's why you need to give plenty of examples, illustrating when a white lie might be acceptable and when it is not. Generally, white lies are used only when making a compliment or a thank-you that is insincere, while ordinary lies are typically used to conceal discovery. Emphasize this to your child, adding that white lies should be used only rarely and that at all other times he should tell the truth. He'll eventually grasp your meaning, but don't be surprised if he occasionally is confused about this.

Bullying and being bullied

Bullying in school (including playgroup and nursery school) is horrible, frightening, distressing, and a reality for some children. If your child is on the receiving end, you'll already know how much it spoils school for him, how much it badly affects him even when he's not actually in school, and how much it lowers his self-confidence. While young children often become wild when playing, that's not bullying because malicious intent is lacking. Deliberate nastiness toward others is one of the hallmarks of the genuine bully; the victim perceives the bully to be more powerful than himself.

Bullying in school can take many different forms. Physical bullying includes punching, slapping, kicking, tripping, jostling, or just the threat of such acts of aggression. A bully often uses intimidation to extort money, candy, or toys from another child and threatens to hurt him if he refuses to cooperate. There is also verbal bullying, for instance, teasing a child about the way he looks or the color of his hair, or making fun of his friends or parents or racial or religious background.

Girls are particularly vulnerable to social bullying in which a child is unfairly and deliberately rejected and excluded from her social group. All forms of bullying are frightening and emotionally harmful.

Children bully for many different reasons. A child raised in a family where aggression to others is commonplace, where little thought is given to the feelings of the others or where verbal abuse occurs frequently, is likely to behave in a similar way outside the family home. That's why bullying parents tend to have bullying children. But bullying can be a means for the child to release frustrations.

A child who is not allowed to express tension at home needs to find an outlet for these negative feelings somewhere, and bullying another child is a perfect vehicle for this. Feelings of inadequacy and general unhappiness can also lead a child into bullying behavior because bullying places him in a position of power and authority. Peer pressure can also be a cause. If his friends are bullies, he may start bullying too in order to retain their friendship.

Recognizing bullying

The chances are that your child won't want to admit to you that he is bullied because his self-confidence has dropped, he is embarrassed about it, and he fears you will think he is making a big fuss about nothing. So he might withstand bullying for several months without saying anything about it at all. That means the onus is on you to watch out for signs that your child is being bullied.

Look for uncharacteristic behavior changes. These can be caused by factors such as trouble between you and your partner, worries about friendships, bereavement of a close relative, and so on. But it can also be due to bullying. It comes down to knowing your child. No single sign (see box) on its own definitely means that your child is being bullied, but you should be alert that this may be a possibility. If in doubt, discuss the matter with him. You may need to persist before he opens up to you.

POSSIBLE SIGNS OF BULLYING

- Your child's fear of attending playgroup or nursery school and resistance when taken.
- Complaints of a sore tummy and a headache when going to playgroup or nursery school
- Unexplained bruises, cuts, grazes, or scratches on her face, hands, or legs
- Regular loss of a schoolbag, lunch box, or books or repeated loss of her money for snacks and/or lunches at school
- Signs of distress such as stammering, or toilet "accidents," and anxiety on being informed that a particular playmate is coming over.

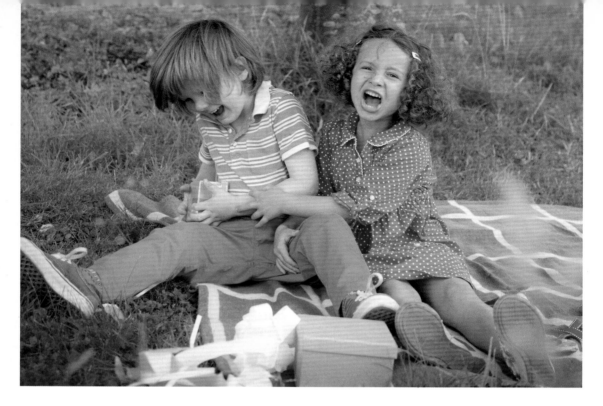

Responding to bullying

You feel so frustrated watching your child suffer this way. His life should be stimulating not terrifying, satisfying not depressing. And to you the solution is obvious—he just needs to ignore the bullies until they go away and annoy someone else. But it's not that easy for a playground or classroom victim. The continual rejection and bullying by a small group of peers (or maybe by only one child) can gradually wear down your child's self-esteem. Feelings of powerlessness will steadily replace his feelings of empowerment, and he will perceive himself as trapped and unable to do anything that can alter the daily grind in school.

That's why you should always treat complaints of bullying seriously. Bear in mind that it takes a great deal of courage for your child to admit to you that he is being bullied; he will be terrified in case the bully finds out he has spoken to you.

Reassure your child that you will keep the matter entirely confidential. Listen to his complaints, don't make him feel silly or babyish, and let him know that you understand the problems he faces. He'll start to feel more confident already, just from

knowing you are there to support him. Then give him some practical advice. Persuade him to walk away unobtrusively whenever the bully moves toward him. Too often this type of avoidance-strategy is mistakenly construed by the victim as an act of cowardice when, in fact, it is really quite sensible. When your child does move out of the line of fire, he should do this slowly without running. Encourage him to show as little reaction as possible to the bully's threats. Teasing and bullying will, probably stop eventually if the victim displays indifference to the actions against him. Ignoring verbal and physical threats is difficult, but it can be done successfully. Practice this with your child through role play at home.

Never tell your child to fight back. Tempting as it may be to encourage him to retaliate, that strategy has a number of drawbacks. First, he may end up getting a severe beating. Second, if you advocate aggression, then your child may think this is a suitable way to deal with all sorts of problems in his life. Instead, advise him to stay with a crowd of other children, especially in free-play situations either inside the school building or outside in the playground. Bullies usually pick on children who are isolated, therefore, a child standing alone is easily identified as a potential target. Being with a crowd reduces the likelihood he will be bullied. And help him develop positive body language. Your child probably looks afraid, because he anticipates the bully's attack. Teach him to stand so that he looks assertive and confident. For instance, he should walk with his shoulders held back, his back upright, and his eyes looking directly in front of him, not toward the ground. He should also try to have a relaxed facial expression, perhaps with a smile.

Ultimately, however, you will have to speak to your child's playgroup leader or the adult in charge about the problem. All institutions have an anti-bullying policy and there should be an established approach for tackling and eliminating bullying. Make an appointment to discuss your concerns in confidence. Staff may not have noticed and therefore you should bring it to their attention, but make it clear that your child should not be publicly identified as the child who complained. Ask the leader about the group's anti-bullying strategy and what he or she proposes to do to halt the bullying. If you already know the bully's parents well, you could consider having a confidential chat with them about their child's behavior, though it may best be left to the staff to handle this.

My child is the bully

You'd feel dreadful if someone accused your child of bullying and your first instinct might be to dismiss such a suggestion out of hand. Yet repeated claims by children, parents, or teachers could force you to take the possibility more seriously. If you suspect your child is a bully or if someone suggests he is, consider the evidence carefully because the accusation could be accurate. Think through some of the possible factors that could be influencing your child's behavior. Tell him that you are aware of the situation and that you want it to stop. Even if he denies the accusation, continue to explain why you dislike all forms of bullying. This discussion alone may be sufficient. Encourage your child to think of the victim. He may never have thought about the impact of bullying on the victim—he might simply see the whole thing as a joke. So explain to him how terrible the other child feels when he bullies him. Then make a point of discussing his behavior with him regularly. It is not a matter of policing your child. On the contrary, it is about letting him know that you care. Your positive attention alone might reduce his need to bully others.

Disruptive behavior

Virtually all children go through disruptive phases. Disruptiveness is related to temperament, parenting style, and environment. Many, but not all, children tend to fall into one of three broad and loosely defined categories: easy, slow to warm up or shy, or difficult or challenging. These labels are a useful shorthand, but none can offer a complete picture of a child. Also, particular patterns of behavior often predominate at different stages. Many parents find it more useful to think about their child in terms of nine temperamental traits (see page 142).

Consistency is very important for a child, both with respect to his daily routine and discipline and in support and involvement in his activities. In addition, providing your child with plenty of encouragement will help foster a positive environment both in the home and away. If you are inconsistent with discipline, are not supportive and/or positive, and do not participate in your child's activities, it will negatively affect his behavior.

If you allow him to watch aggressive behavior on television, or online, or participate in aggressive games, this will also encourage your child to become more disruptive.

How to help your child

Aggression, attention seeking, and lack of empathy are temperamental characteristics associated with disruptive behavior. Even before he started talking, your child communicated feelings he wasn't able to put into words through his behavior. So if your child starts being disruptive, this is likely to be the result of feelings such as anger, fear, anxiety, or frustration. You should, therefore, defuse a difficult situation by commenting on the emotion rather

Disciplining your child

3 years old

Though tending to whine when in a bad mood, your child essentially loves to please, so gentleness should be your guiding principle in procuring better behavior. She will be easily distracted by making a game of something, an activity, or even a simple "bribe." It will be possible for her to have her way sometimes, particularly when it's of no great consequence, and it's important not to make every issue one in which you always have to prevail. Use different strategies: give her choices, avoid rushing her, warn her of imminent changes (countdowns) and, if necessary, use time-outs.

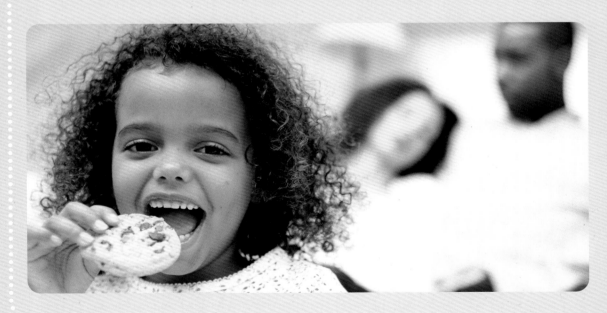

4 years old

Your child will respond well to simple rules and routines and clear boundaries enforced with incentives (rewards and privileges) and withholding them. Strong limits are necessary to protect him from out-of-bounds tendencies, but you should anticipate the probability of unacceptable behavior. Try not to react emotionally to any attention-seeking behavior. Whispering to your child may be more effective than shouting, since it will both calm him and catch his attention. Many harmless actions can be ignored and it's best to avoid confrontation and to use humor and suggestion rather than demands. Your child may be troubled by particular issues, so it's best to talk about them when things calm down to prevent bad behavior in future. Don't forget to praise and compliment him when he behaves well.

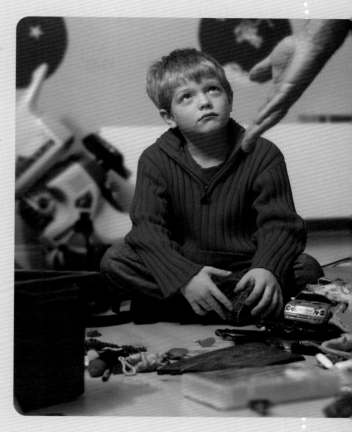

5 years old

Your child won't always be successful at being good so ensure you don't put temptation in her way. Remind her frequently about what is and is not acceptable behavior and what is expected of her—but don't expect too much too soon. Keep your remarks simple and to the point. Don't get into a lengthy discussion about why her actions are unacceptable. Taking away privileges or favorite toys (for longer than previously) may be your best options. If you must reprimand her, do so calmly and using a matter-of fact tone. Time-outs may still be effective. Your child is sufficiently mature for natural consequences (not putting on your mittens in winter means your fingers get cold) to impart their own lessons.

ASPECTS OF TEMPERAMENT

Activity level: How much physical activity, restlessness, or fidgeting your child demonstrates in daily activities (and which may also affect sleep).

- Rhythmicity or regularity: Whether or not your child follows a regular pattern for basic physical functions such as appetite, sleep, and bowel habits.
- Approach and withdrawal: The way your child initially responds to a new stimulus (rapid and bold or slow and hesitant), whether it be people, situations, places, foods, or changes in routines.
- Adaptability: The degree of ease or difficulty with which your child adjusts to change or a new situation, and how well she can modify her reaction.
- Intensity: The energy level with which your child responds to a situation, whether positive or negative.
- Mood: The degree of pleasantness or unfriendliness in your child's words and behavior.
- Attention span: The ability to concentrate or stick with a task, with or without distraction.
- Distractibility: The ease with which your child can be distracted from a task by environmental (usually visual or auditory) stimuli.
- Sensory threshold: The amount of stimulation needed for your child to respond. Some children respond to the slightest stimulation, others require more.

Other things you can do to manage a difficult child include:

- Keeping your child active, with plenty of outdoor activities;
- Praising him whenever he is being calm and helpful, or is playing quietly;
- Giving him some special time each day when he can choose the activity;
- Making sure that he knows the rules about relationships, e.g. politeness and consideration (not easy for a preschooler);
- Teaching problem-solving skills can never start too young;
- Explaining in advance what will happen if he is disruptive (does he know what this means?);
- Ignoring behavior that is boisterous and energetic but not hurtful or harmful;
- Setting a limit on time spent watching TV or DVDs or using the computer or digital devices;
- Making clear what "unacceptable" behavior is, e.g. fighting, hurting a sibling, or damaging toys;
- Using time-out if he oversteps the limits (see page 133);
- Avoiding parental conflict or change in the family structure.

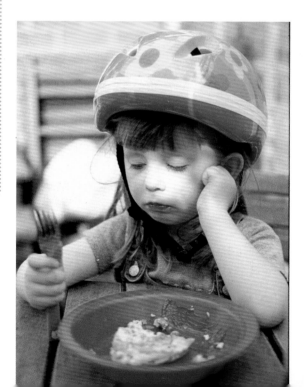

than the behavior. Talk about why he may be angry, worried, anxious, or frustrated instead of why he hit you. You need to try and understand the triggers for various situations and predict in advance when fireworks may arise.

Tantrums

All kids engage in tantrums to release strong feelings of anger and resentment though the severity of the tantrum often has no correlation with the enormity of what is withheld or denied. (There is, however, a correlation between severity and lack of sleep: tired children throw tantrums more often and the tantrums are much more intense and harder to bring to a halt.) When not allowed to have his way, your child may suddenly start screaming. He may lie down on the floor and beat his fists and feet against the ground or may bang his head repeatedly against a wall, throw objects around the room, or begin hitting or biting.

The best way to deal with a tantrum is to prevent it from ever occurring. Once started, however, it is too late to give in or try other techniques. At this point, if at home, the most effective way to end the tantrum is to ignore your child, conveying the attitude that you couldn't care less. "You can do this all you want, but I'm not going to be upset by it." Ignoring your child includes walking away from him, not looking at him, singing a song, and/or not responding to his pleas. If you are concerned that your child may hurt himself, pick him up and convey him to a safer place but try hard not to look at or respond to him.

If a tantrum occurs in a public place, pick your child up and head home. While many of the others present have had a similar experience with their own children and are probably thinking to themselves, "I feel so sorry for that mother/father. I remember how

---

WHEN TO EXPECT BAD BEHAVIOR

- Your child is hungry.
- You are (or your child is) tired or feeling sick.
- You are in a hurry and try to rush your child.
- You are stressed, maybe because everyone needs you at once.
- Daily routines are disrupted.
- At the end of a long day.
- It's important that she behaves well.
- Everyone is watching.

---

embarrassed I felt when my daughter did that," they certainly don't want their meal, movie, or other good time ruined by your screaming child.

It also will be stressful for you if your child is disruptive in playgroup or nursery school as well as at home. In such a case, it is important to maintain close relationships with his carers. Bullying (see page 136) is frequently a factor and can be highly distressing and if it's your child who is being bullied, he may not admit to it, so you may need to draw out the information gradually.

If you are concerned about your child's behavior and need some advice, consult your healthcare provider, who will be able to talk to your child and look for factors that may be involved.

Parenting and the internet

The moment you have a problem with your child, a parenting challenge you have to face, or a question about his progress and development, you don't want to wait for a solution. Whether it's how to manage a tantrum, how to stop him from sucking his thumb, or how many words he should be speaking by now, you want an immediate answer to your question. And that's where the internet comes in. No need to wait till grandma visits, no need to keep ringing your friend until she is available—one click and you have all the information you need. But it's not that simple. How do you know the advice is sound? What do you do when you read different opinions on the same topic? Does it matter if the advice is for a child who isn't even the same age as yours?

Using internet parenting positively

All parents respond to information and advice about their child in their own way, depending on the problem and the personalities involved. Each parent-

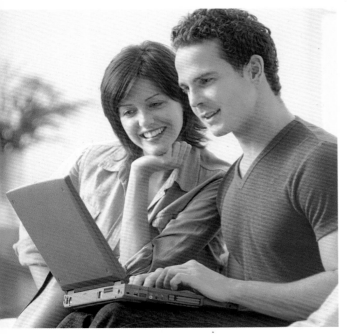

child relationship is unique, just as each parent and each child is unique. That's why when it comes to parenting advice, one size does not fit all. What works for another parent and child might not work for you and your child. Yet that doesn't mean there is no role for "parenting by internet." In fact, you can use it positively in several ways. For a start, the internet is a great way to extend your knowledge base. Whatever parenting question runs through your mind, someone else has almost certainly thought of it before and posted it on the web, so you can learn a great deal about the background, frequency, and causes of your concern. This is especially true when it comes to specific problems, such Asperger syndrome, ADHD, Developmental Coordination Disorder (DCD), or slow speech development.

And parenting on the internet can also help you consider alternative perspectives. It's so easy to get locked into a particular mindset when dealing with your child because of the pressure you are under. Simply reading another person's take on the same issue can open your mind to other explanations and different strategies for managing your child. For instance, some websites suggest managing a child's fussy eating habits by focusing on the food itself (advising small portions, correct temperature, pleasant texture) while others suggest that the parents' attention to their child during mealtimes is what matters most.

Many parents gain reassurance from discovering that plenty of others have had, or are having, the same difficulty. Even if you think you would handle the same parenting challenge differently, it can be helpful to read about another parent's experience.

Avoiding the pitfalls

But all is not completely rosy in the digital garden. For instance, exercise caution when you read parenting advice. While a great deal of web-based information is accurate, helpful, and appropriately detailed, parenting websites are not moderated. In other words, anybody can create a parenting website

USING THE INTERNET

ADVANTAGES

- Instant access to parenting information and advice;
- Very diverse range of parenting resources and opinions;
- Nobody judges your parenting skills;
- Private contact, without involving friends or family;
- Confirmation that others share this parenting difficulty.

DISADVANTAGES

- Quality and source of advice isn't guaranteed;
- Not tailored to suit your individual child;
- You can get overloaded with too much information;
- You don't share your concerns with other parents;
- Parenting websites only tell you first steps and there is no continuity.

and write anything he or she wants. Don't believe everything you read on the internet. Instead, look for common themes across different parenting websites. Whatever the problem you are facing with your child, for example, if he is wetting his bed, compare the parenting information and advice across at least half a dozen different sites. That's not a guarantee of accuracy, but there is more likelihood that the information on a parenting page is suitable if you see the same advice on several websites.

In addition, as a safeguard, use parenting websites with a good reputation. Parenting sites that are, for example, connected with parenting magazines or parenting organizations take their responsibilities seriously. They typically offer mainstream advice that has been tested and is reliable, although that doesn't mean it will necessarily be right for you and your child specifically.

There is a danger that when you look at too many parenting websites, you might start to think you can't deal with any child problem on your own. That's a very typical reaction. It's so easy to lose sight of your own skills as a parent once you start relying too much on internet advice. By all means, use the web for another parenting opinion but have confidence in your own judgment; a parenting website will never be able to raise your child for you!

Making it work

There are some rules you should follow to help you get the most out of parenting by the internet. First, never try to implement parenting advice that makes you feel uncomfortable. If the strategy suggested for managing your child's challenging behavior doesn't feel right for you, then disregard it. Anyway, you won't be able to implement advice in which you don't have confidence.

Second, run information from parenting websites past a friend or relative. No matter how much you like a particular website or web page, there's no harm in having a chat about it with someone you know personally. Listen to this person's opinion, even if you initially don't agree with it. Advice from the virtual world can seem different when discussed in depth in the real world.

Third, don't doubt your own judgment. In the end, raising your child is your responsibility and you should try to have confidence in your own parenting instincts. Bear in mind that before the internet was available, parents used to rely almost totally on their own ideas and opinions.

Fourth, look for research-based parenting advice. Some very sensible parenting suggestions derive from personal experience. However, parenting advice that's based on solid, peer-reviewed, professional research is more likely to be reliable. So check out the evidence that the website draws on to support its suggestions.

Last, resist peer pressure. Some websites have lots of positive reviews from parents. While comments from other users should not be ignored, you can't be sure they are genuine. And even if they are, bear in mind that what worked for lots of other parents and children might not be effective for you and yours.

TV viewing

The chances are that your preschooler spends time most days watching TV, either because he enjoys specific programs or because you find that watching television is a useful activity that keeps him fully occupied while you need to do something else.

Television allows your preschooler access to experiences that would otherwise be unobtainable. He can "visit" other parts of the world, "travel" alongside animals, birds, and fish, and have safe adventures, all without moving from the comfort of his home.

There are also benefits when it comes to developing his thinking skills. For example, a short period spent watching television during the day (approximately ten minutes) helps promote his concentration. A child who is able to sit still for that short amount of time will steadily improve his concentration and this will help him learn once he starts preschool and school itself. In addition, many high-quality preschool television shows help the development of color and shape recognition, naming everyday objects, and elementary counting. Viewing these, therefore, can enhance your preschooler's learning skills. So there's nothing wrong with letting him watch some television, as long as you remain aware of some of the potential pitfalls of your child's viewing habits.

When it's too much

You want your child to become an active discoverer, to seek out information when he wants, and to inquire about things that arouse his curiosity. However, if he spends too much time passively watching television, he might, for instance, be less willing to search for a particular book in the library because he is so used to television shows doing all the work for him. There's also the risk that he may not watch the programs you want him to. Leave him alone in front of the television and you could return a few minutes later to find he has been viewing something aimed at an adult audience.

Every child is different and so there is no "ideal" amount of television time, although most experts would recommend that a preschooler watches no more than two hours of television in total in any one day. Some would say it should be much less, perhaps not at all.

Be prepared to use the off button, particularly if you notice signs that he's watching too much (see opposite). Of course, he will probably protest that this is unfair or that he will miss his favorite show, but keep it switched off if you feel he has had enough for today. (Hide the remote from him if necessary, until he calms down.) Think seriously about the amount of time he watches television.

Decide on the maximum amount you will allow during one day, the sorts of programs you want him to watch, and the spread of viewing time (for instance, one hour when he comes home from day care, or half an hour at lunch and half an hour in the evening before bedtime). Then stick to these limits, no matter how much your preschooler complains. He'll soon adjust to your plan.

Pester power

The attraction of commercials may be so strong for your preschooler that you hear his endless cries of "Mom! I want that!" or "Buy me that, dad!" Pester power can be very strong and draining. The problem is that commercials can transform your preschooler into a consumer addict whose sole concern is the acquisition of as many material good as he can get his hands on. It's as though he believes persuading you to buy him something he saw advertised on television is the only major goal in life worth pursuing and that everything else takes second place.

Television commercials boost your preschooler's pester power in two ways. First, there is his natural tendency to desire what he sees. Commercials present toys and games in a very favorable and imaginative way so that a young viewer's attention is grabbed instantly. You can hardly blame your child for being lured by them. At this age, he is not sophisticated enough to realize that commercials can be misleading, that they can exaggerate, and that the product may not live up to his expectations; he is completely enticed by commercials.

Second, commercials influence the other children he mixes with. So, it's no surprise when he comes home from nursery school one day asking for a new set of running shoes with a particular brand name. To you, his existing pair are perfect, but to your child they are not the ones he really wants because all his pals have a different brand after seeing them advertised on television.

Yet there is lots you can do to reduce the impact of pester power. When your child asks you for something that he saw advertised in a commercial, your initial response should be to ask him why he wants it. Although this strategy seems obvious enough, you may be tempted instead to give an automatic knee-jerk reaction—either saying "Yes" because you want your preschooler to be happy or "No" because you are tired of his endless demands.

Instead of giving such an emphatic reply one way or the other, ask your child to justify his request. Why does he want this toy? How is it different from the ones that he has already? Does he know any other child who owns this toy and who thinks it is good? This forces him to think about his demand and gives you a starting point for discussion—it also lets him see that there is more to getting a new toy than just asking you for it. Even if he is able to justify his request, try to reach a compromise. You might tell him, for instance, that he can't have the game advertised on television because you bought

ways to tell its time to switch off

You can tell if your child has been watching too much television by seeing if she:

1   Is restless and has a bored expression on her face, even though she doesn't ask you to turn the television off;

2   Has been watching for a while and complains that she has a headache and that she feels unwell;

3   Watches her favorite DVD again and again, even though there are plenty of other children's television programs available;

4   Has been put in front of the television so that you can have a break, but she constantly wanders off seeking your attention;

5   No longer enjoys playing with her toys, and complains that she'd rather watch television than play games.

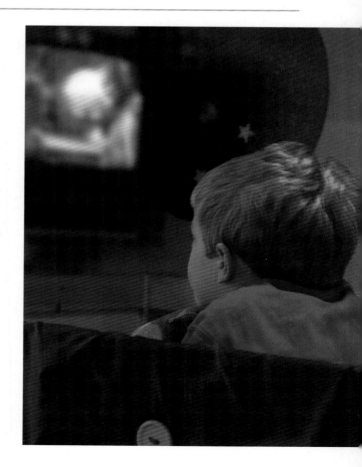

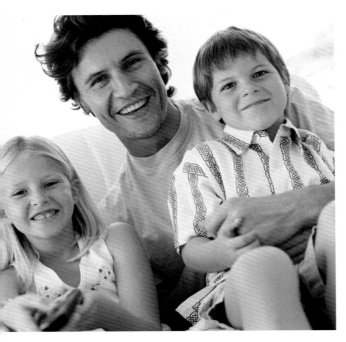

series of scenes in which people are beaten, blown up, stabbed, or come to some other horrible end, but you have also begun to notice that after watching these programs, he can be aggressive toward others, for example, punching or kicking his little brother when he doesn't do what he wants. Common sense tells you that your child has to be influenced by violence he sees on television.

The problem is that although your child knows fantasy from reality—for instance, if you directly ask him about whether or not the violence on television is false, he will probably tell you that the programs are not real—the line in his mind that separates the two can easily become blurred. When he becomes intensely involved watching a television show, fantasy and reality can start to merge. At these peaks moments of intensity, your preschooler can forget that what he is watching is only make believe.

That's why you need to monitor his viewing habits. Fortunately, he is still at an age where you can have direct control over the shows he watches. Don't be afraid to say "No" to programs that contain violence. In addition, discuss with him the content of the programs he watches, specifically mentioning the fact that what he sees on television is not real. Bear in mind that the potentially negative effect of any violent television program is diluted by his watching nonviolent ones, so make sure he doesn't spend his entire time watching bash-em-up cartoons or violence-packed adventure movies. Variety in viewing is good for him. And if you see him behaving aggressively after watching a violent show, discourage this immediately. He needs to understand that violence of any sort is not an acceptable way to deal with conflict, no matter what he sees on TV.

him a new toy last week. Listing all the recent purchases you have made for your child helps him realize that while he doesn't always get exactly what he wants, he does get some things a lot of the time.

You could also suggest to your preschooler that he should pay for part of the item he wants. True, few children that age have an allowance or pocket money they can save, but you can make her think that she is saving. For instance, you could say "Instead of buying you candy today, I'll save the money toward that toy you asked for."

Lastly, there will be times when you react to your child's pester power with a flat refusal, perhaps because you think he has got enough or because you simply can't afford another purchase. Don't feel guilty if you have to do this occasionally. Rest assured that your refusal won't cause your preschooler any psychological damage.

TV violence

No matter how hard you try, the chances are your preschooler will watch television shows or movies with a high content of aggression, and you may be horrified by his reaction to violence on the small screen. Not only does he happily watch an endless

Discussing tragic events

Unfortunately, as well as violent programs, television news can be full of images that your child will find disturbing—particularly because they are often continously replayed. This is another reason why viewing should be limited and why you should always be present when the television is on. Not only is it hard to protect your child from unpleasant news but it's important to acknowledge that your child may be affected by what he sees and hears. He'll probably have questions, which you'll need to answer in a truthful manner, though phrased to suit your child's age and stage of development. It will be important not to speculate or provide more information than is called for.

When a tragedy is played out in front of you and your child, remain calm and reassuring. Make sure you don't overreact or show anxiety or outrage and explain to your child why he is not at risk.

Accept your child's reactions. If he shows uncertainty, fear, or anxiety, explain that this is normal; don't dismiss his feelings. Continue to act as normally as possible at home. Stick to your usual routines for meals and bedtime, for example, but be alert for vulnerability. Some children, particularly those who've previously experienced a traumatic event, will become more stressed than others.

Role models on television

Another factor to consider when thinking about the impact television has on your preschooler is that he may well become attached to a character in a program, which then becomes a role model for him. Suddenly that fictional figure assumes great importance in his life. Soon your child thinks a lot about this character, talks about him, her, or it to you and to his friends, and then starts to imitate some of the character's behavior. Now that's all well and good, if the role model is a sociable, kind, sensitive character, but you won't be so happy if the role model is aggressive, bullying, and violent.

In recent years, for instance, some famous sports figures have achieved fame through the combination of their innate talents and their uncouth behavior. It is almost as though their negative actions toward others on and off the field have helped build them into role models to young viewers. The same applies to some pop singers—they also make the headlines by behaving atrociously in public.

The problem is that your preschooler may admire all the role model's qualities, both desirable and undesirable, and he may think that this is how he himself should behave. If you face this situation, explain to your child that by all means he can

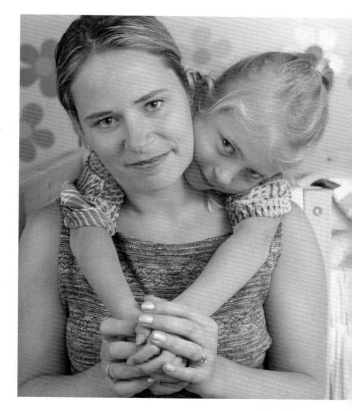

admire this individual, but add that he can like his role model while disliking some of the role model's behavior at the same time. In other words, he can exercise some critical judgement about this person or character; he doesn't have to admire and imitate everything the role model does.

Phone and computer use

We are, by nature, social animals and we love to communicate with one another. That's why you like to chat with your friends, family, and child as often as you can. And your preschooler is the same; he loves to chat with you, his pals, and carers. Verbal or written communication is key for contacting with other people but despite this social need, your child won't be very happy if he sees you spend too much time communicating with others. It's not that he unreasonably wants you all to himself all the time, it's just that he wants his fair share of your attention—and he can't get that if your ear is glued to your cell phone, your fingers are constantly texting or on the keyboard, or your eyes are fixed on your e-reader or tablet screen.

If you would agree to most of the statements in the box, below, it's highly likely your use of phones and computers is getting in the way of communication with your child and that you are spending too much time connecting with others at his expense. You might not like to admit this, but be honest with yourself.

Of course, your preschooler can whine and complain for reasons that may have nothing to do with your social communication behavior, for instance, because he is bored, irritable, or even unwell. But if you spend too much time on the phone, it's likely to lead to your preschooler grumbling and engaging in negative behavior. The fact is that he'll find a way to get your attention, one way or another, if he feels you are too busy with other people—and the easiest way for him to interrupt your calling, texting, or emailing is by misbehaving. He knows that when he creates a scene, you'll hang up or stop typing in order to try to calm him down, and he does not care if this

6 indications your child feels ignored

1   Your phone calls usually last for more than 5 minutes when you are with your preschooler.

2   You often dump your child in front of the TV so that you can send emails or texts.

3   You always answer your phone when it rings while you are playing with your preschooler.

4   Your child occasionally or often whines or misbehaves when you talk on the phone.

5   Your child tries to pull you away from your computer or phone to get your attention.

6   You keep your cell phone on even during mealtimes with your child.

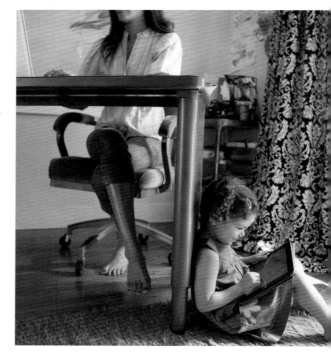

happens at home, in the supermarket, or at a friend's house. While you don't like to draw attention to yourself by behaving badly, your preschooler could not care less. He'd much rather have negative attention from you than no attention from you at all.

Play time not phone time

Changing your use of electronic devices will not be as difficult as you might imagine, as long as you formulate a plan and then determine to stick to it. The first step is to make a realistic assessment of the maximum amount of time (and the maximum number of communication events) that you would feel comfortable with during the time that you spend with your preschooler. There are no fixed guidelines for this—it comes down to knowing yourself and your child. For instance, you could decide that you won't talk, email, or text for more than five minutes at a time and that you won't do this more than four times a day. Unless you work from home, that structure would certainly give you enough time to attend to your daily social communications without disrupting the time you spend with your child. You don't need to cut yourself off from the outside world completely (that wouldn't be good for you or your child), you just need to impose some sensible limits.

In addition, make a decision not to have any of these communications at key times in the day, for example, when you and your preschooler have a snack or meal together, when you are both busy playing together, or while you are reading him a story. Even if a call, text, or email is important, it will wait for a few minutes before you respond to it.

Be open with your child about your new plan. Explain to him that from now on you'll spend more time with him and less time talking to others, so that you will have more uninterrupted time together. Use positive language so he understands you want to do this because you enjoy being with him so much. He'll feel very important and special when he hears this. However, point out that in return for you respecting him in this way, you expect him to respect you by behaving appropriately during the few times you do have make short calls

in his company. Your agreement is more likely to work if you both have a psychological investment and commitment toward it; his participation in the plan is as important as yours.

Then follow your strategy, no matter what other temptations arise. Initially, you may feel quite lost at the thought of not answering a phone call, a text message, an email, or a tweet. But be strong! Your world will continue without instantly responding to these social communications. You'll soon discover that you can call people back later and that you don't have to return electronic messages the moment they arrive.

The benefits of this plan to your relationship with your child will become immediately obvious. His complaints and misbehavior when you are on the phone will decrease very quickly. He'll no longer feel that he has to compete so hard with others for your attention. Your day will be less stressful, too. Tell your child how much happier you are now that you have more time together. And once he has gone to bed, you can chat, text, email, tweet, and surf as much as you want.

There is another long-term advantage to structuring your phone time like this. Although your preschooler is too young to use most of these methods of social communication himself (though he can probably speak confidently on your phone already), he will start to access them in the next few years. That's why it is important to set a good example now, one that he can follow when he is older. If you are able to establish rules about this before he is much older, he'll learn to respect the special times that you have together.

Your child and computers

Your child will see you use many digital screen devices in your everyday life and this learning is important for his future success in school and to enable him to see that IT tools can be used to complete tasks. But similar to television viewing, it's important to monitor your child's use of electronic devices. In January 2012, the National Association for the Education of Young Children (NAEYC) concluded that, when used appropriately, technology

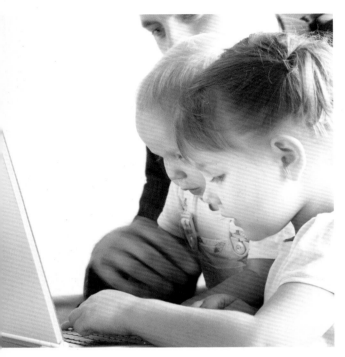

Children in nursery education are often encouraged to work toward understanding how technology is used in the world. It is relatively common for them to have a significant level of computer literacy, which means they can often turn items on and off and record, store, and retrieve data.

That being said, computers and computer games (along with televisions) should not be used in a young child's bedroom. Spending too much time on the computer (or watching television) has been linked with obesity, which can lead to heart disease and other health complications later in life, and can also interfere with a child's social skills. Playing computer games, particularly for long periods of time, has been linked with the development or exacerbation of ADHD in older children (see also page 279) and if they contain violence (as most do), it can lead to aggressive behavior later on. For more information on computer safety, see page 207.

On the plus side, young children who use computers at home are more school-ready and have greater cognitive abilities. Playing computer games can improve fine motor skills; computer game players have noticeably better hand-to-eye coordination than nonplayers. Children who play interactive computer games develop better skills with handling objects—throwing, pushing, and lifting them.

and interactive media are effective tools to support learning and development but limitations on use are important. They recommend keeping track of current screen-time recommendations from public health organizations for preschoolers when setting appropriate limits on technology and media use. Screen-time estimates should include how much time spent in front of a screen of any kind at day care or nursery school, at home, and elsewhere. What kind of media the child is exposed to needs to be considered, and if it is in a group or solitary setting. They further state that effective uses of technology and media are active, hands-on, engaging, and empowering; give the child control; help children progress in skills development at their own rates; and can be one of many options to support learning. Preschool children should be allowed to freely explore touch screens loaded with a variety of developmentally appropriate interactive media experiences that support learning and digital literacy, are well designed, and enhance feelings of success. However, the NAEYC further concludes that the child should be focused on the activity or exploration and not on the technology itself.

Make it a shared experience

Becoming involved with your child's computer use, interacting with him while he uses one, can help him achieve better language and number skills, and improve problem solving, learning and memory than if he is left on his own. Judiciously chosen computer programs use can involve communication, particularly if you ask your child to show you how to do something or if the program involves taking turns or "working" together.

Choose programs or apps that allow multiple correct answers, even if one is better than the others. Such programs and apps will extend his thinking and problem-solving skills while those designed to elicit only one correct answer can limit learning. Do not allow your child access to violent games.

Encouraging your child's independence

Your preschooler has two conflicting developmental trends. On the one hand, he needs to become independent, to manage more by himself without having to rely on your help. At times he seems very determined to be self-reliant. On the other hand, he needs you more than ever, and the moment something goes wrong, he rushes to your side for comfort and reassurance. That's why, for example, he might insist on proving that he can fit all the pieces of the jigsaw together by himself, telling you emphatically that he doesn't need your help. Then the next minute he may howl hysterically and run over to you for a reassuring cuddle, because it is much too difficult for him.

The preschool stage is typified by this dual behavior, namely, your child's desire to become more independent and, at the same time, his reliance on you to make him feel secure when he fails to achieve his self-imposed target. You have to help him achieve a balance.

Parenting styles and their effects

Parents differ in their attitude toward their child's independence. "Autocratic" parents give their child no freedom to express his own ideas and feelings and don't offer any explanation for household rules.

"Democratic" parents explain rules to their child but also listen to his point of view (while still retaining the right to have the final say).

"Permissive" parents give their child total freedom to do whatever he pleases irrespective of the wishes of others.

Typically, a child of democratic parents tends to be more independent than a child of either autocratic or permissive parents. Democratic parenting at home encourages a child's independence for a number of reasons. First, he's given lots of opportunities to try out his own ideas,

with the knowledge that he is safely protected by adults. Second, his self-confidence is increased because he feels cared for, not controlled, and third, democratic parents are themselves usually independently minded and so the child models himself on their attitude.

Bear in mind that increasing independence brings your preschooler many benefits. For example, he enjoys life more. Being able to do things for himself gives him choices. He can make simple decisions each day on his own, for example, to play with his building blocks instead of his model farm, because he can access these items independently. The freedom to make minor choices of this sort increases his pleasure in everyday life. Then there's the positive impact on his confidence—there's nothing like achieving a goal

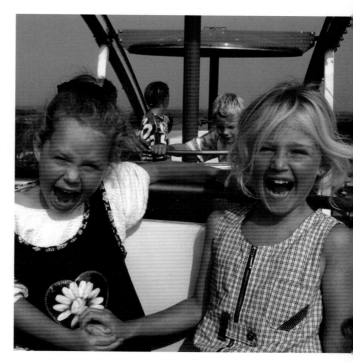

independently to boost a child's belief in his own abilities. He will feel good about himself knowing that he did it on his own.

Independence also helps your child's learning. In many instances, he learns more effectively by doing things for himself than with your help. For example, once he eventually completes a jigsaw puzzle on his own, he'll still remember the solution weeks later.

Safety concerns

When he was a baby and totally dependent on you, you may have longed for the day when your child could do things for himself, and stand on his own two feet without needing you constantly. You may have imagined the freedom his independence would gbring you. But now this moment has arrived, you may be suddenly become afraid for your child.

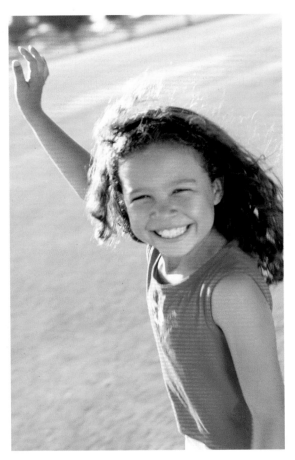

One the main reason why parents are anxious about encouraging their preschooler's independence is concerns about safety. After all, his sense of danger is not fully developed. He still may do all the sorts of things he's not supposed to, like sticking his fingers into electric sockets, spilling cups of hot water, or running out into the road when there is traffic. Your child has to learn to deal with these hazards independently, so that he can look after himself when you are not with him, but that takes time. Right now, you probably place your concern for his safety before your desire for his independence.

Naturally, you want your child to be safe and well, and to avoid upset and injury if at all possible. Sheltering him from life's knocks is a vital part of your job as a parent, and is one of the many ways you express your love for your child. But the line between reasonable safety precautions and over-protectiveness can become blurred. Bear in mind that your preschooler needs freedom to extend his skills, so that he learns how to manage more by himself. That simply cannot happen if you remove all possibility of risk at the very age he needs to interact more indepedently with his surroundings.

However, you do need to be very careful about allowing your preschooler to explore on his own, no matter how independent you want him to be. You should always try to be in a position to keep an eye on him so that you can steer him away from everyday dangers. That doesn't mean you should be overprotective, but it does mean you need to show sensible caution so that he remains safe and well.

Safety should always come first. That being said, your child is unlikely to thank you for thwarting his independence in this way, even though you are doing so in his best interests. Instead, he is likely to be annoyed with you because he can't do what he wants. So explain your reasoning to him. He'll understand eventually.

Helping your child

When it comes to boosting your preschooler's self-reliance, work together with him and keep it fun. Gaining independence requires your child to take a leap in the dark, to risk trying to achieve something that he can't already do. He may be afraid of failure, or that he won't be as capable as his friends or siblings, so give your preschooler lots of reassurance that he can succeed. If he thinks you take a genuine interest in him, his motivation to become independent will be higher. And remind him of the benefits. Spell these out to him clearly. For instance, "If you put your toys away neatly, then you'll be able to find them more easily" or "If you help to set the table, you'll be making mommy's life easier." Your child understands practical examples like these, which adds further incentive for him.

It's also important not to expect too much too soon. Encourage small steps, a few at a time, to achieving greater independence. This approach enables you to pull in the reins if he doesn't seem able to cope. What may seem a simple and obvious task to you (for example, pulling on his sweater) may seem monumental to a poorly coordinated preschooler. He needs time to master each part of the task properly before he can move onto the next one.

Have very clear and specific targets. For instance, "I want you to put this sweater on by yourself" is clearer than simply telling him "I want you to try getting dressed on your own." Tell your child what you expect him to achieve. Then break it down into lots of little stages. For instance, first he gets the sweater out the drawer; then he sets it flat on the bed; then he puts in one arm; then he puts in the other, and so on. And the rate each child learns this depends upon the individual; if you've known another child who found it easy to self-dress early, it doesn't mean your child will reach that stage at the same time. But do praise your child's successes because the more often he masters each small step on his journey to self-reliance, the more enthusiasm he will have for further progress. Reassure him when he's upset by failure and encourage him to try again until he masters the challenge. Eventually, he will.

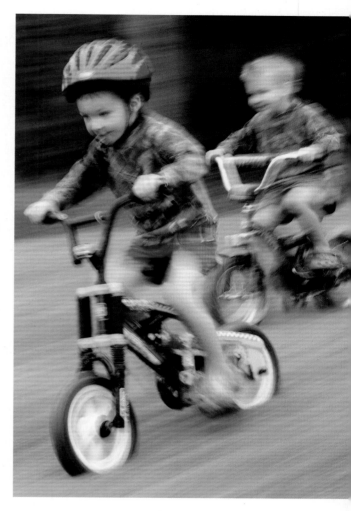

If you are not sure what to expect of your child in terms of independence at each age and stage, have a chat with other parents about what they have experienced or expect of their children; you don't have to follow what they permit exactly but you may find what they say helpful and interesting. You'll also find the information in chapter 3, Developmental changes, helpful.

Getting your child ready for nursery school

Starting nursery school is such a big step for your preschooler. He'll have so many new and exciting play opportunities and so many new children to be friendly with. On the other hand, he might be anxious about meeting so many new children and adults all at once. You can help him adjust to this next interesting phase of his life (which will also be a time of mixed emotions for you). While you will be delighted to have time and freedom for yourself when he is at nursery school, you'll miss him and you'll probably worry about him, too.

Children are afraid of the unknown. In the same way that you like to know what lies ahead of you, so does your preschooler. You can avoid much of the anxiety that is associated with starting nursery school by talking to him about it before he attends regularly. A few weeks before the starting date, tell your child that he will soon be going there. Explain that nursery school is exciting and good fun, and describe some of the activities he'll experience. Encourage him to ask you any questions he has about it. In addition, take your child to visit the school beforehand. Walk around the building, inside and out, including the washrooms. Young children are particularly sensitive about toilets and may be anxious in case they are too large or too dirty. He'll be reassured to discover that they are easily accessible and clean. Likewise, show him the cafeteria or eating area. This increases his sense of security and boosts his confidence about attending there.

Getting to know the staff before the first day also helps; most preschools are happy to let prospective pupils have a tour around the premises. Your child will be less anxious after he has met the adults who will care for him and the other children. Even if he just talks to them for a few minutes, it will be enough to make him feel at ease. In addition, he may already know some children who attend that

IS YOUR CHILD READY FOR SCHOOL?

- Is she comfortable being away from you for an entire day?
- Does she have the ability to express ideas and feelings to adults other than you?
- Can she accept minor disappointments or limits without tears?
- Can she listen to and follow directions?
- Is she able to work independently without constant adult supervision?
- Can she find ways to resolve conflicts and solve problems?
- Can she make simple decisions given a few choices of play activities?

particular nursery school or who will start attending at the same time as him. If so, arrange for your child to play with some of them in the weeks before starting nursery school so that he begins that all-important next stage with some strong social connections. Steps like these familiarize your child with the situation, and reduce his potential anxiety.

Your preschooler looks to you for guidance, and if you appear sad about the thought of him starting nursery school, he'll soon feel miserable about it too. Adopt a positive attitude toward this next exciting stage in his life. First-day tears are quite common, so don't be upset if he cries when he suddenly realizes you really are going to leave him there. (Many nursey schools ask the parents to stay for the first day, but not after that.) Tell your child you will be back later to pick him up and take him home. He will settle down very quickly after you leave.

Readiness for starting school

When it comes to starting school, the same suggestions apply about letting your child become familiar with the school building, pupils, and adults there through visiting before he starts. The advanced preparation that you provided for him when he started nursery school are required again but you can develop his readiness for school in other ways, too. There are key personal and social skills that will enable him have a successful start. Most importantly, he should have a positive attitude.

Talk enthusiastically about school in front of your child, mention specific features about school, which you know he will like, and tell him the things you enjoyed when you started school. Never use school as a threat, or imply that the teachers there are extremely strict. Suggest that he plays "school" with his friends while still in nursery school, and take him with you when you buy his clothing, book bag,

and supplies. If you have older children, have a quiet chat with them to make sure they don't fill his head with the type of horror stories about school that older siblings love to tell a little brother.

Develop your child's self-confidence by reassuring him that he is capable and competent enough to cope with all the activities in elementary school. Point out his strengths (for instance, that he is friendly, that he already knows colors and shapes), and explain that this means he will manage all the activities there. Discourage him from focusing on the things he's not good at. Maintain realistic expectations or he will feel too much pressure to achieve beyond his abilities.

Listening to his teacher and to his classmates is essential, so improve his listening skills while he's still at nursery school. Suggest to your child that he looks at you directly when you ask him a question or give him an instruction; making eye contact

self-help skills needed for school

1   **Your preschooler should be toilet-trained** and be able to go to the bathroom by herself including managing her clothes and washing her hands afterward.

2   **She should know how to sit comfortably at a dinner table,** how to use cutlery properly, and how to eat tidily without making a mess.

3   **She should also be able to take her own coat on and off,** and know how to hang it on a coat-hook.

4   **She needs to be able to cope with temporary separations from you.** If she attends nursery school, she's used to separating from you and that shouldn't be a challenge for her but if she hasn't gone to playgroup or day care, familiarize her with temporary separations, for example, leaving her with one of your friends for an hour.

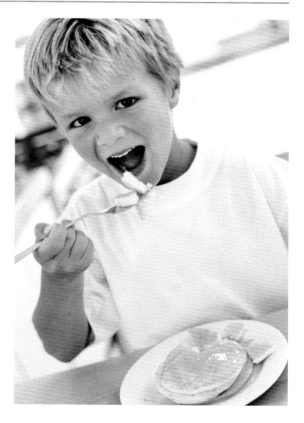

results in more accurate listening. You can also play listening games with him, for instance, clap out a simple rhythm and ask him to copy it. Read short stories to him and tell him to look at the pages while listening; ask him questions about the story when you have finished. Play "Simon says", starting off with an easy command ("Simon says stroke your chin") then moving to a more complex request ("Simon says put your hand on your head and jump up and down").

Curiosity is one of the main driving forces behind your child's motivation to learn in school so do what you can during this stage to foster his inquisitiveness. Always treat his questions seriously and answer them in a way that he understands, without giving too much information that bores him. Once you have provided him with a satisfactory answer, ask him to explain it back to you. Tell your child that in school he will have to wait his turn to ask a question and that he should not shout to get the teacher's attention.

You could also suggest that when possible he should try to find an answer by himself, and only ask for help if he can't resolve the matter on his own.

Since most learning in school takes place in groups, your child will need to be able to cooperate with his peers in the classroom. Practice this with him at home. Join in with your child in activities that you can work on together, showing him how to work with others. Give him chores that he can only complete by cooperating with someone else.

To give him experience of what life in the classroom will be like, involve him in some educational activities that you know he can complete on his own, for example, matching colors. Seat him at a table while he tackles these challenges so that he gets used to working at a desk. There are plenty of useful preliteracy activities that will boost his readiness for reading and writing, for example, listening rhymes, memory games, talking about stories together, recalling sequences, word-matching games, drawing and coloring-in, doing connect-the-dot patterns, tracing over shapes and letters, and maze puzzles. You can boost his readiness for numeracy by playing dice games, discussing time sequences, teaching him number recognition, playing counting games, teaching him about the different coins, and reciting number rhymes to him.

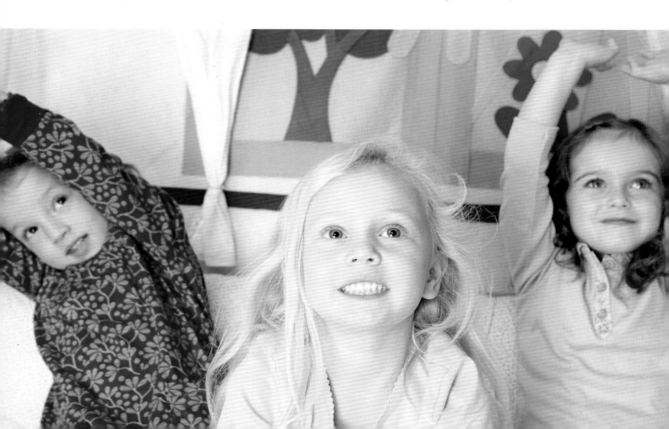

Your child doesn't want to go to school

Your child will thoroughly enjoy attending elementary school because there's so much to do every day, so many exciting learning experiences, and so many friendship opportunities. Yet starting school doesn't always go according plan—you may find that even though he rarely complained about nursery school, he now occasionally refuses to go to school. That is normal; many children would rather stay in a warm bed than get up for school on a cold winter's morning. But if his plea, "I don't want to go to school" becomes regular, you need to take it seriously.

Uncovering the reason

Make sure he is healthy. Your child may tell you he doesn't want to go to school because he has a stomache ache even though he genuinely feels fine, but on the other hand, his stomach ache could be real. In most instances, a day or two in bed is enough to ensure speedy recovery from a minor childhood illness. Should the symptoms persist, take your child to your healthcare provider for a full medical examination. If no underlying physical cause is identified, consider the possibility that his discomfort about attending school is a psychological reaction to something that makes him unhappy. You'd be amazed at some of the reasons why a young child could be unhappy in school, ranging from having had an argument with his best friend to fear of using the school washroom.

It could be that he finds the work too hard. Some children—more than you probably think—have problems with learning, which means they need extra attention from the teacher. In most instances, though, that extra temporary classroom help will be sufficient to enable your child to progress to the next stage in the curriculum. (However, your child might complain that the work in class is too hard just because he finds it challenging, not because it is beyond him. A good teacher should provide educational activities that are sufficiently demanding to interest a child and yet is not so demanding that he gives up too quickly. If your child does complain about this, boost his confidence by reminding him he is just as capable as any other child in his class and give him extra help at home.)

Should a learning problem last more than a couple of weeks speak to his teacher. Don't wait until your child is in tears about his class performance. Explain to the teacher precisely where you think the problem lies (for instance, with reading, addition, writing), and ask for his or her opinion on this. Be prepared to listen to what he or she tells you. Many apparent learning difficulties in the first year at school turn out to be temporary despite the initial concern.

Problems at home can be another factor that cause your child's refusal to attend school. If he feels insecure about his home life, then he may unconsciously be afraid to leave home in case something happens while he is away. Maybe he's worried because you or your partner work away from home or you argue a lot in front of him, or someone in the family is seriously ill or a close relative has died recently, or he has a new baby brother or sister at home. If you think your child is concerned about anything at home, tell him that he has nothing to worry about and that everything will be fine while he's at school.

Sometimes having an older sibling at the same school can create difficulties. Knowing that his older brother, for instance, is in the same building and uses the same playground usually makes a young pupil feel safe and secure. But it can also mean that he is judged by his sibling's previous performance and behavior. If, for example, his brother is very clever and makes excellent academic achievements, then his performance may be compared to his brother's by the teachers, and possibly by your relatives and friends. That's unfair. Comparisons with an older sibling serves no positive purpose. So make a specific effort to avoid such unproductive comparisons, and speak to the teacher if you discover comparisons of this kind are being made at school.

Then there's the relationship your child has with his teacher to consider. That has a crucial influence on his enjoyment, progress, and attainments in school. A positive teacher-pupil relationship encourages your child's positive attitude to learning, relationships, and behavior. You are right, therefore, to be concerned if your child says "I don't want to go to school because I hate my teacher." Of course, he might say that just because the work is too demanding, or because the teacher won't let him sit with his friend all the time. He might even complain to you about his teacher because he has been misbehaving in class and his teacher has threatened to contact you about this—your child makes a preemptive strike by complaining about his teacher before the teacher has a chance to do the same about him.

However, on rare occasions, there can be clash of personalities between a teacher and a pupil.

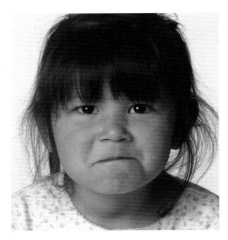

Unfortunately, not every single teacher likes every single pupil or vice versa. It is possible that your child's teacher has a preference for, say, quiet children and your child is outgoing, or for independent pupils and your child frequently asks for help.

That's why it is important to talk to your child about his classroom experiences. All the time reassure him that the problem will be resolved and that he'll soon get to like his teacher. If you think his dislike of the teacher is genuine, you'll probably need to speak to the teacher about this. Use tact and diplomacy. Don't tell the teacher exactly what your child said about him or her. Instead, explain that your child seems unhappy and troubled in school and that you want to help him become more settled. Seek the teacher's view. A calm discussion like this can shed a great deal of light on the problem. The teacher might reveal information that you were totally unaware of. Whatever emerges from your discussion together, your child can only benefit by having his parents and teacher being aware of his distress. Certainly, the teacher will be more sensitive toward him from then on and you'll feel happier knowing that he or she is aware of the difficulty, which in turn will probably put your child's mind at ease as well.

In some instances, the cause of a child's refusal to go to school isn't obvious and he may not be able to give you an immediate explanation a to why it is. Yet you have to do your best to find out what's troubling him anyway. So ask him directly if something is upsetting him. Even if he can't think of anything specific that he dislikes about school, talk to him about the key areas of his school life including his classmates, school work, playground activities, school meals, the washrooms, and his teacher. The answer to his reluctance to attend school lies in there somewhere, and your challenge is to find it. Avoid "closed" questions (that can only have a "yes" or "no" response) such as "Are you unhappy in school?" or "Do you like your teacher?" Children this age are reluctant to say anything that might upset their parents and so yours will probably give you a monosyllabic answer that he thinks you want to hear. Instead ask "open" questions (that can be answered in an infinite number of ways), such as "How are you getting on with your teacher at the moment?" or "Which of your friends do you play with in school each day?" Encourage your child to give reasonably long replies.

When you think about it, you may realize that there has been a change in his behavior recently, for instance, he no longer talks about a particular friend any more, or he makes only negative comments about his teacher. This can point you to the source of trouble. You should certainly talk to his teacher because he or she is the best source of information regarding his progress in school. Make a special appointment to speak to the teacher, explain your concerns, and listen to his or her observations. This also makes the teacher aware of your child's unhappiness, something he or she may not have been aware of. Sometimes, a problem like this can be resolved quite easily. For instance, a change to another group within the class, or additional help from the teacher for a few days, may be all that is needed to make your child feel more settled. If there is an obvious practical solution like this, try to have this implemented as soon as you can.

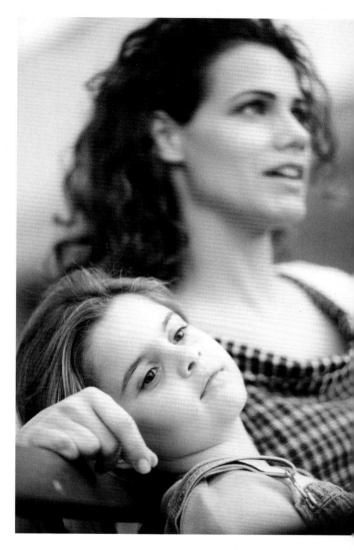

Ensure attendance

However, no matter the cause of your child's reluctance to attend school, or how long it takes you to resolve it, you must make sure he goes to school regularly anyway. Take him each day even if he is tearful and protests along the way, all the while calming him and telling him that everything will be fine. Almost certainly, he will stop crying and settle down once he enters his classroom, so you can leave him there without worrying that he'll cry all day.

It's very important that your child understands school attendance is not negotiable—explain clearly to your child that you'll do everything you can to make him happy in school, and to solve any

problem he has there, but that he must go to class every day while you do this. The longer he is absent from school, the harder it will be for him to return to a pattern of regular attendance.

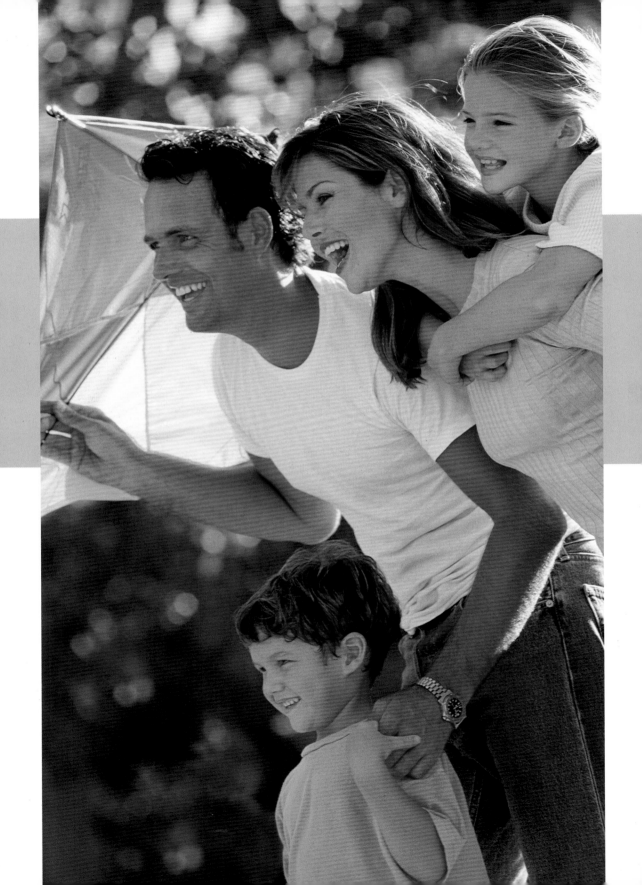

CHAPTER 5
FAMILY MATTERS

Having a secure family life is vital for preschoolers. Mom's input has been taken for granted for years but now more dads are becoming the stay-at-home parent. Help may also be on hand from grandparents and if nurtured, the extended family. Protecting your child from unnecessary worries is vital when there are financial worries, a new baby is expected, you anticipate moving to a new house, or illness, separation, or a death occurs. And what's a parent to do if adopting a preschooler or when living with a child with special needs?

When dad is the caregiver

Our generation of families is more flexible than any previous, and more fathers than ever before are taking responsibility as primary caregiver for their preschool children. Sometimes this happens for unavoidable reasons (for instance, when dad is laid off from his job or is otherwise unable to find steady employment) or for financial reasons (for instance, if mom's income is higher than dad's). But more often than not, dad becomes the main caregiver through conscious choice; he wants to be the principal parent raising his child during her preschool years.

Yet this arrangement, which enables dad to become the main caregiver, is not simply a case of both parents switching roles, with family life going on exactly as it would if the parental roles were reversed. When the father is main caregiver during the preschool years, this has implications for everyone in the family and these should be thought through carefully. The more both parents are aware of the potential challenges in this arrangement, the more effective it will become. Even in families where both parents are the same gender, the decision about which one becomes the main caregiver has an impact on everyone involved.

Effect on your preschooler

No matter how strong the relationship is between a mother and her child, a preschooler usually has a special connection with his or her father. Psychologists studying the relationships between parents and their children have found significant differences between the father-child relationship and the mother-child one and, when dad is the main caregiver, these differences will influence your child's upbringing on a day-to-day basis. For example, although both parents like to play with their child as much as they can, dad is more likely to encourage boys and girls to take part in rough-and-tumble play, whereas mom is more likely to prefer sedate activities. Moms tend to play in a way that encourages a child's sensitivity, is nurturing, and

brings the two of them in close physical contact; dads, on the other hand, tend to favor play and activities that are intellectually challenging for their children.

Moms and dads often have a different attitude toward their child's independence. Although both parents usually want their child to become self-reliant so that she can mix confidently with other children her own age, more mothers than fathers worry about leaving their child when she starts nursery school, and more mothers than fathers expect their child to cry in that situation.

When dad is the main caregiver, your child will talk more with him and although your preschooler still chatters away to mom, telling her lots of personal things—perhaps more than to dad—being able to talk to dad as well means your child has someone else to listen to and be advised by. In addition, your preschooler will typically be less challenging behaviorally with her father than with her mother. Most preschoolers are less likely to push limits laid down by dad than by mom, and are probably more willing to accept discipline and rules from him.

The more time a preschooler spends with her father, the more she learns about relationships from him. The relationship both boys and girls have with their father often acts as the standard by which they judge the quality of relationships they will have with other male figures later on in life.

Effect on dad

The task of providing full-time care for a preschooler is demanding for any parent, mother or father, and the practical demands are the same irrespective of the main caregiver's gender. However, given that the majority of stay-at-home parents are women, despite changes in social and familial attitudes and opportunities, it is reasonable to assume the stay-at-home father has particular hurdles to get over during the preschool years. By far the major challenge is making child-care decisions on a daily basis. Even if mom is heavily involved in child-care issues despite her full-time employment, dad is the one that has to deal with everything as it arises from one moment to the next. That's why it's important for the stay-at-home father to have confidence in his own parenting skills, yet still be able to discuss and share child-care decisions as much as possible with his partner. Dad shouldn't assume all decisions are his sole remit, much in the same way as a stay-at-home mother wouldn't assume all the decisions were hers.

Another major challenge is the daily grind of coping with child-care and domestic chores. This can wear down the enthusiasm of the most determined stay-at-home father, particularly if previously mom was the one with responsibility for managing household chores—and the chances are, this burden may be shared more with the working parent than if mom was the one who stayed at home. So for someone who might have been accustomed to independence as a working man, the transformation into the main caregiver is likely to be daunting. On the plus side, a stay-at home father often attracts empathy, admiration, and plenty of offers of support and that all helps. On the negative side, however, he can also be on the receiving end of prejudice from those who consider that traditional parenting roles are best for raising children.

Then there is the self-doubt that often arises. A father who is the main caregiver is bound to have moments of uncertainty about his skills as a parent. The thought that he has the main responsibility for raising his preschooler can shake the foundations of his self-belief. Encouragement and praise from his partner can help boost dad's confidence. In reality, however, most dads actually do a very good job as the main caregiver.

Effect on mom

Even when it's decided that dad assumes the role of main caregiver after full discussion between both parents, and even when both are in total agreement with that decision, the chances are that mom will have at least a few twinges of guilt and regret—and

for many mothers working full-time, these feelings are much, much stronger. That doesn't mean a woman distrusts her partner's ability to raise their preschooler, nor does it mean she thinks her child will suffer psychologically in that home situation. It's just that guilt and regret may be an instinctive reaction, particularly if mom would rather be the stay-at-home parent and has traded roles simply for practical or economic reasons.

One of the common fears a mother experiences when leaving her child in dad's care during the day

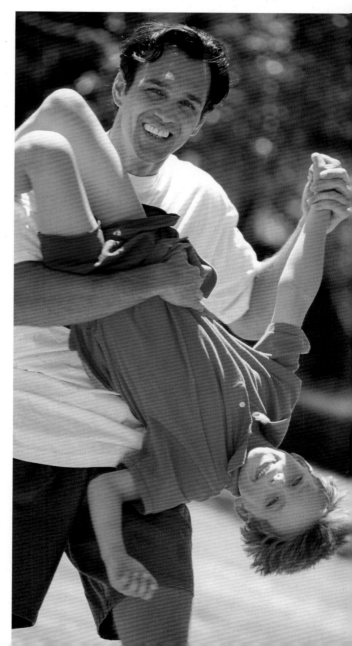

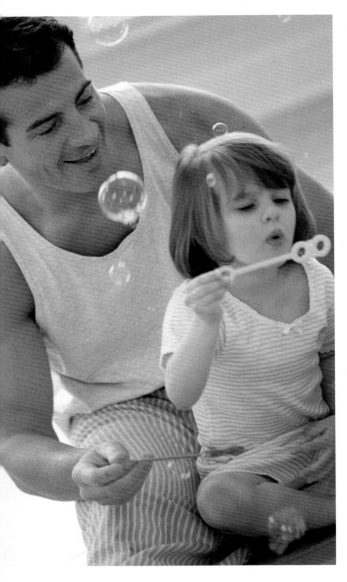

approach, and values those precious moments together with her child before and after the working day, the emotional attachment between them will remain strong. Of course, time management becomes extremely important. When dad is the main caregiver, mom needs to manage her nonworking time effectively so that she spends as much free time in the company of her child as possible. Instead of worrying about how much time they are apart, she should enjoy the times they spend together, whether talking, playing, or eating.

Every parent wants to be there for all the important "firsts" in her preschooler's life, whether it's when she first names colors accurately, rides a bicycle with training wheels, or reaches the top of the climbing frame in the adventure playground. When these "firsts" are missed, it is quite common to feel guilt. But a working mom shouldn't beat herself up about it. Aside from the fact that she'll eventually see her child do what she missed seeing the first time around, what matters most to a preschooler is that she is loved, valued, and cared for by her parents. She won't mind that her mother missed a "first," as long as mom shows excitement and interest later on when she hears about it.

A bright future

There is no reason to assume that your preschooler will lose out psychologically in any way whatsoever by her father taking on the job of main caregiver. In fact, she'll probably benefit in many of the ways already discussed. Nor will her relationship with her mother automatically suffer. Have confidence in both yourself and your partner as parents. There is ample evidence from research and from everyday life that confirms preschoolers in this situation thrive normally.

is that the bond between her and her preschooler will weaken—but that is unlikely to happen. What matters is not the amount of time a mother and her child spend together but the quality of their relationship with each other. A preschooler who spends all day with a distracted mother who would much rather resume her career than be a stay-at-home mom, for instance, is less likely to bond than a child who spends only a few minutes at the start and the end of each day with her loving, attentive, caring mother. If a working mother has a positive

Making the most of grandparents

If you are fortunate to have a close, warm, loving relationship with your preschooler's grandparents, you'll already be aware of the potential benefits this special attachment can bring your child. Every loving bond in your child's life adds something distinctive, and makes its own unique contribution to her development. So a strong grandchild–grandparent connection is good for your child.

However, grandparents can give added value to you as well. For example, they can act as trustworthy, reliable, and willing childcarers. You don't need to check out their credentials or ask for references before leaving your preschooler with them. They raised you or your partner and you have confidence in their ability to look after your child carefully and sensibly when required. This can be especially useful when you need to arrange childcare at very short notice. Of course, you can't expect your child's grandparents to be on call 24/7—they have their own lives, schedules, and possibly work commitments, so they may not be as available to support you with childcare arrangements as you might like. But your negotiating skills and the way you present your requests can make a difference. If grandparents are made to feel that the childcare they provide is special, they are more likely to help you when asked. On the other hand, if they think that they are your second choice or that you take their availability for granted, the chances are they won't be so responsive. A tactful and sensitive request such as "We'd love you to look after ... on Monday because she has such a good time with you" is better than saying "We need you to look after ... on Monday because we can't get anybody else."

Grandparents can also be a great source of advice. The reassuring comments from a grandparent who has raised several children of his or her own into adulthood can be very comforting for a parent who lacks self-confidence. Don't be afraid to seek such guidance. To approach your child's grandparents in this way is certainly not a sign of weakness. In fact, many people would argue that it's a smart parent who recognizes his or her own weaknesses and then tries to do something about them.

Yet bringing grandparents on board the parenting team does need careful management. On the one hand you want advice and support, but on the other hand, you may end up feeling disempowered. Always keep in mind that grandparents want the best for you and your preschooler, and they also want to maintain a positive relationship with you. Tell yourself that they are not deliberately trying to undermine you, but that they are only trying to help.

That being said, unless you give the grandparents clear guidelines, they may spontaneously give you as much help as they think you need, so it's best to keep your requests specific in order to reduce ambiguity. For instance, if you tell grandparents "I can't cope. I need your help," this suggests you are struggling on all fronts, so don't be surprised if they respond by trying to do everything for you. This is a normal, loving reaction. It's far better if you say something like "Can you take ... to the park this afternoon? I don't think I'll get home in time." It's a question of balance. As long as you don't become overdependent on your child's grandparents, you'll maintain confidence in your own parenting skills.

Another way grandparents give added value is that they typically think their grandchildren are perfect. It is often said that parents "love" their children but that grandparents are "in love" with their grandchildren. In other words, they may be so totally infatuated that they can't see anything wrong in anything the children do. That means grandparents are likely to tolerate more from your children than you do, and will probably be very willing to help out when you feel stressed. Bear in mind, though, that this could result in your preschooler receiving mixed messages about discipline. She'll be very quick to pick up on differences between carers when it comes to rules and limits and you may even hear her indignantly announce "But grandma lets me do that when she looks after me." Tackle such assertions immediately and directly. Make it clear to your preschooler that when she is with you, you set the standards for her behavior, no matter what she is allowed to do when she is with grandparents. And have a gentle word with the grandparents, too. If you express your concerns in a caring child-centered way ("I'm worried that she is getting confused over the mixed messages she gets about discipline") and not in a critical grandparent-centered way ("I'm worried that you are far too soft with her"), the chances are they will treat your worry seriously. Put all of these ingredients together and you will have a recipe for grandparents who have the potential to provide a rich source of support, advice, and practical help. The challenge for you is to make the most of them.

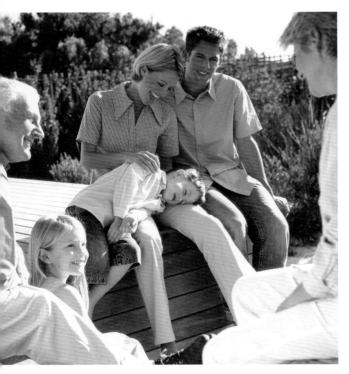

Grandparents as carers

Consider childcare options for your preschooler very thoroughly before even mentioning this to your child's grandparents. You may decide that although the grandparents are available and could provide cost-effective (free) childcare, you would prefer your preschooler to have a more stimulating experience during the day while you are at work. If so, you'll find it easier to explain this to the grandparents if you haven't already told them that you were considering whether or not to ask their help with childcare. They won't be comfortable thinking that they were considered then rejected!

Some preschoolers are fortunate enough to have two sets of loving grandparents who are eager to provide some, or all, day care when one or both of you are at work. That could be wonderful for you too, because you know your child is going to be well looked after during the day. If both sets of grand-parents can offer excellent care, you truly are spoiled for choice!

Think carefully about each offer, though, and consider how realistic it is for each set or individual to look after your child. Bear in mind this is a very demanding task, physically and emotionally. If a grandparent has health problems, or is particularly frail, then caring for your preschooler may be too much for him or her. There are other practicalities too. Either you will have to take your child to and from her grandparents every day, or the grandparents will have to do the daily traveling. Consider what would be involved with each set.

The ideal option would be to split the childcare responsibility so that one set of grandparents cares for your preschooler two days a week and the other set three days; they can trade days on alternate weeks. That would keep everyone happy. But if childcare can't be split equally this way, explain the reasons for your optimal choice, and make it clear that it is for practical or health reasons only, not because you think one set of grandparents will provide better care for your child than the other (even if you do think that). Make sure that the grandparents who aren't picked as the ones to provide childcare are given lots of opportunity to see their grandchild on weekends.

This offer should go a long way to help ease any potential feelings of rejection.

Favoritism

It's very common for grandparents to form an especially strong emotional connection with their first grandchild. And when the next grandchild comes along (whether yours or your sibling's child), they will form a strong psychological bond with him too. But in some instances, the oldest grandchild becomes the grandparents' favorite; they have known her longer, think she's cute and smart, and she does more than her younger siblings. "Playing favorites," however, is always divisive. Young children are quick to pick up on this, and no grandchild likes to think grandma prefers a sibling over her.

To head off a potential crisis, tell the grandparents how much you and your siblings appreciate their input with and affection for their grandchildren. Then tell them that you think perhaps they prefer the oldest, that you understand why they feel this way (because they are so close with her and because she is so bright and beautiful), but that you worry this could have a negative effect on the younger ones. Explain that no child wants her grandparents to prefer one grandchild over all the others and that ultimately, this leads to low self-esteem and a sense of rejection. All their grandchildren deserve their love. Be ready for them to try to convince you that you are wrong, that they don't have a favorite, and even if they did, the grandchildren wouldn't be aware of it. Point out again that favoritism is always unfair on children, and is always destructive. Whether or not the grandparents agree with you—and expect them to be slightly upset by your observations— suggest that they need to take the matter of favoritism very seriously.

You can't make your child's grandparents feel differently; even if they admit to favoritism, they probably won't be able to change their emotions. Yet they can change how they act on their feelings. In other words, just because they have a favorite doesn't mean that they have to behave as if they have a favorite. Suggest, for example, that they spend the same amount on birthday presents for each of their grandchildren, that they take the same interest in all of them, that they praise all of their achievements, and that they have loving physical contact with each one. In addition, suggest they make a special point of spending time with each child alone every visit, if possible, even if only for a few minutes. Those practical steps will encourage each grandchild to feel that she is special to her grandparents.

Positive approach

It's up to you to keep the relationship with your child's grandparents positive. True, some grand-parents are very forceful, totally convinced that they know best and may be overzealous in offering their opinions. But most are reasonable, loving relatives with the best interests of their children and grandchildren at heart.

Bear in mind that grandparents, like everyone else, like a pat on the back every now and again. They like their help to be recognized and to feel appreciated. The best way, of course, is to express your gratitude verbally. For instance, you might say "Thanks for helping me get ... to sleep this afternoon; I feel more confident about managing on my own with her tomorrow."

If you asked a grandparent for advice, give some feedback; if grandparents know that you are coping better with the situation now, they are less likely to get involved subsequently. Therefore giving positive feedback avoids the potential for them to interfere and undermine you.

Make sure, too, that your preschooler understands that you value her grandparents. If, for example, she hears you groan or take a sharp intake of breath when they arrive at your home, she'll start to adopt those negative attitudes as well. Keep all criticisms of her grandparents—and any disagreements with them—well away from your young child. Make her grandparents feel welcome in your house and let her see that you value them. In most instances, that special bond with grandparents adds something uniquely wonderful to a young child's life and to your life as well; as such, it should be welcomed and encouraged where possible. That's the best way to get the most out of grandparents.

Involving your extended family

You may have heard from your parents or grandparents how, when they were young, everyone (that is, grandparents, parents, aunts, uncles, cousins, nephews, nieces, and grandchildren) usually lived in close proximity to one another, and it was common for many family members to live in the same city, even on the same street. That network brought huge potential benefits, such as having a host of helping hands for parents to draw on for practical support and childcare advice. Parents never needed to feel they were alone when it came to managing their children. Grandparents in particular were viewed as having the wisdom derived from raising children from birth to adulthood and consequently were frequently called on for ideas and suggestions, which was made easier by the fact that they lived nearby. Frequent contact with so many adults gave children a set of roles models to respect, admire, and learn from.

Of course, this close-knit extended family had its potential downside too. With so many people dropping in every hour of the day, parents hardly had a chance for any privacy. Rarely were they alone with their child for any length of time. The house always had to be kept clean and tidy to avoid criticism from uninvited visitors. Then there was the endless—often unsolicited—advice. Everyone had an opinion and they didn't need any encouragement to share their thoughts about child rearing with the parents. And if there were disagreements in the extended family, there was no way they could be ignored or allowed to simmer until everyone calmed down—disputes had to be dealt with as they arose because people saw so much of one another. However, most people then agreed the benefits of a warm, loving extended family outweighed the potential disadvantages.

But that traditional model of the extended family is rarely found today. We are much more mobile now, and rarely expect to live in the same location in which we grew up. Nowadays, it's likely you, your parents, and siblings live in different parts of a city, if not in different cities altogether. And even if your family members live near one another, it is likely that the adults (including grandparents) all work and that you often have jobs with different hours, which decreases even further your contact, even though you use email, texts, phone calls, and Skype. In theory, contact should be easier because you can now be in touch with your extended family any time of the day. Yet indirect contact isn't the same as speaking to someone who is right in front of you. It's harder to discuss a problem or concern about your preschooler through emails or text messages so you may come to rely on other sources of information, such as parenting books, magazines, or websites. While these can be extremely useful when it comes to helping you decide the best course of action to take as a parent, their advice isn't geared specifically to you and your individual needs and background, as is that from your extended family.

Families usually have shared values, which is why, if your child is to model and incorporate them into her way of living when she grows up, it's important that she have meaningful contact with her family so that these values can be fostered and nurtured. Unfotunately, however, because extended family gatherings are commonly infrequent and typically limited to recognized occasions such as over the holiday season or for special birthdays or anniversaries, when they do occur, they can be stressful because all those attending don't know one another as well as they would if they were all in more regular contact.

Rekindling family ties

When you think back to your own childhood, you may have a sense of loss, a fear that your child is missing out on something that should have been an important part of her childhood. You worry that she won't have the same rich family upbringing that you had when you were a child. While you can't force your extended family to live closer to one another, compel your parents to live beside you, or even move closer to them possibly because of employment

4 ways to create a wider support system

1 **Become a member of a religious congregation** and attend social gatherings there as well as services.

2 **Become close to another family,** and allow your child to spend time with them.

3 **Seek out groups in the community** such as family support programs or even neighborhood activity centers where your child can meet like-minded families.

4 **Ensure your child has godparents** or designate some close friends as special "aunties" or "uncles."

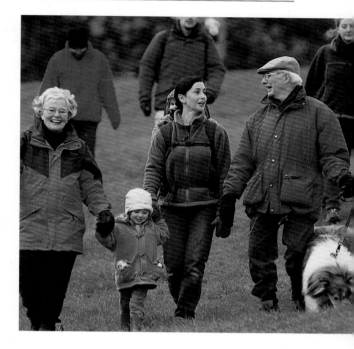

demands and opportunities, there are things you can do to strengthen your child's sense of family. Make sure she keeps in touch by calling or writing them (even if the letters or emails are only dictated to you), and encourage the exchange of photos.

Above all, maximize every family occasion to make sure your preschooler gets the most out them. For instance, talk to your child about the next planned family get-together well in advance. Try to develop her anticipation and excitement about the upcoming event and point out all the fun and excitement she'll have at that time. Mention the different people she'll meet, describe them positively (even if in reality you may not be that fond of them), and involve her in choosing a gift, if possible. All of these strategies make her feel connected to her extended family.

On the day of the gathering, dress your preschooler in her best clothes so that she feels this is a special occasion; remind her of all the fun she will have there, and set out in plenty of time. Once there, introduce her to everyone. Keep an eye on her as she starts to play with her cousins—she may be a little nervous and need some reassurance from you at the start. Do your

best to ensure she doesn't become too wild, excited, or overtired. If you think it is all getting a little too much for her, settle her down to a quiet activity so that she can regain her emotional stability. When it's all over, ask her to tell you what she enjoyed most about the day, who she liked best, and so on. In this way, your preschooler will develop an appreciation of her extended family.

Bear in mind that you can also take the initiative. Instead of waiting for the next formal date in the calendar to trigger a family get-together, arrange one sooner to take place in your family home. While that could be a lot of work for you, and not everyone might be able to come along, it's better than waiting a long time for your child to see her relatives once again. The more frequently she meets them all, the more she'll enjoy their company and the more she'll gain from having closer relationships.

Financial considerations

You probably won't be surprised to learn that the main cause of arguments between a couple in a first marriage is money. (In a second marriage, it's how the children should be raised, mainly because second marriages often involve step-parenting). There are many reasons why money problems are especially stressful during the preschool years.

For a start, all the clothes and childcare equipment that were given as presents at the time of the birth have long since been outgrown, and preschooler equipment is expensive. Your child now eats more, is harder on her clothes, breaks more toys, and loses more pieces from games, so she is a bigger financial drain. In addition, especially when she is around the age of four, she starts to become more product-aware from watching television or playing with her friends. Pester power can be hard to ignore. Second, many parents decide that the stay-at-home caregiver can safely resume his or her career now that the crucial first couple of years have passed. Unfortunately, the costs of outside childcare can be very expensive, leaving the family worse off financially. Third, preschoolers often enjoy attending activity classes, such as dance, drama, or athletics, and these lessons are expensive. Finally, family vacations are more expensive. Your child will now be charged a higher fare on flights, which could put the hoped-for vacation out of your reach.

Like most parents you probably want to give your child the best of everything, and to offer the most stimulating opportunities possible. Even if you are independently minded, you'll probably still feel the pressure to give your child the same high-quality enrichment experiences that other parents provide for their children. These activities may be very expensive and the thought of them might make you feel even more stressed about money. You don't want to make unwelcome decisions about what clothes and food, leisure activities and experiences you can and cannot provide for your growing child. Even when you think you have your family budget finely balanced, an unexpectedly high utility bill or expensive car repair can appear. All these factors combine to keep worries and arguments about money high on the agenda for many couples with a preschooler.

Resist debt

Before his or her first child is born, every parent has an idealized view of how he or she wants to be as a father or mother. In most instances, that includes being able to comfortably provide for all a child's material needs, and maybe even making sure she has everything that parents themselves did not have when growing up. No wonder then that economic difficulty in the family creates such psychological pressures for mom and dad—it's not just worry about paying the bills, it's also about your having to accept the need to modify your aspirations as parents.

The easiest solution, and most tempting, is to go into debt. After all, you might reason, family income is likely to increase year on year as each of you moves farther up the career ladder, and this means you will be able to repay that bank loan or line of credit in a year or two. While that can happen, very often increases in income don't match the costs of debt repayment. It can happen that one of you will have to accept a pay cut, or be laid off or will not have your temporary contract renewed. That's when stress about family economics can be so high that it goes off the scale, creating a strained atmosphere at home that is bound to be felt by everyone in the family, including your preschooler. It's very hard for parents raising a young child to clear large debts, so avoid overborrowing in the first place.

Realizing what matters

By all means, try to increase your family's income without borrowing if money worries start to pile up during your child's preschool years. You might be able to increase the number of hours or shifts you work or switch to a higher-paid job but in most instances, that solution isn't available. And

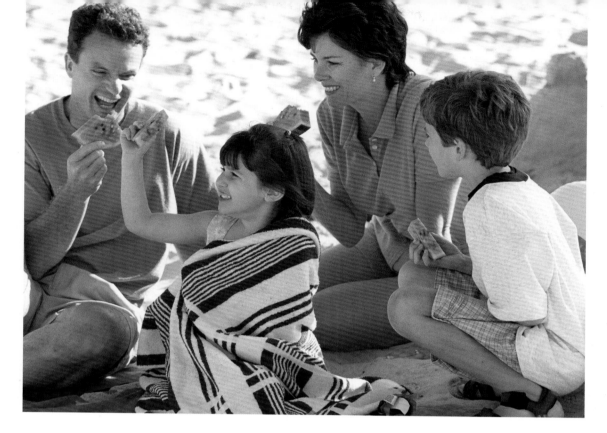

even if it is, working more hours simply replaces financial stress with other negative factors, such as fatigue, resentment, and having less time to share with your child.

A better strategy is to step back and think for a few minutes about yourself, your partner, and your child as a family. Try to identify the key factors that will enable your child to have a happy and fulfilling childhood. Write them down on a piece of paper. Almost certainly, that list will include, say, providing unconditional love and care to your child; offering her a range of play opportunities that allow her to develop her individual skills and talents; raising her in a warm, loving home environment; giving her lots of individual attention to encourage her all-round development, and helping her acquire social skills so that she mixes well with her peer group. None of these key features of a happy childhood need to include buying her the latest toys or gadgets or the most expensive clothes or taking her on exotic vacations. Play opportunities don't need to be expensive; going to your local park or playing in the

backyard don't cost anything and can be just as stimulating as a paid-for activity.

Of course, as parents, we partly judge our effectiveness by the level of material comfort we provide for our children, and we probably do this because this is easy to measure; it's visible to everybody and we are, by nature, competitive. Yet that is such a small part of parenting. When your preschooler grows up and reflects back over her childhood years, she is more likely to remember when she sat on her own bicycle for the first time than the cost of the bike itself, and she is more likely to remember the fun she had splashing in the water with you at the seaside than a fancy meal she ate in a deluxe hotel overseas. In this material world, you can easily lose sight of what really matters to your child. Always remember that what she wants and needs are loving parents who show care and interest in her progress and who spend time encouraging her development. She won't judge the quality of her childhood by the size of her parents' bank account.

INEXPENSIVE ACTIVITIES

Thrift store expeditions: Particular good if the weather is bad, visit your local thrift store and give your child a small amount of money (50 cents or a dollar) to spend on a used book or toy or something for the dress-up box. Your child will enjoy both the rooting around and getting to spend "his" money on what he wants.

Nature hunts: There is bound to be a park or woods nearby and many have nature trails. Even if yours don't, they are ideal places for your child to collect leaves or pine cones or to "study" various flora. Once home, have your preschooler create a "woodland" album or collage—pasting in the leaves and adding any appropriate captions (such as the name of the tree, where and when found). It's a good idea to collect the leaves at various stages so your child can learn about seasonal changes.

Garden centers: As long as you are not overly intent on shopping, these often contain many things of interest to a child such as plant and flower displays, aquaria, and aviaries. Many have play areas and nice cafes.

Library and museum visits: Today's libraries lend books, DVDs, computer games, and often toys (though the three latter may be at minimal charge). Many offer activities for kids, including craft days and story hours. As well as a wealth of things to see in a museum—think dinosaurs, Egyptian relics, Roman coins, and spacecraft—most offer fun-filled children's activity days or culture trails; some have special areas for children, with books, toys, and other activities. More sedate art galleries are best saved for older children but most museums have a relaxed policy toward children. Moreover, many museums are free of charge or some offer free entry deals to holders of certain types of credit cards.

Finding a way forward

Once you have achieved a more balanced perspective, try to have a positive attitude in front of your preschooler. When she asks for the latest toy or gadget, for instance, you can say "No" to her without giving a long explanation about how difficult things are financially or about how sorry you are that you can't buy her everything that she wants. That's the best way to resist pester power. Likewise, don't fall for her "But everyone else has got one" argument. If you have an upbeat attitude, your child will accept "No" with less complaints. You wouldn't buy her everything she asked for even if you did have more money (because you don't want her to be spoiled) and that's just what you are doing now as well (though for a different reason).

There is no need to feel guilty or apologize every time you refuse to buy her something.

If you start to look around, you'll discover that there are other ways to keep your child happy without spending more than you can afford. Family outings, for example, don't have to be expensive to be enjoyable—a picnic in the park costs very little and could be as much fun for everyone as a visit to a theme park. What makes an activity satisfying and pleasurable, as far as your preschooler is concerned, is that she spends time with you and that you are in a good mood. Likewise, toys and gadgets can be bought secondhand; your child will be just as a happy with a used slide that costs a fraction of the price of a new one, once it has been cleaned up, polished, and repainted.

Moving home

Psychological surveys consistently reveal that moving is usually a very traumatic life event for adults—top of the list of stressful life events comes the death of a partner, second comes divorce, and next comes a moving to a new house. That's hardly surprising when you think about it. Aside from the anxieties and pressure associated with making the decision to sell your current home and having to choose your next one, there are all the practicalities involved when moving, such as packing, organizing utilities to be transferred, arranging the movers, and the moving day itself. Then there is the pressing need to sort the living arrangements inside your new home as quickly as possible. Even when moving is done for positive reasons (a new job with increased income, access to better schools, more space for family members) rather than negative ones (excessive debt, separation from partner, being laid off or unemployed), the psychological pressures are there all the same.

It's important, therefore, to recognize also that moving will be difficult and psychologically challenging for your preschooler too. True, she doesn't have to deal with the organizational issues that you have to sort out, but she may experience emotional stress for a number of reasons. For a start, she'll have to adjust to sleeping in a new bedroom, playing in a new living room, eating in a new kitchen, and using a new bathroom. No matter how lovely your new home might be, your child will probably be sad to leave familiar surroundings where the sights, sounds, and smells are such an important part of her life. Familiarity is comforting to a preschooler, and consequently the loss of familiarity is unsettling.

In addition, your older preschool child (aged four years and up) may be afraid of losing contact with her friends once she moves to another area, and if a move to a new playgroup or nursery school is contemplated, she'll also be worried about having to make new friends there as well as the neighborhood. Social relationships become increasingly important to preschoolers as school age approaches.

Many home moves necessitate a change of childcare arrangements. Your child likes the playgroup or nursery school she already attends and she doesn't want to move to a new one, because that will mean getting used to new teachers, a new building, a new peer group who already know one another, and new travel arrangements to and from nursery school each day. That's why she'd probably prefer to stay exactly where she is.

As moving day draws closer, these worries will intensify. So all the pressures and excitements felt by you, as an adult, as a result of moving home, are also felt by your preschooler. In some ways it is even harder for her because she hasn't any previous experience of moving to draw on. It's therefore important to make a special effort to support your child in ways that help her adjust to moving to a new home.

Before moving day

Talk to your child about the move long before it happens so that she has advanced warning. Her reaction is hard to predict, though the chances are that she'll be very excited initially when she first hears the proposal. Almost certainly, though, once her initial enthusiasm for the move dies down, she'll start to ask you questions, which reveal her concerns over the effect that the impending change will have on her life. Tell her about the move once you have bought your new home, so that she can be told specific details rather than just a general idea. But don't wait until packing-up day is nearly upon you. She needs time to adjust to this transition in family life.

Once you have told your preschooler that she'll be moving to a new home, the most helpful next step is to reassure that she'll be able keep in contact with her old friends—you can't tell her this enough times, especially if she is aged four years or older. If she is only two or three, worry about friendships won't be as strong, but make a point of telling her she'll make new friends very easily because she is such a popular child. Give your older child some practical suggestions about

Being helpful around the house

3
4
5

3 years old

Your older toddler has sufficient kitchen skills so he can help to stir batters or use an eggbeater, fill and level off a measuring cup, and assemble salad ingredients.

Around the house, he can help to load the dishwasher and washing machine and help put away utensils and clothes. He also can collect litter to throw into wastepaper baskets or newspapers to put in the recycling bin at home. He can gather up his toys and put them away according to type. He can hold a dustpan and help with your sweeping up.

Outdoors, your child can assist with planting seeds and plants, water plants with a small watering can, and help sweep up leaves.

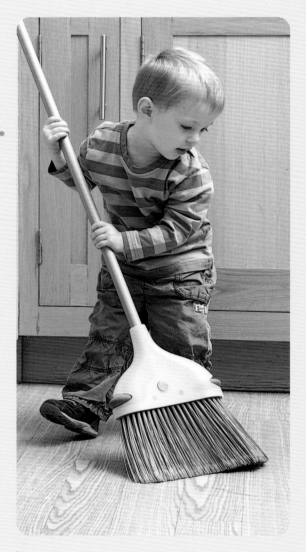

4 years old

Your child's kitchen skills now include setting the table, putting away groceries, making simple snacks (a slice of ham on bread), cutting out cookies from dough and decorating them.

Around the house, she can sort clothes by color for the laundry, pair socks, fold bath towels and face cloths, help get things to care for younger siblings (go get a diaper), and may be able to use a small broom effectively.

Outdoors, she can pull weeds (if shown which ones), bring in toys or seat cushions when rain threatens, and use a hose on plants and grass.

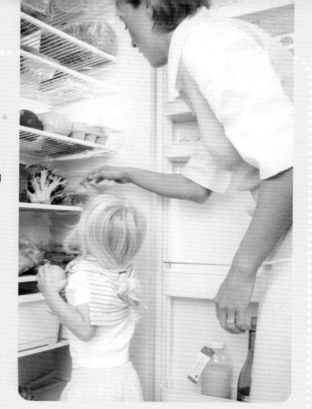

5 years old

Your preschooler's kitchen skills include making a simple meal—sandwich, potato chips, and fruit, producing simple baked goods from scratch (under supervision), pouring his own juice or water from a pitcher or carton, and clearing plates and utensils from the table.

Around the house, he can dust and polish furniture, help make his bed (put on a fitted sheet and pillowcase), sort out and stack magazines, put stamps on the outgoing mail, tidy his room, help feed family pets, and amuse younger siblings.

Outdoors your child can pick and deadhead flowers (under supervision), put fallen leaves into sacks, place household garbage bags into trash cans, help wash the car, and help unload groceries from the trunk.

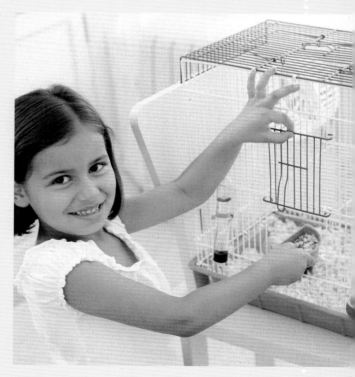

how this could be achieved, for instance, she can invite her friends over to visit her in the new home on weekends, she can call them after nursery school during the week, or they can phone her, and she can see and speak to them on Skype. She'll be pleased if you are able to tell her that her new room is big enough for a friend to sleep over. Explaining all these suggestions in detail—with the promise that you'll do all you can to help her keep in touch with her pals—reduces your child's potential anxiety about the change of family home. Let her see you write down her friends' phone numbers and contact details. It's also a good idea before the move for you to make a specific arrangement for her to get together with her best friend very soon after the move. She will look forward to this. Keeping these links with her past relationships, however tenuous, makes her feel more secure.

As soon as is practically possible after you have bought your new home, take your preschooler to see it. Point out all the advantages it has compared to your existing home, such as a larger backyard, more rooms, closer proximity to the shopping mall, and better play areas. Involve her in decisions about decorating and furnishing her bedroom. Ask her opinion about the color of the paint and wallpaper. The more involved she feels in the transition to her new home, the easier it becomes for her.

The same applies to her new nursery school, if the home move makes such a drastic change necessary. Expect her to be apprehensive about meeting the staff and her new peer group, so do this sooner rather than later. Once you have found your new home, but before you have moved, arrange to visit the new nursery school with your child. Talk to her enthusiastically about it, telling her all the activities she'll enjoy there. You could arrange with the nursery school that she visits several times before she starts, possibly mixing with the children for a few minutes each time. This enables your preschooler to build up her self-confidence and familiarity before leaving her current place, and helps the adjustment process.

You'll be extremely busy in the days leading up to moving day, try to find the time to hold a special "moving home" party for your child and her friends, a few weeks before moving day itself. Don't call it a "goodbye" party, because that has negative associations. Your older preschooler will particularly appreciate the opportunity to host this occasion for her friends. On the invitation, ask the children to bring a small memento, such as a photograph or small toy, and at the party, your child and her pals should trade them with one another. Encourage her to store these precious keepsakes in a special box that she can easily access whenever she wants.

After the move

The move itself will be a hectic time for all of you, and your preschooler may still be upset despite all your preparations for the change. Spend time with her each day, talking to and reassuring her. The typical preschooler can be very fragile emotionally when under pressure and needs extra love and attention during difficult phases. These chats with you allow her to express her worries and anxieties, rather than bottling them up inside. At all times, maintain a positive attitude about the relocation of your family home—this will encourage your child to have an upbeat approach too.

Do what you promised about helping your older preschooler keep in touch with her old friends. She may need some prompting from you, not because she doesn't want to speak to them but because she is afraid they will have lost interest in her. Encourage her to pick up the phone, and ensure that she makes an arrangement to see them the first weekend following the move. At the same time, however, get her socially involved with children in her new area. Look for opportunities for her to form new friendships with your neighbors' children, and enroll her in your local preschool facility if you haven't already done so—this is probably the most effective way for your child to meet new peers.

Give her plenty of reassurance that these new children will like her just as much as her old friends do. You'll probably find that in time, your child's new pals become more important to her than her former friends, largely because she spends much more time with them. New pals will gradually compensate for the loss of the old ones.

A new brother or sister

Suddenly finding out that there's a new family member on the way can come as a shock to a young child. Most commonly, a younger brother or sister appears two years after a firstborn child—exactly the age gap that research has shown most likely to result in tension, jealousy, and resentment. It's no wonder that the typical older child becomes a handful when the second baby arrives in the family. And when you think about it from her point of view, such difficult behavior is hardly surprising. After all, your firstborn is used to having you all to herself, and she wants that way of life to continue forever. She worries about having to share your time with someone else. She might also be afraid that you will love the new baby more than her, and that she will be less important to you, or even that you want a second child because she herself is not good enough for you or that you are having another baby just to punish her. In other words, she feels insecure.

Looked at this way, you can understand why she will be unsettled by the news that a new baby is on the way, as well as the actual arrival itself. And she can show her anxiety in different ways. She might become clingy, tearful, and whiny, or aggressive, hostile, and uncooperative. It's the change in her behavior that tells you something is wrong. As a parent, you know that loving your second baby won't decrease your love for your older child—but she doesn't know that. She has to learn by experience, which takes time. In the meantime, she may feel hostility toward you and jealousy toward the new baby.

However, if family life is to be as rewarding as possible for you and your children, it's vital that your children are strongly connected. You should try and create this connection before your second baby is born and continue from the birth itself (see page 180). What happens in the early days and months can set the tone for your children's relationship with each other throughout their lives, which is why it helps when their tie is positive right from the start.

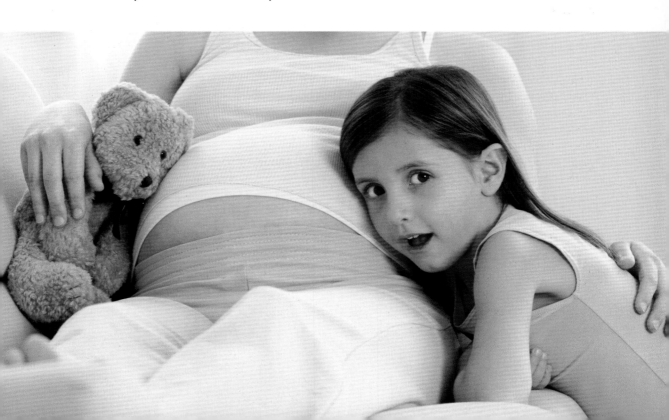

Introducing the idea

You should tell your child in advance that she's going to have a new brother or sister—don't wait until the last moment when labor has started, but don't tell her about the new baby when you are only a few weeks into your pregnancy either. A child's sense of time is different from that of an adult's; yours may see no difference between a week and a month, or between one month and six months and she may become bored with the long wait!

Start talking about the new baby when your abdomen is so large that even an inexperienced child would notice it, perhaps around the fifth or sixth month of pregnancy.

Tell your child calmly, without feeling embarrassed about it. Pitch the conversation at a level suitable for her age and understanding, and avoid giving too many pieces of information to her at the one time. For instance, it's better to say to her "I've got a terrific surprise for you. We're going to have a new baby soon" than to say, "I'm pregnant and in three months time I will have a baby."

From the moment you first mention to your child that a new baby is on the way, use positive terms. Tell her the new baby loves her already and thinks she is a terrific older sister.

Dealing with her reactions

You might find that your child reacts with total indifference. Or she may seem very interested and want to talk about it further. Or she may simply burst into tears. Be prepared to let her ask you questions, either at the time you tell her or later—and always give her an honest, sensitive reply that will provide her with information and reassurance. For instance, if she asks "Where will baby sleep?", it's better to say "We will get him a crib; you will still have your own bed," than to say "We'll find somewhere. Don't worry". Those early predelivery discussions and information-sharing sessions start to build your child's involvement with her sibling. If you plan on breastfeeding your new baby and your older child was weaned from the breast at an early age (so she has no memory of the process) or

6 ways to help your preschooler anticipate the new baby

1 **Read him books about new babies.** Your local bookstore or library should have a good selection of books on this topic, written specifically for young children.

2 **Get him used to new babies.** Try to arrange for your child to meet, for example, your friend's new baby so that he is comfortable in the baby's presence.

3 **Let him play "we have a new baby."** Buy him a baby doll and encourage him to pretend to be a big brother to the new arrival.

4 **Show your child his baby book or family album.** Spend time together looking at pictures of when he was a baby. Seeing pictures of him crying, being bathed, or having his diapers changed can prepare him for what will happen when his new sibling arrives.

5 **Involve him in choosing the baby's name.** You decide on the name, but present it to your child in a way that makes him think he has made the choice with you.

6 **Let him help select baby items.** If you need to buy new clothes, toys, or equipment, take your child with you and ask him to help you select the things. Make it easy by narrowing the choice—which of two toys, for example.

you hadn't breastfed her, make opportunities for your child to see babies being breastfed. Explain that you will make milk for the baby, that breastfeeding is how a baby eats, and that it also helps a baby feel that he is loved and protected.

It's common for children to be curious about breastfeeding and it is not something you should hide from your older child. When she sees you breastfeed later on, she will learn that breastfeeding is the normal, healthy way to feed a child rather than something that needs to be hidden.

In on the delivery?

As well as at home, it also may be possible to have your child with you if you deliver your baby in a hospital. But as well as ascertaining whether the hospital will allow your child to be present, and even if you plan to have your birth at home, it's also important to consider some other factors when deciding whether your child should see the birth. Things to consider are:

- The age of your child;
- The maturity of your child;
- The interest your child has in seeing the birth.

If your child is under four years old, she may be too young to appreciate the experience, but more importantly, she may be scared by what is happening. If you are in pain, bleeding, or have a drip attached to your arm, it may frighten your child rather than making her feel a part of the process in a positive way. If your child is older, it is reasonable to ask her if she wants to be there.

If your child expresses real interest and enthusiasm at the idea of being present, then you can sit down and explain to her exactly what she should expect. It is a good idea if you are giving birth in a hospital to give her a picture of what the room looks like and where you will be. You will also want to explain how you will be examined and how the baby will actually be born. Make sure you let her know that sometimes unexpected things can happen, and that it is possible you could be taken to the hospital from home, or if already in the hospital, be wheeled to a different room to have the baby (for example, if a cesarean section is needed).

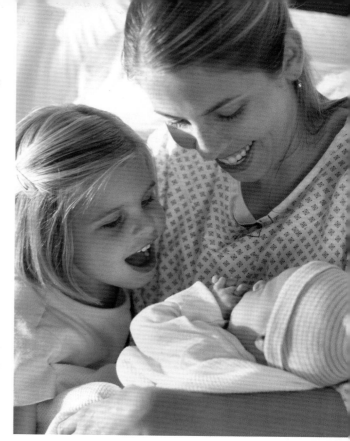

Your child may benefit from seeing pictures in books or watching an educational movie about the whole birth process. Also, when the big event happens, remember that labor can take a long time, so be prepared by making sure she has plenty of activities to keep her busy.

Keep in mind that no matter how mature or excited your child seems, she may not ultimately react the way you anticipate. Sometimes the delivery room is too intense and scary even for a very mature child. You should have an additional adult available to take her out of the room if she starts to feel uncomfortable, and also reassure her that you will not be disappointed if this happens.

After the birth

When your child sees her new sibling for the first time, try to arrange that you are not holding the new arrival. That way you can give your full attention to your firstborn. Give her a big cuddle, tell her how pleased you are to see her and ask lots

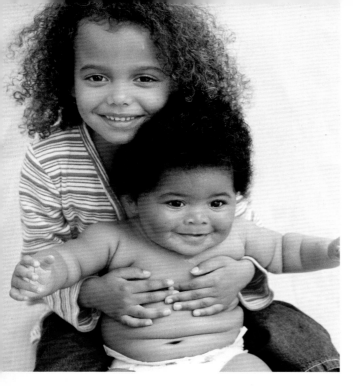

of questions about what she has been doing since you last saw her. After a few minutes, introduce her to her younger sibling. Make sure the new arrival has a present lying beside him in the cradle for his older sibling (one that you purchased previously and took into the hospital with you or have at home) and arrange for your first child to have a present for your second baby. This exchange of gifts is stage-managed, yet it can help form an emotional bond between the two children right from their first meeting, and reduces the likelihood of tensions between them later on.

During the early days

Once that initial meeting is over, get your older child involved in some of the minor chores of baby care. She'll be full of self-importance when you ask her to bring you a clean diaper from the pile in the corner, or when you thank her for rubbing in some cream on the baby's legs after bathtime. Basic, responsible tasks make her feel part of her brother's or sister's life.

The first few days when you are back home with your family after the birth of your second baby will normally be a very busy time, with visitors keen to see your new arrival. They can help your existing

child keep any feelings of jealousy in check by bringing a present for her as well as one for the baby. Wherever possible, ask your visitors to do this and do try to encourage them to spend a few moments with your older child before they go charging in to see the baby. True, the main purpose of their visit is to inspect the new arrival, but there is no harm in quietly asking them to spend a moment or two talking to your older child first. And appoint your firstborn as tour guide. She'll love to be given the job of leading visitors into the baby's room, and will take great pride in explaining all about him. This particular role ensures she gets lots of attention, too, and emphasizes that she is the "big one" at home—you'll find that she responds very positively to your request.

It's also important for you to maintain your relationship with your firstborn at the same time as encouraging her to have a strong relationship with her new sibling(s). One of the best ways to do this is by making sure you spend some time alone with your older child every day, perhaps while your partner is bathing your second baby or when the youngest is sleeping. A few minutes of individual attention from you every day will make her feel that she is still as special to you as she was before her sibling came along. If your first child can continue her usual daily routine without the baby's schedule interrupting, for instance, going to playgroup or visiting her friend, then so much the better.

It may also be a good idea for your child to spend more time with your partner and/or other relatives and friends. Generally speaking, fathers spend more time on parenting and household chores once a second baby arrives, but you don't have to wait until your second baby arrives to encourage your partner's participation (see also box page 188).

It also makes sense to have the grandparents on hand more, too. The more your child is used to being looked after by others, the better it will be for you once the new baby arrives. And, if you are planning to have a nanny or au pair, make sure he or she is familiar to your child before the new sibling arrives.

Two children at home

In the months and years that lie ahead, you'll have the delight of watching your first and second children grow up together. But that's not a passive process. How you manage them and contribute to their lives is the biggest single influence on the outcome of their development. Recognizing and responding to their individual differences will be a key challenge for you—but if you achieve this, it will be highly rewarding for you and for them.

Even if your new baby is of the same gender, don't expect that he or she will be similar in temperament, personality, or likes and dislikes to the elder. If you're lucky enough to have an easy and relaxed preschooler who deals calmly with everything that comes her way, your new baby might be hard to settle and easily upset. You'll be surprised at times at how two children from the same family, with the same home environment and the same upbringing, can appear so entirely different from each other! And even when they appear to be initially similar, their dissimilar abilities and personalities may produce widely differing results later on. This characterizes the nature of child and family development.

Aim for fairness

The most important thing when there is more than one child in the family is to respond to each child as an individual. Aim for fairness in your parenting rather than equality.

Perceived lack of fairness is a common complaint of siblings; the cry of "She always gets more than me" is heard in most families at one time or another and it is one the main causes of sibling jealousy although there are other factors, too. In fact, sibling rivalry is so common in virtually every family that

 ways a second baby changes your life

While having a second baby means that there's one more person to love and who loves you, it's also true that you will

1 **Be much more tired.** This is particularly true if your older child is active or if he regresses and if your baby is not yet sleeping through the night.

2 **Have less spare cash.** While you may be able to save money on some equipment and clothes, your second baby may end up costing you a lot more than your first— you may not be able to accommodate a new baby into your existing home as easily as you did the first and may have to stop working to care for both.

3 **Have a lot more work to do.** Looking after the needs of two children will take up most of your day. As well as seeing to your preschooler's daily care routines, providing activities and outings for him, and tidying up after him, you will also have to manage feeding, dressing, caring for, and changing a young baby.

4 **Have less time in which to do things.** Feeding, bathing, and dressing two children takes a lot of time as does taking them places and sorting out their squabbles. Moreover if one child becomes sick, you have the extra burden of care.

Your child and his siblings

3
4
5

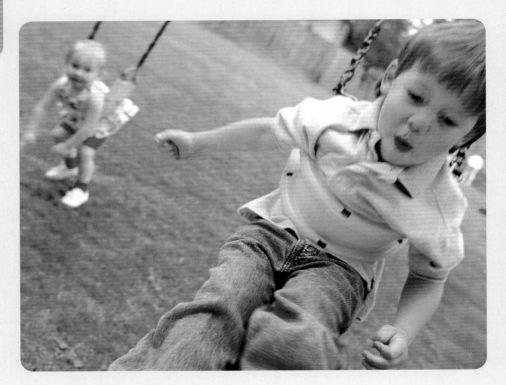

3 years old

As an older toddler, your child may be unpredictable with any brothers or sisters, particularly those close in age. Older siblings may boss him around while he will dislike younger ones getting a lot of attention or taking his toys or interfering with his games.

4 years old

Your child's developmental abilities mean she can hold her own more with older siblings, being more assertive with them and instigating disruptive behavior, while with younger ones, her desire to be "sisterly" or "brotherly," which she may show evidence of, can be thwarted by her jealousy so that she becomes nasty and even violent toward them.

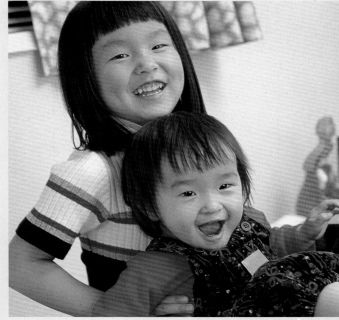

5 years old

Your preschooler feels more master of himself and extends his beneficence to his siblings, becoming less demanding and bossy. He can show much kindness and generosity to younger siblings while being able to share and take turns with older ones.

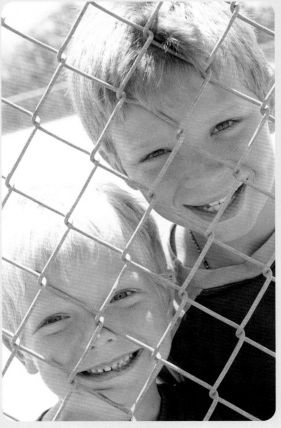

most psychologists now regard it as normal. You can rest assured that your children are not the only ones to fight with each other—you would have great difficulty finding two young siblings who never fought.

Your young child is very sensitive to your comments (and your younger baby soon will be), so never make comparision between your children. When you lose your temper, you may inadvertently compare your older child with the new addition, perhaps pointing out that her younger brother never complains when his toys are tidied away or when it's time for bed. Such comparisons are always divisive and will only make your firstborn resentful of you and of your second baby. Likewise, make allowances that recognize your first child is older, for example, by allowing her a later bedtime; a basic measure like that demonstrates to her that you regard her as older and more mature, and this helps maintain your positive relationship with her.

No matter how hard you will try not to compare your children with each other, however, the chances are other people will (friends and relatives, for instance). If it is remarked upon, for example, that your older child is more boisterous and attention-seeking than her sibling, she may start to resent her overly good sibling (or even try to harm him) and their relationship may suffer. Each child must feel valued and not have his or her achievements compared to those of a sibling, and you may need to point this out to others.

When making major decisions as a parent, you instinctively act in the best interests of your children. Yet that doesn't mean your children will like your suggestions, for instance, when you don't let the elder play with another child because you think that child could have a negative influence on her. And neither do you probably like being a parent who has to say "No" to your child. Have confidence in your decisions, even in the face of opposition from her or when having to balance long-term considerations against a disagreement with your child in the short term.

You may find that you want to change some aspects of parenting with your second child, having learned from experience with your first. For example, you may become more exacting about rules for bedtime. Whereas you were relaxed about time-keeping with your first child, you now take a stricter approach with your second because you value the extra time you may be able to spend with your older child or by yourself. There's nothing wrong with that. You don't have to feel guilty because the way you respond as a parent has changed over time. You don't have to feel badly because you now have to do things differently. At the time, you did what worked with your first child but now there are two, if you see alternative courses of action for managing your second child's development and behavior, that's a positive sign of your personal growth—it would be much worse if you didn't learn from experience.

Dealing with sibling rivalry

The intensity of sibling jealousy varies from family to family, and even within the same family; some children are more antagonistic toward a particular sibling. Usually, it simply comes down to the individual differences between siblings, whether in personality, talents and abilities, gender, or even birth order.

Sometimes you'll feel that you cannot win, no matter how hard you try. There will always be moments when your older child will be jealous of her sibling or the time you spend with him.

Although you cannot eliminate sibling rivalry altogether, you can try to control it. Treat your child seriously. If she thinks that you regard her with amusement rather than genuine respect, then she will soon become even more jealous. Listen to her complaints—even though the endless list of gripes and groans about her sibling can be extremely irritating. It is better to make time to listen to what she has to say because if you try to ignore her, she will force you to give her your attention by acting aggressively toward her sibling. When you have heard her complaint, suggest a solution. For instance, if she wants to be fed while you are feeding your baby, suggest that she snuggles up to you if you are breastfeeding or holds the bottle for the baby. Later on, when your new baby is older, you might find that he will resent the greater freedom his older

GENDER DIFFERENCES

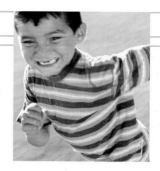

Boys (compared to girls) tend to...

- Enjoy risk-taking and be adventure-seeking;
- Take part in rough-and-tumble play;
- Use their hands as a first response to conflict;
- Take longer to develop language and independence skills;
- Compete with one another when playing together;
- Have a better developed right side of the brain (hence advanced spatial skills).

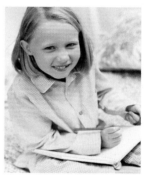

Girls (compared to boys) tend to...

- Consider risks carefully before taking action;
- Like sedate activities, such as puzzles and creative play;
- Resolve disagreements through talking;
- Start talking and achieve bladder control earlier;
- Cooperate with one another during play;
- Have a better developed left side of the brain (hence advanced speech).

sister has. Like it or not, he has to face the fact that his sister is older and is therefore entitled to do some things that he cannot, such as going to bed later than him or being given more individual responsibility at home. Point out the significance of their age difference.

As your children get older, enhance their positive relationship by encouraging the elder to take more responsibility for her younger sibling. One way to do this is to provide opportunities for sharing. Ask your child to pick out a suitable toy for baby to play with or to portion out something meant for both of them. Heap praise on her when she hands over the toy to him or helps with his care. Don't make all the decisions about sharing for her; it's important that she learns this from practice.

Partner considerations

Having a second baby also has an impact on your relationship with your partner. True, you already have experience of the massive change that took place when your first baby arrived—you shifted from being a couple without children, able to make lifestyle and

work choices that suited you and your needs, to a couple with children, now having to make child-centered decisions. So you know what it is like to put a baby's needs before the needs of you and your partner, and presumably you have adjusted accordingly.

With your second baby, there will be further change, perhaps not as dramatic as with your first baby, but change all the same. The practical demands of caring for two children multiply exponentially and there will be less space at home and less money to go around. Any career or work plans may be on hold once again. All of these have an impact on your relationship with your partner. Family stresses can strengthen the connection between parents but can also create barriers between you. Successful parenting is heavily influenced by, among other things, resilience and a capacity to adapt to change.

A settled family life does not depend on the practical arrangements you make, for instance, whether it's you or your partner who gives your children their bath tonight, or whose turn it is to make dinner. Neither is it a question of your financial arrangements, for instance, whether you have enough money to afford to pay for a babysitter and a meal in a restaurant, or what you need to sacrifice in order to pay the utility bill. Nor is it reliant on your agreeing about your extended family, for instance, whether you should go to his parents with the children this weekend or to yours, or which relatives you should invite to your child's forthcoming birthday party. All these factors play a part in your home life, but the central component when it comes to partner consideration is honest and open communication between the two of you.

If you are able to express your ideas and feelings openly to each other as parents, adults, and partners, then resentments are unlikely to build, misunderstandings are unlikely to occur, and your relationship is more likely to remain positive and optimistic. Making time to talk is crucial. Avoid the trap of becoming so absorbed in the demands of parenting that you and your partner lose sight of each other as a couple. When communication with your partner becomes low on your list of priorities, the chances are that problems will emerge. In contrast, good communication means most potential problems can be resolved before they reach crisis point.

When partners disagree

Perhaps the most worrying type of disagreement about parenting is when you and your partner are in dispute about the best way to handle your children. As you will have already discovered, managing children is not an exact science! Everybody has his or her own opinions about areas such as discipline, bedtime routines, how to deal with tantrums, and so on, which is hardly surprising given that there is usually more than one way to do anything.

ways to improve shared care

1 **Be specific about what is needed.** Instead of generalizing about how tired or overworked you are, agree with your partner specific tasks you each will perform. Ask him which tasks he prefers to do instead of assigning him chores.

2 **Try not to criticize** what your partner does. Everyone has his/her way of approaching things and if your partner handles your baby or older child differently than you, just accept it, otherwise you'll give him or her reason not to do the task at all in the future.

3 **Remember to thank your partner** and to offer praise for a job well done.

4 **Keep him or her in the loop.** If your partner works away from home, it's important to tell him or her about what your children did during the day, so that your partner feels part of family life when he or she is not around.

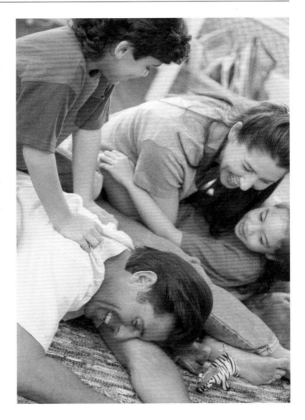

Adopting a preschooler

After waiting for what probably seems far too long, your adopted child has finally arrived. Now the excitement really begins as you start to build your new family structure. Like all new parents, though, you'll be anxious. You want to do everything right for your new arrival, and your confidence as a parent may be fragile. But don't expect everything to fall into place instantly. Both you and your child need time to adjust to this new arrangement. The age of your adopted child matters to some extent. For example, a three-year-old may seem more of a mystery to you than an older child because a young child is not as capable of telling you what she thinks and feels, and so you'll probably want to read as much as you can about the psychological needs of the typical child that age and about ways to manage her. In contrast, a five-year-old is better able to express her thoughts and emotions, and may also be more resilient than a younger child. Similarly, a younger child may not have strong memories of life before becoming part of your family, whereas an older child may have more vivid recollection of her past experiences.

Some adopted children who have had a difficult upbringing have learned not to trust adults, while others become so needy for parental love that they are overly demanding. So take your time. Have realistic expectations of you and your preschooler. Be patient with her and with yourself. Give your new arrival lots of love, reassurance, and attention and remember that all children thrive best within a loving, consistent family discipline.

It's also important to know as much as possible about your child's previous medical history to ensure that she continues with or starts any treatment required at present. But you also need to know about allergies, whether to particular foods or to particular prescription medicines.

Make sure that you don't fall into the trap of thinking every single thing your preschooler does is due to her previous experience before she became part of your family. Of course, some aspects of her personality and behavior are linked to what happened before, but some have nothing to do with it. You are her parents now, and what you do from this moment on matters more than anything that has taken place in the past.

More than parents who have raised their child from birth, you may worry that bonding with your new preschooler will be difficult because of her age and background. Rest reassured, there are no insurmountable psychological barriers to prevent a strong emotional attachment between you and her. Every child has the ability to form many emotional attachments with loving adults—there isn't a fixed number of close relationships she can manage in her life. Therefore, the fact that your preschooler has been close to someone else when she was younger does not stop her from growing emotionally close to you. Similarly, if she hasn't had a warm, loving relationship with an adult by the time she has reached this age (perhaps because of poor parenting or because she has been moved so frequently from one carer to another in the first few years of life), she still has the emotional capacity to bond with you.

Telling her she's adopted

Depending on your adoptive preschooler's age, she may not retain strong memories of her life before she became a part of your family. So, you cannot assume that she knows she is adopted. That means you have to decide when (and how) to tell her. Explaining about her adoption as early as possible is in her best interests because that way she grows up knowing that the adoption took place; she simply considers it is part of her life which she just accepts. Deliberately concealing this information from your adopted child suggests that there is something wrong about the adoption process. Anyway, if you don't tell her, the chances are that someone else will—secrets are hard to keep—and it would devastate her to hear this news from another person.

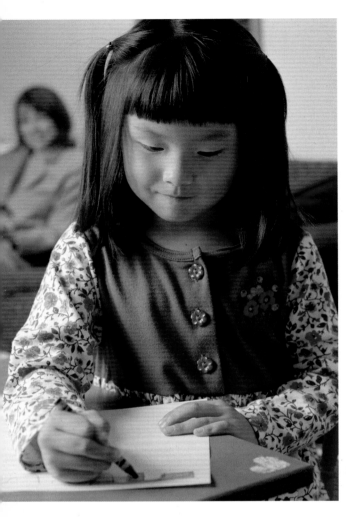

some tell their child that she is so special she was chosen to be part of the family, some have "adoption day" celebrations as well as birthday parties, and some use photographs to explain the day their child arrived in the family. When discussions about adoption are out in the open early on, there is no embarrassment or strangeness about the topic.

Expect your preschooler to ask detailed questions about her adoption. Answer these honestly, calmly, and at a level appropriate to her age and understanding. Give only enough details to satisfy her curiosity; avoid telling her too much all at once. There are many child-friendly books about adoption, pitched at children of different ages, and you might find one of these helpful in supporting your discussions. Talking to other adoptive parents also helps you learn from their experiences.

When she is from a different background

Your adopted preschooler may face additional challenges if she comes from another country or is of a different race or ethnicity, because people can see immediately that she is not your biological child. They may start to ask you or her lots of questions about your child's origins and country of birth. This makes it even more important that your child understands her background from the earliest possible age.

While making it clear that she is your child, that you love her, and that her place in your family is totally secure, try to develop her knowledge about her birth country (if it is not the one you live in), culture, and parents. If available, show her pictures that show her before she came to be part of your family. And if no such photos are available, show her pictures of her native country. This helps strengthen her identity and self-confidence. With a good understanding of her past and origins, your preschooler will have a stronger understanding of who she is and where she comes from.

The majority of adoptive parents introduce the topic of adoption to their child when children are around the age of two years. Of course, a child cannot possibly understand the implications of adoption at that age, but using the word "adoption" starts to bring the concept of adoption into her consciousness. While you might choose to put off introducing the topic, if you still haven't told your child by the time she is four or five years old, don't delay any longer. Bear in mind that the older your child is, the more of a shock it will be and the more she will wonder why you did not tell her before.

Some parents talk about "when you were adopted" instead of saying "when you were born,"

When you already have a preschooler

Some parents who already have a preschooler adopt a baby, perhaps because they are unable to have a second child or they want to offer a loving home to a baby who wasn't born into such an opportunity. Whatever your reason for adopting, a singleton preschooler may resent a new arrival, not because her sibling is adopted but because your existing child is no longer the center of attention. To be honest, your preschooler probably couldn't care at all about the baby's background—all he cares about is that your time, love, and resources will now be divided between two.

To make your adopted child's entry into your family as smooth as possible, tell your preschooler in advance about the new arrival. Talk positively from the start and tell her the new baby loves her already and thinks she is a terrific older sister. It's only natural your older child is anxious the first time she sees the new arrival, so do your best to ensure that you are not actually cuddling him the exact moment your preschooler first sees him. In addition, buy a gift for your older child and put it beside your new baby in his cradle when your preschooler meets him. She'll be delighted that her new sibling bought her a special present; arrange it so that she has a gift to give to the baby too.

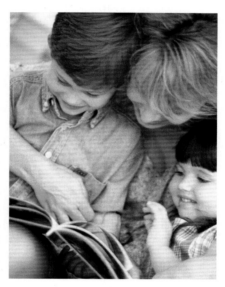

The more your older child is involved in the care of the baby, the more she'll feel connected with him. That's why you should try to give her minor responsibilities—asking her to bring you a clean diaper, for example. Hands-on jobs like that help form an emotional attachment between her and the new arrival. The first few days at home with your family after your adopted baby has arrived is a busy time, with visitors keen to see him. They can help your preschooler keep any feelings of jealousy in check by bringing a present for her as well as one for the baby. And give your child the job of bringing visitors into the baby's room. This particular role ensures she gets lots of attention and emphasizes that she is the "big one" at home. As a result, she will feel less threatened by the presence of the new arrival.

Although you will need to give your new baby loads of attention even if only feeding, changing, and bathing him, try to introduce your preschooler to this idea gradually. Potential tension between her and the new baby will be greatly reduced if you manage some of these tasks when your older one is kept busy on some activity of her own. It's also important that you never compare your children. In anger, you may inadvertently compare your older child with your adopted baby, perhaps pointing out that her baby brother is much calmer than her. Such comparisons are always divisive, however, and usually create even greater tension between your preschooler and the baby. Last of all, treat your children as individuals. Each of them is unique with his or her own particular personality, likes, and dislikes. Resentment between them is less likely when you allow that individuality to show through. Encourage their differences. Spend time alone with each of your children every day so that each feels special.

Sometimes parents adopt a child who is older than their existing one. In that situation, sibling rivalry can appear in both children, because each of them may be jealous of the attention the other gets from you. However, as long as each of them feels you love and care for him or her—and that you demonstrate this in practice by giving each of them their fair share of your time, attention, and other resources—their relationship will become steadily more positive.

Living with a child with special needs

At this stage in your child's life, if she has special needs, you probably have developed a good understanding of the nature of her difficulty. If your child has been specifically diagnosed (for example, a hearing or vision impairment, spina bifida, cerebral palsy, or Down syndrome) you'll have read a great deal about it, will have spoken to many professionals with experience in that area, and have made the necessary adjustments at home to ensure her continued development. However, if your preschooler's special needs are more general and

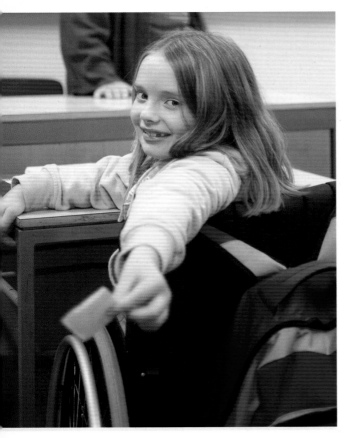

nonspecific, without a clear diagnosis (for example, general developmental delay, general language delay), or she may be too young for a firm diagnosis (ADHD or autism), you may still not have a clear grasp of the underlying cause. Either way, whatever your child's difficulty and however much or little you understand it, you face a number of key challenges during the preschool years.

Living with uncertainty is extremely frustrating. Every child is an individual, and even if she has a diagnosed difficulty in common with thousands of others, her development will be distinctive and unique. That means significant developmental outcomes, such as her eventual intellectual growth, physical progress, learning potential, and sociability, will still be unclear at this point in her life. Lack of certainty is demanding for you as a parent, but try to maintain an optimistic outlook and expect the most from your child, just like every other parent—that's the best way to maximize her potential.

Choosing a suitable nursery school

This takes careful consideration. You know her strengths and weaknesses now and the type of stimulation that best suits her, and must match her special needs and talents with the available preschool provision. (The same decision will need to be made when she reaches school age.) Consider the available choices, and listen to advice from the professionals involved with your child. You'll make up your own mind, but there's no harm in listening to their opinions. Visit each potential establishment, speak with the staff there, look around the classrooms, and check out specifically what the nursery school will be able to offer your child. You'll probably spend months reaching a decision.

Then there's managing the impact of your preschooler with special needs on your other children. She requires much more of your time and attention because of her particular difficulties, yet that doesn't stop her sibling from feeling left out at times or even from resenting that she is your main focus for much of the time. This type of jealousy is perfectly normal—try to see family life from the perspective of your other child. No matter how much his head tells him that he has more advantages than his sibling with special needs, his heart tells

him that he still wants more of your attention than he gets at the moment. Compensate for this perceived lack of attention by making special time for your other child, time when you and he can be together without any interruption. Five or ten minutes each day will be more than enough to ease his hard-done-by feelings. What you do together during these moments doesn't really matter—you can talk together, play games together, eat together—it's the fact that you give him your attention that counts. Choose times when your child with special needs is asleep or is being cared for by someone else so that you can give him your undivided attention.

Living with an ADHD child

As well as following the guidelines for managing general disruptive behavior (see page 139), there are additional things you can try to encourage the positive aspects and control the negative. You must also keep your child under constant supervision.

- Join in your child's activities. Talk to her about what she is doing and any toys she is playing with. Try to keep a back-and-forth interaction going;
- Point to interesting objects and reward your child with praise when she makes appropriate responses;
- Teach your child to point at things that she wants or things that interest her instead of crying or leading you by the hand. Make sure to acknowledge it when she shows you something of interest to her;
- Repeat rules frequently, concentrating on "Do" rather than "Don't." If possible, avoid confrontations.

Children with ADHD need to have clear limits set and be constantly reminded of them. You should, therefore, create and adhere to a timetable at home, setting specific times for waking up, mealtimes, playtimes and/or activities, and going to bed—and ensure that your child knows when they are and is given plenty of warning if you need to change any of them. Make sure your child is given the opportunity to work off some of her excess

TWINS WITH SPECIAL NEEDS

For various reasons—prematurity, uterine conditions, etc.—one or both of your twins and may have special needs (the rate is higher for multiple births than singletons). While you will have great difficulties in managing two children of the same age with special needs (so it's vital that you have familial and professional support), there may be other problems if only one child is affected and it's important to be aware of them.

The affected twin may:

- Need to understand why he has different abilities than his sibling and may require different "rules" of behavior, etc.;
- Want to achieve at the level of his twin and may resent low expectations of his behavior and abilities;
- On the positive side, find his more able twin motivating and stimulating.

The nonaffected twin may:

- Need to understand why his sibling behaves differently and is treated differently;
- Be conflicted about his sibling's situation, feeling guilty he doesn't have the same problems or embarrassed by his brother's needs;
- Display jealousy and disruptive behavior if he is unhappy about the time and attention given his less-abled sibling.

energy by getting more exercise and spending less time watching television, using computers, or playing computer games.

Restricting sugary drinks and foods is also important, as is preventing your child from eating highly processed foods containing additives and preservatives; many of these (identified on labels by E numbers, see page 42) have been linked to hyperactivity in sensitive children. Food colorings, especially tartrazine (E102) and erythrosine (E127), which is not commonly used in the US, and antioxidants such as BHA (E320) and BHT (E321) are known to cause problems (BHA and BHT are not approved for use in the US). Alway check labels.

Living with an autistic child

A child with autism finds it hard to understand what is going to happen next and change of any kind can make her highly anxious. For this reason, autistic children can be inflexible and prefer to stick to a rigid routine. This inability to imagine what will happen next can also make a child oblivious to danger so she requires a far higher level of supervision than her peers.

Many children with autism have difficulty processing their senses, making them either over- or undersensitive to things they see, hear, taste, or smell. When a child is exposed to more sensory information than she can process, particularly in highly stimulating environments, such as a supermarket or swimming pool, she experiences sensory overload, which can result in explosive tantrums or outbursts. If your child reaches meltdown, she will no longer be able to process information, so the only option will be to remain calm, make sure she is safe and cannot harm herself—preferably away from other people—and allow her to cool off.

It helps to make your home environment as placid as possible. Paint your child's bedroom in pale

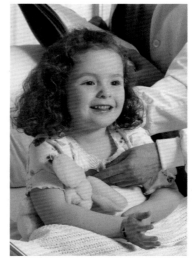

colors and keep the number of toys and other clutter to a minimum. Make her a den or tent to retreat into when she feel overwhelmed by her surroundings.

Verbal information may be difficult for her to process. However, most children with autism are very able visual learners, so you can use pictures or photographs to teach life skills, such as potty training and getting dressed, more easily. Keeping to a routine is very important because it makes your child feel secure. Plan her days and weeks ahead with a visual timetable.

Children with autism also tend to enjoy spending time in front of a computer and television since they allow a child to zone out from external stimulation. You should allow your child more screen time than usual (see page 146) as long as her choice of viewing is carefully supervised. Movies or shows need to have a G rating because autistic children can be more sensitive than a typical child of a similar age, but it's best to avoid high-octane action-packed viewing because this can overstimulate her.

Physical activity such as jumping on trampolines or sensory activities such as playing with sand or water can have a calming effect and should be incorporated into your child's daily schedule.

Children with autism often lack the hormone melatonin, the chemical the brain produces to trigger sleep, so your child may have difficulty either getting to sleep or staying asleep. If so, speak to your healthcare provider or a specialist pediatrician who can prescribe melatonin, which can be given to your child before bedtime.

A child with a long-term illness

Most children experience occasional bouts of sickness. Fortunately, these are usually short and temporary, and a preschooler generally gets back on her feet within a few days. Sometimes, however, ill health persists and

TEACHING DIVERSITY

Your preschooler will have trouble understanding differences—whether of abilities, appearance, or behavior.

- 3-year-olds can describe skin color but don't understand the idea of race;
- 4-year-olds venture guesses as to why people are different (color, ability, sexual orientation, for example)—"she broke her leg so she has to sit in a wheelchair"—and may use "socially unacceptable" terms learned from others;
- 5-year-olds recognize that skin color and other attributes relate to race and that this is a permanent situation. They may also repeat prejudiced stereotypical remarks.

It is important to help your child understand that people are different, and to do so in a positive way. Whenever you hear your child tease or name call, or make comments about disability, culture, race, sexual orientation, or appearance, make sure you insist that he stops, and explain that such comments are hurtful and in the case of stereotypes, untrue. Point out what's wrong with stereotypes and try to discern where your child is getting his misinformation. If at nursery school, you may want to discuss this with the teacher.

Try and answer any questions your child has about differences in a helpful way; don't reinforce any misconceived ideas. When possible, point out differences, again in a positive way, so your child is given accurate information and not left to figure things out on his own.

chronic long-term sickness can have a huge psychological impact on a young child. Aside from the physical discomfort of ill health and all the medication she has to take, your preschooler's natural tendency is to be on the go the whole time, to play actively, and to seek stimulation wherever she can find it. That instinctive drive pushes a child this age. Ill health blocks that, resulting in boredom and restlessness; your child will hate being stuck in one place the whole time. So don't hold her back on the grounds that you are afraid for her. By all means follow the medical advice offered by those who are treating her, but don't insist she remains in bed all the time if she could be up at least for part of the day. Resist the urge to keep her tucked up in bed until she reaches perfect health.

True, when your child is sick, she looks so vulnerable that all you want to do is cuddle, protect, look after, and keep her safe from every germ and disease possible. You will do anything to restore her good health, to keep further illness at bay. While that is part of your job as a parent, you have to strike a balance between sensibly protecting her and unnecessarily stifling her.

An added problem is that a preschooler with long-term ill health is used to someone looking after her all the time. She expects to be the center of attention. Understandably, she likes being spoiled. That extra attention you give her makes her feel good and those special presents you buy to cheer her up are very effective. Naturally you should do everything you can to return your child to good health and there is no question that you should make a fuss of her. But don't overdo it. Try to return her life to normal, even if she hasn't made a full recovery. For instance, if she is able to walk at all, encourage her to stroll around when she has sufficient strength; then she can return to bed and rest once her brief walk has finished.

The same applies to letting her mix with her peers. Assuming her ill health is not caused by an infectious disease, and assuming that she is not especially vulnerable to infection, she would still benefit from playing with her pals. Invite them to your house. Your preschooler will cope better than you expect, as long as she has enough rest beforehand and the playdate is not too long. The fun and excitement of playing with her friends can be a very effective boost to her long-term recovery.

Illness, separation, and divorce

When mom or dad are unwell

Raising a preschooler isn't easy when you have ill health or have special needs yourself that significantly restrict your physical movement or lifestyle. You have plenty to do just managing your own needs, never mind having to worry about looking after your child. Where possible, try to limit the impact that your illness has on your preschooler's life—she wants to have as much fun and stimulation, and as many opportunities, as anyone else her age. For example, enlist the help of your partner, friends, or relatives if necessary when it

comes to taking her to nursery school or playgroup, if you are unable to take her there yourself. The more her life is like that of the typical child her age, the better.

You may worry that your own incapacity has an adverse affect on your preschooler's outlook on life, that she feels sorry for herself, and perhaps resents your limitations. But that won't happen. She won't grow up thinking that all her friends have a better life than her, or that she wishes she had different parents. Instead, your child accepts as normal what she sees around her each day. So she just gets on with her daily routine without feeling sorry for herself. When she is an adult, she might look back and begin to understand her family dynamics differently. For now, have confidence in yourself as a parent. As long as you do your best to give your child a full and satisfying life, she will be content without any resentment about your health issues.

Separation and divorce

If you have gone through (or are going through) separation or divorce, you'll already know the massive emotional impact that a family breakup has on the adults involved. The long buildup of disputes that led to the separation, the difficult decision to separate permanently, and then the huge upheaval that inevitably follows such a major relationship change, all take a powerful emotional toll on each partner, leaving you both drained. Your preschooler, too, has been caught up in all this turmoil. No matter what measures you took to protect her, never make the mistake of telling yourself that "She's too young to understand what's going on" because that would be a gross misjudgment. From the age of two or three, a child is very aware of her family surroundings and is finely tuned in to the verbal and nonverbal expressions of tension in her parents' relationship. By the age of four or five, her understanding is much better than you probably give her credit for.

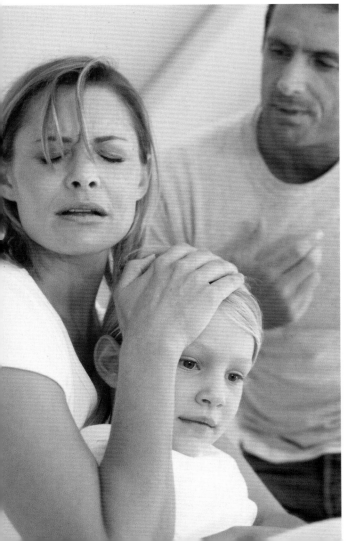

It's only natural when you are under emotional pressure associated with separation and divorce that you want to believe that your young child is oblivious to the disharmony. After all, that would give you one less thing to worry about during this stressful period in your life, and you would feel that she was safe and secure. However, the true position is vastly different. Far from being in a state of blissful ignorance about parental breakup, your preschooler follows each day's events closely. She may not talk about what happens, but she watches closely all the same. That's why you need to take her feelings seriously.

So if you find yourself in the unfortunate position of breaking permanently with your partner, you not only have to deal with your own emotional trauma, you also have to think of your preschooler because she will be affected by the family split too; she may even mistakenly blame herself for the breakup.

Telling your child

Research shows that the preschool children of divorced or separated parents are twice as likely to show signs of behavioral and emotional difficulties in playgroup and day care, and this is often caused in part by the parents' failure to consult their child about the family split and by their failure to provide an opportunity for her to express her feelings. In many instances of separation and divorce, neither parent talks directly to his or her preschool child when the breakup happens, some simply tell her that "Daddy's leaving," and others give no details to their preschooler at all.

There's no one "right" way to explain to your child that you and your partner are getting divorced, that you will no longer be living together as a family. Much depends on her maturity, understanding, personality, and previous experience of managing emotional stress. Sit with your preschooler so that she and you face each other, and calmly explain that mom and dad are separating because they don't get along any more. Make sure she understands that it is not her fault, that she is not to blame; it's worth repeating this several times because children often irrationally feel responsible for their parents' divorce.

YOUR CHILD'S WORRIES

Here are some of the questions that he might ask when you explain that mom and dad are not getting along and that one of you is leaving:

- Will I see my mommy/daddy again?
- Where will my mommy/daddy live?
- Will my mommy/daddy be safe and well?
- What will happen to me?
- Will I have to change my nursery school?
- Who else knows about this?
- Will I have to tell my friends?
- Am I getting a new mommy/daddy?
- Was this my fault?
- Have I been a bad boy?

A child usually adjusts better to her family breakup when she continues to keep in contact with both parents. So reassure yours that her mother and father still love her very much, and that she will continue to see both of you even though you will live in different houses from now on. Resist any temptation to ease the emotional impact of divorce by giving your preschooler false hope about a possible parental reconciliation unless that is a genuine possibility; well intentioned promises that are misleading will only cause more confusion in her young mind.

Emphasize to your preschooler that her home life will continue as before, that she won't lose her friends or have to change nursery school or childcare arrangements, and that you (the custodial parent) and she will continue to live in your present home (unless, of course, your change in domestic circumstances forces a such a change). She wants life to continue as before, as much as possible. Comfort and cuddle her and let her ask any questions she wants—answer her honestly while trying to be optimistic about your future life as a single-parent family. Your confidence will further reassure her.

Be ready for a range of possible reactions from your preschooler when you reveal to her that you are separating. Maybe she'll burst out crying, or maybe she'll just stare blankly at you. Each child responds in her own way to this type of news. Try to anticipate some of the questions she might ask and have a good answer prepared. Bear in mind that she'll probably harbor a secret hope that her parents will get back together again after this upset in your relationship has settled. These discussions can be very difficult to handle and you may find that you become tearful yourself, but that's much better than avoiding such a discussion altogether.

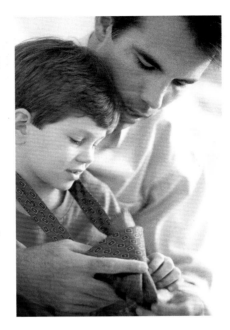

Next steps

Watch your child's behavior very closely in the following days, weeks, and months, being sensitive to any indications that might signify her deeper unhappiness, for instance, becoming withdrawn, fighting more with her playmates, or a lack of interest in her toys. Talk to your child regularly about her nursery school, friends, and family so that she has plenty of opportunities to express her feelings to you. Of course, you need to be careful not to overdo this or she will just clam up with boredom—it's a matter of striking the right balance.

As life after the separation or divorce begins to settle down, encourage your child to see her father (or mother). Resist any temptation to make her take your side against your ex; if she is forced to choose one parent over the other, that would only create tremendous pressure and distress. She loves both of you and wants to remain loyal to each one—she doesn't want to choose between you, so don't make her. And no matter how bitter you might feel about your family split, avoid using your child as a weapon to get back at your partner (for example, criticizing your partner in front of your preschooler). The temptation to gain revenge for the mess you are in

right now can be very strong, but don't involve your preschooler since that is likely to undermine your child's sense of security even further.

Finally, do your best to ensure your child maintains regular contact with your ex even if your own relationship is strained. Bear in mind that children who adjust best to the divorce of their parents are the ones who have regular contact with their noncustodial parent. No matter how difficult life becomes for you and your ex, your child's dad is still her dad; her mom is still her mom. So help arrange contact visits and do everything that you can to encourage your child to attend.

At some stage in the future, you are likely to want to introduce a new partner to your preschooler, perhaps sooner than you expect. Do this gradually, to give your child time to adjust to the fact that you are friendly with someone else other than her father or mother. Your child will remain loyal to her parents and may resent any new relationship. Don't worry about that, just take your time. Probably the biggest mistake made in this situation is for the new partner to assume parenting responsibilities too soon. Many months will pass before your preschooler is ready for that.

Living in a family broken up by separation or divorce is never easy, especially in the early stages. Yet the long-term prospects for the children can be positive. When a child's psychological needs are met by her parents, the chances are that she'll adjust to her new family structure without any long-lasting emotional damage. Reassure yourself with the thought that life will eventually get better for you and your child, despite the possibly bleak outlook at the moment. Your positive attitude to the future will rub off on her.

Helping your child cope with bereavement

Sadly, many preschoolers have to deal with the loss of a loved one, most commonly the death of a grandparent but sometimes the death of a parent, a sibling, or even a close friend. Your young child can even be deeply affected by the death of her pet, and her own ill health (or the ill health of a close relative) may cause her to start thinking about mortality. Unfortunately, learning to cope with bereavement and grief is often part of childhood.

Don't make the common mistake of assuming that your preschooler is too young to grieve—that's wrong. At her age, she can experience many of the emotions that a mourning adult feels. Even though the initial shock on hearing about a bereavement is often less intense in a young child than in a teenager or adult, the grieving process can still be strong and lengthy. However, your preschooler probably understands death differently from the way you do.

She may not fully grasp the finality and irreversibility of death, and she may react in ways you don't expect. For instance, one minute your four-year-old might tell you that she knows grandma has died and gone to heaven, and the next minute she might add that she is going to draw a picture to give to her.

Grief reactions

Each child reacts differently when becoming aware of the loss of a loved one. Some preschoolers are very tearful when the news is broken to them, while others just shrug their shoulders and get on with whatever they were doing at the time. Don't assume that your preschooler copes well with bereavement just because she smiles a lot; she may hurt beneath her facade of contentment. She needs time to adjust. A preschooler who appeared to be completely unmoved when told

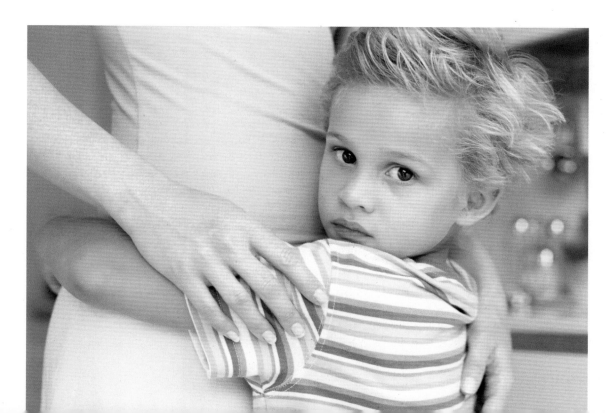

IF A PET DIES

Very often, a pet dying is a preschooler's first experience of grief. Even if the pet is naturally shortlived (a gold fish, for example) or has been sick or aging for some time, your child will still feel the loss keenly.

Help by explaining that all creatures have a particular life span and that it can be cruel, too, to try and prolong the life of a pet if it is sick or simply too old to enjoy its normal life (a dog, for example, likes to run around and sniff things, not lie down in its bed all day).

Spend time together recollecting the good times you had with the pet and reassure your child that he did everything he could to look after it. Then suggest your child help you to bury the pet or otherwise perform a formal "farewell." Perhaps your child wants to create a memorial of sorts. Afterward, don't rush to replace the pet but wait to see whether your child expresses a desire to have another (of the same type or a different one).

You could use the death of a pet to explain death in general. While it's true that the death of even a beloved cat or dog might not prepare your child completely for a grandparent's death, it can go some way to teach your child that death occurs to all and that grieving is part of the process. Make sure you emphasize, however, that good times do continue.

might start to show an outward reaction several days later. Keep a close watch over her in the days and weeks following a family or friendship bereavement.

The most common response is shock, that is, an overwhelming surge of stunned sadness when your child is first informed of the death. It may be that she had never considered the possibility of death before that moment. She could be tearful, passive, quiet, angry, or even aggressive. In some instances, a preschooler might act as if the death hasn't taken place at all, for instance, she talks about her dead relative as though that person is still alive—if so, let her, because she'll face the facts when she is psychologically ready. Bear in mind that any loss of a loved one can make a child frightened and insecure because she worries that others may die too. That's why she may become clingy and needy, desperate for your constant attention.

Another way you can help your young child cope is by encouraging her to say what she feels. Pick a quiet time and chat with her in private about what she thinks about the dead person. Listen carefully.

A warm cuddle from you may just be what she needs to help her through this difficult time; a loving gesture like that makes her feel better. Very young children are able to release their inner feelings through creative or imaginative play, especially when they have difficulty verbalizing their emotions. Your preschooler might like to talk about the dead person, perhaps looking at photographs and other momentos in order to discuss the deceased with you. Most local libraries have books about bereavement, which have been especially written for children either to read or to have read to them.

If your child is four or five years old, she may search for a deeper explanation from you and may ask probing questions about death. One of the major difficulties you face when discussing the topic with her is that you probably haven't worked out your own feelings about death, and you may feel that you don't have an adequate explanation for your child. After all, nobody fully understands death. The situation becomes even more difficult if you need to have this discussion because someone close to your child has died; then you have the added problem of coping with your own grief at the same time. That's why some parents prefer to introduce the subject before their child has to face it in reality.

Your child's reaction to a conversation around bereavement will be linked in part to the way you present your ideas. So if you become distressed during a discussion about death, and show her that you are afraid, there is every possibility that she will also become confused and afraid. Try to be calm and

ways to help your child grieve

1. **Prepare him for the inevitable:** if a family member or someone close to him becomes terminally ill, share your concerns about the situation (in an appropriate way) and let your child, if circumstances allow, visit the person and later on, say "goodbye."

2. **Be sensitive to his need for security.** This is particularly important if a parent dies, because your preschooler will worry that his remaining parent will die, too and may become overly anxious if you are late arriving home or get sick. Sticking to his regular schedule and routine will help reassure him.

3. **Address any unexpressed emotions.** Every child occasionally experiences jealousy and hateful thoughts toward a sibling, so if one dies, your preschooler may feel he is to blame.

Assure him that any bad behavior or feelings between the two are natural and were quickly forgotten. Or, your preschooler may be angry that his sibling has "gotten himself killed." Such feelings are legitimate and shouldn't be supressed.

4. **Share your feelings.** Your preschooler may find it easier to share his grief if he sees your unhappiness, rather than you trying to "be brave for him." Talk about the person who has died—both the good things and those you found annoying (don't create a saint from a sinner) and keep a photograph of him or her on display. Involve your child, too, later on, when the anniversary of the death comes around. Ask him how would he like to mark the occasion?

sensitive on the outside, despite any possible inner feelings of anxiety.

Reassure your preschooler that she shouldn't worry about this, just in case she becomes anxious that people in her family will also die. Explain to her that everyone she loves will be safe and well for a long time to come (even though you can't actually offer such a cast-iron guarantee). Before you start giving your own explanation of death, ask her what she thinks about it already—you may be surprised at what she says. And be aware that children aged five or younger have great difficulty understanding complex concepts whether it's "death," "justice," or "artistic beauty." Explanations of death, therefore, should be kept as basic and as simple as possible.

The actual way you express your views about death, and the words and concepts that you use, will depend on your understanding, religious beliefs, and personal experience. Some parents tell their child that the dead person has gone to heaven and is with the angels. Others says that death is like going to

sleep and never waking up, and that there is no pain involved. Again, it is up to you to select your own particular approach. Whatever slant you adopt, you should cover two aspects of death. First, talk about the deceased's body, because most young children focus mainly on that. You could explain to your child, for example, that a dead body doesn't feel anything anymore, but that your child can still love someone even though that person's body has no feelings. Second, talk about the spirit. This will be influenced by your own religious beliefs. You could explain that the dead person's spirit lives on because those living remember him or her, or say the person's spirit dies with him or her, or even that the person's spirit is in heaven. There is no one "right" or "wrong" approach to this sensitive area. Be ready to admit to your young child that you don't have all the answers—that's much better than getting yourself all tied up in knots.

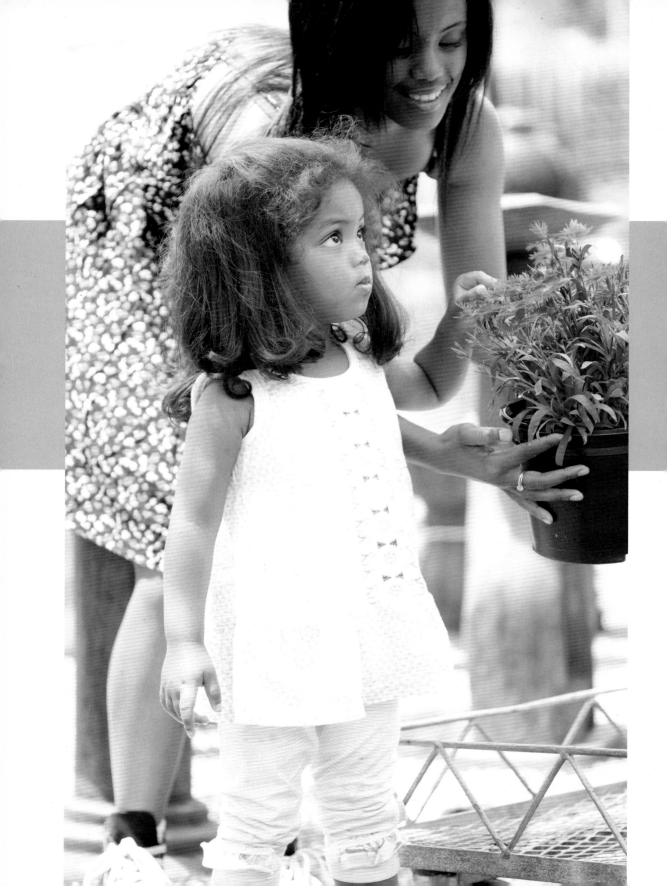

CHAPTER 6
YOUR CHILD'S WELL-BEING

What do you need to know to keep your child in good health, to childproof your home, and to care for your child if he gets sick or has an accident? How can you recognize ill health and emergencies and keep your child safe when he is away from home? Here is the vital information you need to know in all such situations—and it's a good idea to become familiar with this chapter's contents before anything untoward happens.

Keeping your preschooler safe at home

Young children are naturally inquisitive, and fascinated by everything around them. It is your task as a parent to allow your child to explore his world as much as possible, but at the same time to keep him safe and well, and to teach him to become aware of likely hazards. These "lessons" can help keep him safe as he grows up. Most children have accidents because they develop so quickly that parents can't keep up (how many times have you heard the phrase, "I didn't know he could do that!"?) and have no sense of danger. You need to ensure your child doesn't have an accident because he exercises newly found skills unsafely.

You will already have had a good look at your home as your child developed from a baby who lay in his cradle to a crawling, walking, and climbing toddler and put a number of safety measures in place. However, it's important to review any measures you have taken on a room-by-room basis

every few months, to take account of any newly acquired skills. In addition, your preschooler will be involved in more and more adventurous activities outside his home, for example, learning to ride a scooter, pedal a bicycle, swim, try roller skates, or even take part in group activities or sports. There are important safely issues with each activity.

Supervising your child

The only way to be sure that your child is safe is to be aware of what he is doing at all times. The level of supervision your preschool child needs changes as he matures. Three- to four-year-olds require constant supervision; four- to six-year-olds may be able to play on their own but within earshot. For most younger children, supervision entails a parent or responsible adult being in the same room while they play, being aware of their activities, but not questioning everything they do; a few children,

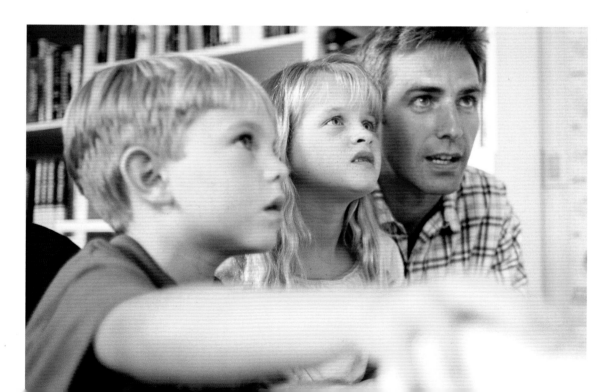

however, may require much closer monitoring. Older children will need some independence, so it will be even more important to ensure that your preschooler's surroundings are safe when he plays on his own.

When you are out and about, at the playground, park or local sports center, for example, make sure the equipment is in good condition, and stay with your child at all times. Teach him safe playground practices like not walking behind swings, waiting to go down the slide until the last child gets off and then getting off quickly himself, and holding onto ladders and climbing frames with both hands. If he's leaning to ride a scooter or bike (or to skate), make sure that it is well serviced and that he is protected with a helmet and/or knee and elbow pads as

necessary (see also page 212). Bear in mind, however, that whatever precautions you take, no situation is ever completely hazard free. Familiarize yourself with the first-aid technques on pages 230 to 245 so that you can act quickly and confidently if an accident does occur.

Accident-proofing your home

Most accidents do happen in and around the home, but by eliminating as many of the obvious dangers as far as you can, and carefully supervising your child, you can reduce the risks.

Keep your home as uncluttered and clean as possible (easier said than done with young children) to protect your child from infections and food poisoning—but don't be overanxious. Contact with some bacteria and viruses help a child build up his immunity to disease. Store food safely and don't consume items beyond the manufacturer's recommended use-by dates.

Make sure all keys (for the door, car, garage, mailbox, and shed) are kept well out of your child's reach; this will not only stop him using them, but also stops him from picking them up and hiding them so you can't find them when you need them.

Hall, stairs and landing

Keep stairs and corridors clear of toys and other objects and make sure they are well lit. Never leave anything on the stairs; this will become a trip hazard. You will still need to keep stair gates on the top and bottom of the stairs. If your child likes his bedroom door open at night, it is worth putting another gate across his bedroom doorway in case he sleepwalks in the night.

- If you have rugs, make sure they have a nonslip backing and that the edges are not folded under; its all too easy to trip on them.
- Fit night lights on the landing. This is especially useful once your child is old enough to go to the bathroom by himself at night.

Doors and windows

- Wedge doors open during the daytime, or fit door-slam protectors to prevent a child's fingers from becoming trapped as the door closes. Don't let your child play on doors—swinging on the handle, for example—because there's a risk of his fingers getting caught.
- Put a chain on the front door of your home so that your child can't open the door. Put the main lock as high as is safe and put the chain above it.
- If you have a bolt or lock on the bathroom door, put it toward the top of the door so that your child can't accidentally lock himself in to the bathroom.
- Make sure patio doors are made from toughened glass, which does not break into sharp pieces if someone falls against it or something is thrown at it. You also can place stickers on the glass to ensure your child can see that the glass is there.

- Put safety catches or locks on windows on the upper levels of your home so that the window only partially opens and your child can't open it and climb out. Don't put furniture under windows either, as children can use it to climb up to a window.
- If you have cord-operated blinds or curtains, or rope tie backs, hook the cords or ties well out of reach of your child; any cord longer than 7 inches presents a strangulation risk.

In the kitchen

You still need the protective devices you installed when your child first became mobile, such as stove guard shields and stove knob covers, as well as childproof cupboard latches. But now, your child may insist on "helping" you in the kitchen. If so, give him safe tasks like stirring the cake batter or measuring dry and liquid ingredients; keep him well away from hot pans and knives.

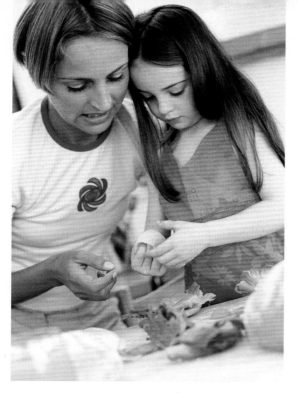

- Make sure kitchen trash cans always have a firmly fitting lid. Empty the main garbage can regularly. Always wrap sharp objects in paper and tape the parcel before putting it into the garbage. If you have a number of recyling bins taking different contents, encourage your child to learn about what goes in each one, but discourage him from taking things out of them! Ideally keep all bins in a storage cupboard or out of easy reach.
- Make sure your child is always sitting down when he has anything to eat or drink; there is a high risk of choking if he walks around with a snack or beverage.
- Keep all cleaning materials well out of his reach and buy products that have child-resistant tops.
- Don't carry hot drinks around yourself when there are young children running around the house. And don't leave them near the edge of a table or countertop for your small child to reach up and grab.

BE ALERT!

ONLINE SAFETY

Children learn to use computers, tablets, smart phones, and even interactive televisions from a very young age. While the internet can be a wonderful resource for you and them, it also can be a source of unwanted material, and children can accidentally download expensive or inappropriate games.
    To prevent this you should:

- Talk to your child about any concerns you may have.
- Create a "favorites" folder with your child's name on it and add some safe sites to it; that way she does not need to look anywhere else on the computer.
- Monitor your child's use of a computer. Keep the computer in the main living room where you can see what she is looking at; don't let your child have the computer in her bedroom.
- Install parental control software that lets you block your child's access to websites with adult material, track online activity, and help protect your child from internet predators.
- Avoid selecting "remember password" panels, and don't let your child know your passwords.
    In addition, tell your child to:
- Let you know if she sees something that makes her feel uncomfortable.
- Never give out passwords or personal details to anyone.
- Always check with you before downloading or installing software or moving to a new level of a game.

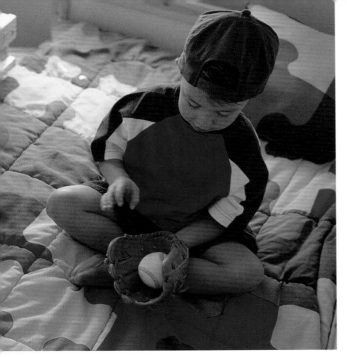

trip hazards if he gets out, or for you to trip on when you check on him last thing at night. You can store his toys on a shelf, or in storage boxes that slide under the bed. If you want him to stay in his room but don't want to shut the door, put a safety gate across the entrance instead.

Protect your family from fire risks

Install combination smoke/fire detector and carbon monoxide alarms that comply with fire-department approved safety regulations on every level of your

Electricity

Keep cords and extension cords tucked away behind furniture so there's no temptation to pull on the cords or any risk of tripping over them. Don't overload sockets because this can be a fire risk.

A wide range of very inexpensive but efficient child-resistant adapter and plug covers are available in many styles, along with power strip covers, some with a key that is sold separately or in sets with locks to fit a normal-sized surge protector. Some styles of outlet covers keep the exposed electrical outlets and plugs covered even when they are in use.

Your child's bedroom

Most preschoolers sleep in a full-size bed or one that starts short and can be extended to its full length when they are older; some small children feel lost in a full-length bed. If your child hasn't been in his long, position it against the wall, if possible, and put a fold-down bed guard along one side while he gets used to it. Choose a bed that is not too high because it won't be so far to fall if he happens to roll out of bed in the night.

Once your child is in a bed he is more likely to get out in the night, so encourage him to put his toys away before he goes to bed so that there are no

WHAT TO DO IF THERE IS A FIRE

- Call 911 for the fire department, then guide everyone out of your home following your agreed plan; carry your children if necessary.
- If making a call will cause delay, get everyone out of the building first, then call 911.
- Keep as low as possible while making an escape; as smoke rises, the air at the floor level will be clearer.
- If you can't get out of the house, or get to a phone, shut any doors between you and the fire and shout for help from a window, ideally at the front of the house. If you need to breathe clearer air, lean out of the window. Keep drawing attention to yourself. If the window is locked try breaking it with a heavy object. Strike the corner of the window to break the glass.
- If you are trapped in a room, put a heavy rug or blanket against the bottom of the door to stop the smoke from coming in.
- Always feel doors with your hand before opening them. If a door feels hot don't open it as you may fan the fire.
- Once out of the building DO NOT go back in for any reason.

home—ideally in central areas such as the hall and landings. Check the alarms at least once a week and, if they are battery operated, replace batteries as necessary, but at least once a year. If the alarm nearest your kitchen keeps going off when you're cooking, either move it farther away or replace it with one that has a hush feature or one that's "toast proof." Never take the battery out while you are cooking because you may forget to replace it.

Work out and agree a realistic escape plan—it can can save vital minutes and help ensure you get your family out. It is also advisable to have a room in which you could all stay if for some reason you cannot escape. Make sure everyone in the family knows what to do and practice the plan with your child, whatever his age. This will not only reassure him but without one, if there is a fire, your child will be scared and may be tempted to hide, taking him longer to escape or for you to rescue him.

Turn off all appliances every night before you go to bed—don't be tempted to run the dishwasher or washing machine through the night. Close doors and windows, make sure cigarettes and candles are completely extinguished. Keep matches, firelighters, or gas stove lighters well out reach of children. If you have an open fire or wood-burning stove, make sure there is a secure fireguard around it that is fixed to the wall on both sides.

Install fire extinguishers in key places around the house, especially in the kitchen. Make sure you choose the appropriate type: some are universal, some only work on electrical fires. Check the National Fire Protection Association's website (www.nfpa.org) or ring the local fire department safety officer for advice if you are in any doubt. Keep a fire blanket in the kitchen.

Check that the hall and stairs are clear at night because you don't want to be tripping over things in the rush to escape if a fire breaks out, especially if the house is filled with thick black smoke.

Pet and animal safety

Teach your child to treat all animals with respect from the outset. Many pets are child-friendly and love children, but boisterous, young children can frighten even the most placid pets if they are not used to children. Children under the age of four are most at risk from dog bites.

Animals can spread infections. For example, reptiles spread salmonella and dogs and cats can have dirty claws that carry infection. A bite or scratch from a cat (most commonly a kitten) can cause cat scratch disease (see page 231). Dogs and cats that spend a lot of time outside, especially in woodland, can pick up ticks, which spread Lyme disease (see page 232). If you have a dog or cat, it should be checked for ticks regularly in addition to receiving regular preventative tick treatment.

Tell your child not to touch dog or cat feces or vomit as they carry infections. Cat feces also carries a disease-causing parasite, *Toxoplasma gondii*, which can be left in garden soil. The parasite causes toxoplasmosis, which produces mild flulike symptoms, such as high temperature, sore throat, and aching muscles, but in those with a weaker immune system, such as a young child, it can lead to complications. If you have a cat, you should wear

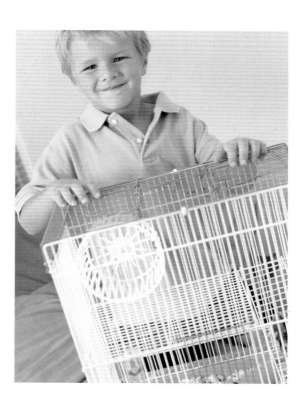

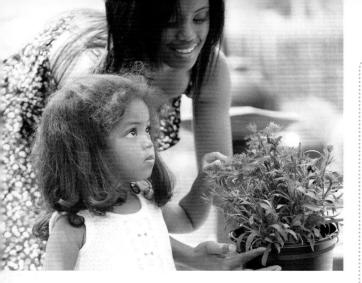

COMMON POISONOUS PLANTS

The following contain particular compounds that have been known to cause adverse reactions in people and animals.

Amaryllis	English Ivy
Anemone	Holly
Azalea	Hyacinth
Buttercup	Hydrangea
Calla lily	Iris
Chrysanthemums	Jerusalem Cherry
Cyclamen	Lily of the valley
Daffodil	Mistletoe
Delphinium	Philodendron
Dumb cane	Rhododendron
Poinsettia	Swiss-cheese plant

gloves when gardening, and encourage your child to do the same if he helps you.

Contact with animal fur can cause allergies. If your child develops an allergy to fur, consider having a pet that does not shed its fur, such as a poodle, for example. Keep pets out of bedrooms, just in case.

Teach your child not to approach animals he doesn't know well, even if it's a friend's pet. Always ask an owner if a dog is safe and if so how it likes to be stroked. Learn about animal body language yourself so that you can help your child: never approach a dog that has a stiff body posture; it is not comfortable—relaxed dogs are much safer. If a dog walks away or backs away from you, it does not want you close. When a dog is afraid it cowers and may hide under furniture. It might even put its ears flat back, show its teeth, snarl, or growl.

Show your child how to handle pets; it may be some time before he completely understands, but it's worth starting young. Explain to him that he should never squeeze an animal, drop it, fall on it, pick it up too quickly, tease it, pull its tail or ears, disturb it if it is eating, sleeping, or tending its young, or take a toy or bone away from a dog. He also should wash his hands after handling a pet, and never encourage a dog to the dinner table.

Plants, flowers, and gardens

It's fairly common for young children to eat household plants or cut flowers, so make sure none of yours are poisonous (see box). Put vases of cut flowers or pot plants well out of your child's reach so that he can't drink the plant water or pull them over (plant pots can be heavy and could cause a head injury). Check your yard, too. Remove plants that have poisonous leaves flowers or berries, or fence them off so your child is not tempted to pick or eat them. If you are unsure about the plants in your garden (you have just moved house, for example), look online for lists and images of poisonous plants that grow in your horticultural zone.

- Fix a childproof lock to each garden gate and put them as high as you can.
- Take great care around water. Swimming pools should have a fence that's at least 4 feet high with a self-locking, self-closing gate. Ponds and water features should also have a high fence around them, or better still be removed; wait until your child is much older before reinstalling one. Paddling pools should be emptied immediately after use and turned upside down.
- Lock the tool shed. A shed may be full of tools, machinery, and chemicals that are highly dangerous in a child's hands. If there are toys that your child uses in the garden, keep them in a separate, designated shed.

Keeping your preschooler safe away from home

You and your child can have fun exploring the world outside your home. You are his teacher not only about the things she will see and experience but also about keeping safe when away from home. It's important to make sure that the places you take her are as safe as they can be but also to supervise her at all times. Hold her hand when you are out walking. Make sure she stays with you in stores. Teach her safe practices in the playground and if she's doing something sporty, ensure she has on the right protective gear. If you are traveling, make sure that you and she have all the right immunizations before you leave (see page 217).

Cars and roads

It is essential to keep your child as safe as possible in and around cars. If you have a driveway and need to move your car, make sure your child is in the house under the supervision of an adult, or strap her into her car seat while you maneuver the car. Always hold her hand when walking in a parking lot; other drivers can't always see small children.

Child passenger restraint requirements vary from by state based on age, weight, and height. The Governor's Highway Safety Association website (www.ghsa.org) lists the web address of every state highway office, so you can check local regulations.

Preschoolers must use booster seats, and that includes other people's children in your car or your child in someone else's car. Adult's seat belts are not safe for children because they sit too high on a child's chest and a child could be injured in an accident if wearing one.

Make sure that the booster seat fits your car, and choose car seats that are easy to fit, especially if you have to move them from one car to another, for example when a babysitter or grandparent looks after your child. Most cars have attachments for car

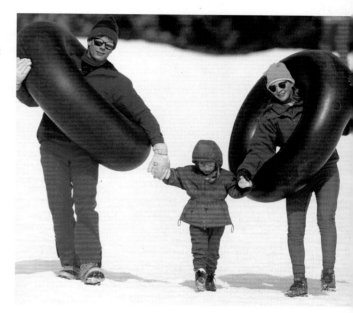

seats, which is the safest way to secure the car seat. Many states require all children to ride in the rear seat. It is safer to put car seats on the back seats of the car; they can only be put on the front passenger seat if there is no airbag, or the airbag is switched off. Activate the child locks so that your child cannot open the doors while you are driving (it's amazing how many children try to do this).

Some airlines let you take your child's car seat onto a plane and she can sit in it during the flight, then you can use it in a rental car, though most car rental companies will provide car seats. However, always check the seat carefully before you use it.

Tricycles and bicycles

All children love ride-on toys and they are an excellent way to help them develop the essential important motor skills such as coordination (pedaling) and balance (on a scooter, balance bike,

LEARNING TO CROSS THE ROAD

You play a key role in educating your child about road safety, even though it will be a long time before he will understand the dangers and can do it on his own. Start showing him how to cross the road safely as soon as you can—this can even be while he is still in his stroller. If you are walking together, hold his hand, and tell him you are looking for a safe place to cross the road. It should be well away from parked cars, and ideally on a designated crossing. Tell him to stop, look both way, and listen. Explain that he must only cross when the cars have stopped at a crossing or the road is completely clear. You can also set an example by not wearing earpods or headphones or talking on your cell phone or texting while crossing the road.

Bear in mind when teaching your child how to cross a road that children under the age of 10 years are:

- Easily distracted and focus on only one aspect of what is happening;
- Small and so drivers can't always see them;
- Less predictable than other pedestrians;
- Cannot accurately judge the speed and distance of moving vehicles;
- Cannot accurately predict the direction sounds are coming from;
- Don't understand abstract ideas such as road safety;
- Can't identify safe places to cross the road.

ride-on toy for your child to reduce the risk of accidents; some scooters and bikes are adjustable and can be extended as your child grows. Put a cycling helmet on your child every time she rides a scooter, tricycle, or bike, whether it's in your backyard or out in the park. A correctly fitted helmet can reduce significantly the risk of head injury; check the fit regularly and get a new one as soon as she grows out of it. Buy a new one if she ever has an accident and lands on her head; she may be fine but the helmet could be damaged. If your child wants to try roller skates or wheelie shoes, make sure she wears elbow, knee, and wrist protectors as well. Once she progresses to a bicycle, fit training wheels initially to help her balance, and reduce the risk of injury. If your child is on any ride-on equipment always stick to the sidewalks, or the park. If you have to cross a road, make her get off and push it across with you.

Children also enjoy riding on your bicycle with you and it's a great way for you to stay fit. Always

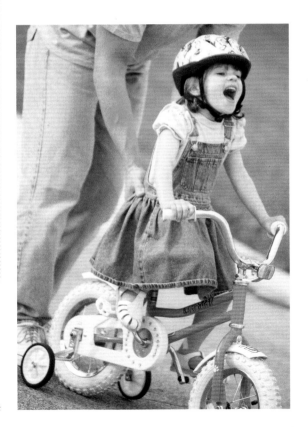

or later a bicycle). But children can also fall off in the learning process.

Children start riding scooters and tricycles from about the age of two, but don't progress to a bicycle until the age of five—although pedal-less balance bikes can be ridden earlier. Always buy the right size

STRANGER DANGER

Parents always say to their children: "Don't talk to strangers." But sometimes children actually need to talk to strangers—they need to know what to do if they become separated from you in a shopping mall, for example. Who else will they turn to if they're lost and need help?

The best advice is to tell your child that if a stranger ever approaches him and offers him a ride or asks for help with a task (like helping find a lost dog or child), your child should step away, firmly shout "No!", leave the area immediately, and call for help to draw attention to the situation. Tell your child that if this ever happens to him, he must tell you or another trusted adult (such as a teacher or caregiver) immediately. The same applies if anyone—whether a stranger, family member, or friend—asks your child to keep a secret, tries to touch your child in an inappropriate way, or asks your child to touch them.

Teach your child to judge people by their actions not looks. Children will be naturally wary of mean-looking strangers. However, most child molesters and abductors go out of their way to look friendly, safe, and appealing to children.

Tell your child that if he is ever separated from you, he should try to find a person in uniform, like a police officer, security guard, or sales assistant, or go into a store and ask at the first counter he comes to. If there are no uniformed people, then older people, other mothers, or people with children may be able to help. And again, remind him about instincts: if your child doesn't have a good feeling about a certain person, he should approach someone else.

strap your child into a secure child bike seat that meets 1625-00 standard, and put her cycling helmet on; and always wear a helmet yourself. Wear high visibility reflective clothing, but also remember to put something fluorescent on your child as well.

Stay safe with water

Supervise your child at all times when you are near water, whether you are in the backyard in a paddling pool, at the local municipal swimming pool, on the beach, by a river or lake, or on a boat—even when she is in the bathtub at home. Don't take your eyes off her for a second.

◆ Take your child to swimming classes as soon as she's old enough. Swimming is a life skill and the earlier a child learns the better, and the less likely she is to develop a fear of water. Many pools and sports clubs start with water awareness for parents and babies, progressing to "proper" lessons from the age of three or four years old.

◆ Choose pools where she can stay in her own depth initially until she is confident in the water; give her arm bands or long foam floats to help support her until she can swim.

◆ If you are going to the seaside, choose public beaches with lifeguards and stay in the area designated as being overseen by the lifeguards.

• Don't let your child use inflatable toys or water buoyancy aids in the ocean because they can quickly be swept out to sea; the current can be deceptively strong.

◆ Don't let your child swim in canals, rivers, or lakes, unless there are designated, lifeguard-supervised beaches along the edge. Water depths change very quickly, the deep water can also be very cold (even on a hot day), and it is often difficult to see what lurks at the bottom. Many rivers and lakes also have dense reeds or objects hidden just below the water's surface..

◆ If you are going out on a boat on a lake, river, or at sea, everyone on board must wear a personal flotation device, such as a life jacket, at all times. Make sure children sit in the center of the boat away from the edge.

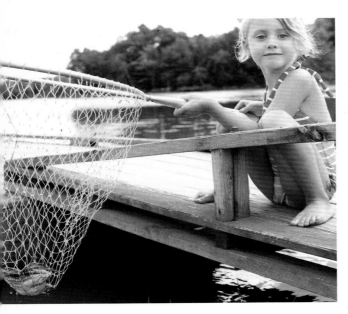

using, check that there are no dangerous materials, like broken glass or twisted metal, on the ground.

The playground should be fenced off and dogs not be allowed in the area. Swings, seesaws, and other equipment with moving parts should be set away from the rest of the playground. Toddler swings with bucket seats should have their own bay.

Always supervise your child in a playground and make sure she does not engage in unsafe behavior. Young children can't distinguish distance or foresee dangerous situations and they often want to test their limits.

Playgrounds and play centers

Whether indoors or in the park, children love playgrounds, and climbing and sliding on the equipment are excellent ways for them to develop motor skills. Make sure the equipment is in good condition and clean before letting your child loose on it. All equipment must comply with Consumer Product Safety Commission regulations. If you see any defective equipment always let the local authorities, or play-center management know.

The safest playgrounds have areas designated especially for younger children, which are away from those for more boisterous older ones. Younger children should not play on equipment designed for older kids because the equipment sizes and proportions won't be right for them, which can lead to injury.

Ideal outdoor playground surfaces are cushioned with wood chips or rubber, for example, not tarmac, grass, soil, or packed earth, and should extend at least 6 feet beyond the equipment. No surfacing materials should be considered safe if the combined height of playground equipment and the child (standing on the highest platform) is higher than 11 feet. Playground surfaces should be free of standing water and debris such as rocks, tree stumps, and roots, which could cause children to trip. Before

TRAMPOLINES

Children love trampolines and they are a great way to work off excess energy but they are also the cause of a lot of accidents, particularly in children under the age of six years.

- ◆ Choose a trampoline suitable for children under the age of six years;
- ◆ Consider models that have safety net as part of the design, or purchase a safety cage when you buy the trampoline;
- ◆ If you have the space, dig a hole in the ground the size and depth of the trampoline so that it can be at ground level;
- ◆ Place the trampoline in an area clear from hazards such as trees, fences, clothes lines, poles, or other equipment. Ideally there should be a safe fall zone around the trampoline of at least 8 feet;
- ◆ Supervise your child at all times and never allow more than one person on the trampoline at the same time;
- ◆ Make sure your child only bounces in the middle of the trampoline, and never let him bounce out of the trampoline cage when he gets off.

Indoor soft-play play centers should provide supervisors, but you should also remain aware of your child's activities. Many of these centres are large and on several levels so it can be difficult to see your child all of the time. There should also be trained first aiders available in case of an accident. Surfaces should be mats made of safety-tested rubber or rubberlike materials. If the playcenter has a multi-story frame, the exposed support beams should be padded as well. Find out how often the play center is cleaned; this is especially important if there is a ball-pit section in the play area.

Organized activities

There are many clubs and organizations that run team activities, such as soccer or gymnastics, for children as young as three years of age. Coaching children under the age of eight presents its own unique set of challenges primarily due to the children's developmental immaturity, short attention span, and less developed muscles. If you take your child to one of these groups make sure that all the coaches are trained and understand the sport and the limitations of young children. They must also adhere to all child protection laws as well as health and safety guidelines—especially if some of the leaders are volunteers. There should always be personnel trained in first aid present. If your child is injured make sure all symptoms have been resolved before returning to the activity; a child who sustains a head injury should not be allowed to return to the activity unless a doctor has checked her.

Check the playing surfaces the children are using: indoor flooring should be splinter-free, and field turf outside should be clear of hazards and animal feces. Ensure that there is drinking water available; always make sure your child is well hydrated before she starts playing.

Winter activities

Snow and ice provide the opportunity for doing many activities that young children enjoy: playing in the snow, throwing snowballs, tobogganing, ice skating, even skiing if you are near mountains. But as with everything it's important to stay safe.

- ◆ Your child needs to wrap up in sensible winter clothing to prevent hypothermia (see page 244); she'll need a warm coat, gloves or mittens, and a hat. Scarves can become caught in toboggans, bicycle wheels, and playground equipment, so are not a good idea.
- ◆ If your child is skiing, skating, or tobogganing, she should also wear a winter sports helmet; it's all too easy to slip on ice and snow, which can result in a serious head injury (see page 241).
- ◆ If you take your child skiing, she will also need goggles or sunglasses and plenty of sunblock on her face. She can be burned by the sunlight that reflects off the snow even on an overcast day.
- ◆ If you take your child tobogganing choose a short gentle slope. Avoid slopes that end near ponds, trees, fences, or parking lots, and check to make sure that the hill is free of obstacles. Choose places that are snowy rather than icy; icy slopes make for hard landings.

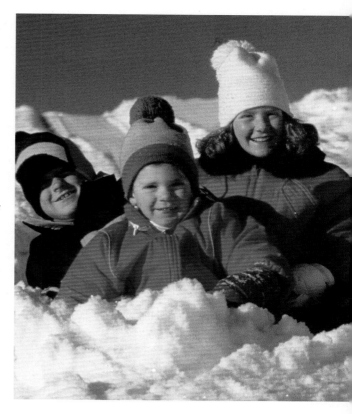

Sun safety

Everyone needs some sunshine because it's a main source of Vitamin D, which helps the body absorb the calcium needed for healthy bone growth; but you don't need that much. Young children especially should stay out of sun as much as possible since their skin is very delicate. There are dangers to too much sun exposure. Sunlight emits invisible ultraviolet rays which, when they reach skin, can tan it but can also burn it.

There are three types of ultraviolet ray: UVA rays cause skin aging and wrinkling and contribute to skin cancers, such as melanoma. UVB rays cause sunburn, cataracts, and can affect the immune system and contribute to skin cancer. Melanoma, the most dangerous form of skin cancer, is thought to be associated with severe UVB sunburn that occurs before the age of 20. Most UVB rays are absorbed by the ozone layer that surrounds the Earth, but enough pass through to cause serious damage. UVC rays are the most dangerous but they don't reach Earth because they are blocked by the ozone layer. Skin produces melanin to protect it from UV rays. However, the fairer a person is, the less melanin there is in her skin, and therefore the risk of burning is greater.

If your child is out in the sun cover up as much of her skin as possible (sunproof clothing is ideal) and always put a hat on her head. Put high sun protection factor sun cream, or sun block, on her skin and reapply at least every two hours (more often if its windy) and always immediately after swimming. She should stay out of the sun when it's at its peak between 11 A.M. and 3 P.M.

Travel

Although the saying goes that "it's the journey that counts [rather than the destination]," traveling is not without hazards. On long journeys—whether by car, bus, train, ship, or plane—there's the boredom of being confined to one's seat for extended periods and (particularly if a sea trip) the possibility of motion sickness. Wherever you go, there's a chance of being exposed to different "foreign" germs and bugs. If it's not a vacation where you buy and cook your own food, you must take precautions to reduce the risk of food poisoning or drinking dirty water.

Immunization

Before you leave, make sure your child's immunization program is up-to-date (see page 218). Talk to your healthcare professional or local travel clinic to find out if you need any additional vaccinations for your destination. Do this well in advance of your trip because some of these vaccinations need to be given in two stages several weeks before you travel.

Trains

Encourage your child to sit down beside you, or on your lap. If she really wants to stand up, insist that she holds onto the hand rails because trains often stop and start suddenly. If she's not holding on there's a risk of injury. If you are on a longer journey you can explore the train together but always hold her hand and don't let her wander off on her own.

Planes

Over the age of two years children must sit in their own seat. If you are going to be renting a car and driving at your destination, you may want to take her booster seat on the plane for her to sit in (if this is possible). It is a good idea to encourage your child to use a lightweight stroller, which you should keep with you while in the airport, because there can be a lot of walking to do and a lot of people around.

Make sure too, that you have a supply of drinks and snacks with you in the event of your flight being delayed.

Preserving your child's health

It is very important that your child continues to be monitored throughout her early years. Your healthcare provider will want to check on her from time to time, but as the person who is with her everyday, you are the one with the greatest responsibility for ensuring she gets the proper care or to notice if things are not as they should be. In terms of development, your child's genes and environment can influence the age at which key milestones are reached but it's worth being aware of what these are and when they are usually achieved. But bear in mind that some children achieve them later than what is widely considered "normal," while others do so more quickly. If you are in any doubt, always talk to your doctor or primary healthcare provider.

For optimum health, your child must have a balanced diet to ensure she is getting the right nutrients, plenty to drink so she is well hydrated, lots of play and exercise, and finally, sufficient sleep.

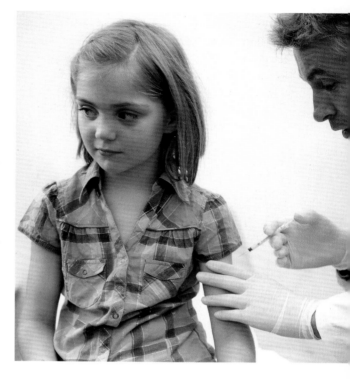

Regular health checks

Your child should have already had developmental assessments from birth, another, at around age four, or before she starts school. The American Academy of Pediatrics sets out recommendations and guidelines for checkups (www.aap.org), but in general, all aspects of your child's development (weight and height, posture, gross motor and fine motor skills, vision and hearing, speech and social interaction) should be assessed. Your child's height and weight will continue to be monitored. However, at this stage height is more important than weight as a guide to growth rate. If there is any cause for concern you may be asked to measure your child at regular intervals over a period of six months. Development, in particular of fine motor and language skills, relies heavily on normal visual and hearing skills, so it is imperative that any problems in these areas are picked up early and (treated appropriately) see below and page 262.

Immunizations

Vaccination is one of the greatest breakthroughs in modern medicine. No other medical intervention has done more to save lives and improve quality of life and it is vital that your child receives them all. The vaccination schedule is broken down by age:

- MMR—the combined vaccine that protects against measles, mumps, and rubella (German measles) given as a second dose
- DTaP/IPV—the vaccine that boosts your child's protection against four potentially serious childhood diseases (diphtheria, tetanus, pertussis [whooping cough], and polio).

After this, no more vaccinations are needed (apart from annual flu protection) until your child is around 12 years of age, unless you are traveling to countries where there is a risk of infectious diseases such as hepatitis, tuberculosis, or yellow fever. Some travel vaccinations are not recommended for very young children so consult your healthcare provider before you book to travel as a family.

Some parents have been concerned about possible complications associated with the MMR vaccine, and whether it results in the development of autistic spectrum disorders (see page 194) and inflammatory bowel disease. The MMR vaccine does not cause autism and the fact that the MMR is given to children at or before 18 months, when the first signs of autism can appear, is coincidental. However, not having the vaccination can lead to measles (the US experienced a record number of measles cases during 2014), which can result in disability and/or death.

Going to the dentist

As well as ensuring daily brushing, it's important to take your child to your dentist for regular checkups. Most dentists recommend a checkup every six months from the time the front teeth erupt, at 12 to 18 months. At the initial visit the dentist will identify any dietary or dental problems; an early intervention can help prevent more complex procedures later on.

Visiting the dentist or hygienist is a good way for you and your child to learn about oral hygiene including the choice of toothbrush and tooth paste and effective brushing techniques. You'll also be

IMMUNIZATION HISTORY

VACCINATION	PROTECTS AGAINST	WHEN GIVEN
5-in-1 DTaP/IPV/Hib vaccine	Diphtheria, tetanus, pertussis (whooping cough), polio, Haemophilus influenzae type b (Hib, a bacterial infection that can cause severe pneumonia or meningitis)	2 months 4 months 6 months 12 to 15 months
Pneumoccocal (PCV)	Bacterial pneumonia caused by *Streptococcus pneumoniae*	2 months; 4 months; 6 months; then 12 to 15 months
Meningoccal group C	Meningitis C	11 to 12 years of age
Hib booster	Haemophilus influenzae type b	2 month; 4 months; 6 months; then between 12 to 15 months
MMR	Measles, Mumps, and Rubella	given in 2 doses between the ages of 12 and 15 months
Rotavirus	The most common cause of severe diarrhea among young children	Given as an oral vaccine at 2 months; 3 months; and 6 months
Nasal flu	Influenza virus	6 months of age; then annually as a nasal mist

given advice on a diet that promotes good dental health. At a checkup, your child will have her teeth cleaned and may be given fluoride treatment or have a supplement recommended.

Your dentist may recommend applying dental (or fissure) sealants to the chewing surfaces of the back teeth, where decay occurs most often. These clear or colored plastic coatings fill in the grooved and pitted surfaces of the teeth, which are hard to clean, and stop food particles from getting caught, possibly causing cavities. They are quick to apply, and can effectively protect teeth for many years.

Pediatric dental problems

If, however, your child develops a cavity in a tooth, it's important that it be filled. Primary, or "baby," teeth are important not only to help children speak clearly and chew naturally, but also to maintain the space for the permanent teeth. Although your child won't start losing her baby teeth until the age of six, her primary molars won't be lost until she's 10 to 12 years old, and if a cavity is not treated, she can suffer pain, infection of the gums and jaws, impairment of her general health, and premature loss of teeth, which, can create future orthodontic problems.

Dental problems can start at an early age. Because of the amount of refined and hidden sugars in our food, according to the Children's Dental Health Project, nearly 25% of American children aged 2 to 5 have experienced tooth decay, and also states that "tooth or gum pain can hurt a child in many ways, including her ability to learn, play, and eat healthy foods." Some parents erroneously believe that baby teeth do not have a nerve supply, and so do not need to be filled.

The truth is that baby teeth, being small, have less space between the outer enamel and the nerve, and therefore decay does not need to progress far in the tooth before the nerve of the tooth is exposed causing an abscess. Treatment of a tooth with an abscess is far more challenging for a child than a simple filling. However, your dentist may decide to simply keep an eye on the decay if there is no pain and the tooth is going to fall out naturally within six months.

YOUR HEALTHCARE TEAM

The following people will help you monitor your child's health during the preschool years.

FAMILY PHYSICIAN

Your family physician will be your first port of call if your child is unwell. He or she will advise you on measures to alleviate symptoms of illness and prescribe any necessary medication. Certain doctors specialize in child health, and may even run child health clinics where you can discuss any concerns.

PEDIATRIC SPECIALISTS

If your family physician or healthcare provider feels your child needs additional medical assistance from a specialist, he or she will refer you to a doctor—generally at a hospital—with extra training in that particular aspect of children's (pediatric) health. These doctors specialize in anything from child development to heart disease.

NURSE PRACTITIONER

Pediatric nurse practitioners work with infants, toddlers, preschoolers, school-age children, and adolescents, and focus on education and guidance to promote wellness children and to prevent illnesses and injuries. In primary care settings, nurse practitioners conduct well-visit checkups and diagnose and treat common childhood illnesses. They work in a range of well-child or primary-care settings, as well as in acute-care hospitals, schools, community health centers, or specialized practices.

PEDIATRIC DENTIST

This is a dentist who has specialized training in looking after the oral health—teeth, gums, and mouth—of your child from infancy through to her teens.

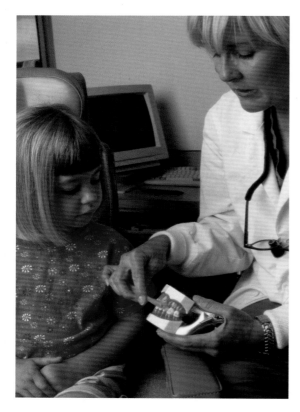

Dental trauma is also common in children up to four years old, because this is the time they start to walk and have no fear. If your child is familiar with her dentist, she'll be less likely to be anxious or frightened should she need to be seen for an emergency visit.

Because injuries to baby or primary teeth can potentially affect the development and health of the underlying permanent teeth, if your child displaces or fractures a tooth, it's important that a dentist assesses her promptly. This normally involves a taking a thorough history, and detailed clinical and radiographic checks. Pediatric dentists are skilled in saving injured teeth.

Hearing and vision checks

If there is a family history of eye and ear problems, talk to a nurse practitioner and/or your family doctor. You should be alert for signs that could indicate your preschooler has developed a problem.

Hearing

A reversible short-term hearing problem may be the case if your preschooler is:

◆ Not speaking by the age of 3;
◆ Speaking, but always mispronounces words;
◆ Struggling to keep up with conversations;
◆ Talks loudly and/or listens to the television on full volume;
◆ Does not turn toward a sound.

If your child has a cold, her hearing could be impaired because the tubes between her eardrum and nose are temporarily blocked with mucus, but an inability to hear can also be caused by otitis media, a middle ear infection also sometimes called "glue ear," (see page 267). If the problem persists, your doctor will refer your child for a hearing test. The tests may be repeated over a few months before any action is taken because the problem may clear up on its own.

Vision

At each developmental check, your child will be given simple tests to make sure her sight is developing normally because there are defects, such as long or short-sightedness, lazy eye (vision in one eye does not develop properly), and a squint (where eyes don't move together) that do not develop until later (see also page 269). Moreover, seek advice if your child:

◆ Does not make eye contact with you;
◆ Has erratic eye movements;
◆ Is unusually clumsy (children with lazy eyes have difficulty judging how far away objects are).
◆ Does not turn toward a sound (children won't bother to look if they think they won't be able to see something).

Younger children are often unaware that they have a problem with their vision, though as many as one in five children has an undiagnosed problem. A simple test may confirm that your child's eyes are normal. Young children will not be able to read letters off a chart or say which lenses are better, but an ophthalmologist can examine your child's eyes with a retinoscope to measure the eye's ability to focus. Some children need glasses, or in some situations, minor corrective surgery.

When your child is unwell

One of the most worrying aspects of being a parent is when your child gets sick. A young child may not be able to tell you what is wrong and it can be hard to tell whether to treat her at home, call the doctor's office, or treat it is an emergency. Familiarizing yourself with the signs of illness and the simple measures needed to relieve symptoms and knowing how to monitor your child (all described here) will help you gain the confidence to care for her.

Coughs and colds will be very common as your child grows up and it may help to bear in mind that her immature immune system becomes stronger as a result. Although she may be "under the weather," as long as your child is still interested in playing, eats, and drinks, is alert and smiling at you, has a normal skin color, and looks well when her temperature comes down, any illness is probably not serious.

Nor should it worry you if your child has a fever and doesn't want to eat much. This is very common with infections that cause a fever and as long as your child is drinking and urinating normally, that is fine; her appetite will return when she is better.

What you do need to do is treat any symptoms, such as fever, and monitor any change in your child's condition. If you are concerned, however, call your doctor and/or healthcare provider and he or she will let you know if your child needs to be seen.

What causes illness?

Viruses, bacteria, and fungi are all "germs" that can cause illness and infection. Most human illnesses are caused by viruses and bacteria that are spread in droplets of moisture produced by infected individuals when they sneeze or cough. A viral disease is caused by a virus—an infectious agent that replicates inside the cells of a living being. Once a virus enters the body, the immune system normally develops antibodies that can fight it.

Bacteria are single-celled microorganisms that are often already present in the body. Many are helpful and harmless, but infectious or disease-causing bacteria (known as pathogens) can make a person sick. Their infections can cause symptoms similar to viruses, but they can be "killed" by antibiotics that break down the bacteria, curing the person and preventing the spread of the disease. Antibiotics kill bacteria by breaking down their cell walls, but they have no effect on a virus. Some bacteria are becoming resistant to antibiotics because of the overuse of such drugs, so doctors will not prescribe antibiotics unless they are certain there is a bacterial cause.

Fungi are simple parasitic life forms that can multiply through tiny spores that thrive in warm, damp conditions. Most are either harmless or beneficial to your health, but some cause disease. Spores can land on the skin or are inhaled so infections often start on the skin or in the lungs.

---

more **about** | **Preventing spread of infection**

Droplets in the air spread most infections. Teaching your child good hygiene habits from an early age can mean he suffers from fewer infectious illnesses.

Catch it *Make sure your child always has a tissue. If he wants to blows his nose or sneeze, encourage him to put a tissue in front of his mouth and nose first—to catch the droplets. You will need to do this for him at first.*

Discard it *Tell your child to fold the tissue inward and throw it away after he's used it.*

Kill it *Have him wash his hands thoroughly to kill any remaining germs.*

Fever

Normal body temperature for a child is 96.8 to 98°F. Anything above 100.4°F indicates a fever. Fever occurs when the body's internal "thermostat" raises the body temperature above its normal level, often as a response to an infection, illness, or some other cause. You will know if your child has a fever simply by feeling her forehead with the back of your hand but you must use a thermometer to get an accurate reading. If your child's fever is high, she may say she feels cold and shivery, or her skin may look flushed.

Body temperature varies naturally throughout the day. It is likely to be lower in the morning or after a rest and higher in the evening or if your child has been active. If your child is unwell, check her temperature at regular intervals throughout the day. Don't take her temperature, however, if she's just eaten hot or cold food, had a drink, or been running around because you will not get an accurate reading.

Treating a fever

To help bring a fever down, give your child infant or pediatric acetaminophen or ibuprofen at the prescribed intervals, see below. Don't over- or under-dress her, keep the room warm, but not too hot, and

FEVERS AND MEDICAL ADVICE

Trust your instincts and call your healthcare provider if you are at all worried. Seek medical advice if your child has a fever:

- Of 102.2°F or higher (but if 105°F or above, dial 911 and ask for an ambulance);
- Without an obvious cause, particularly if it lasts more than three consecutive days;
- Accompanied by a sore throat that lasts more than 24 to 48 hours;
- Accompanied by vomiting and/or diarrhea lasting more than 24 hours, or 8 hours if he has not been able to hold down any fluids;
- And displays signs of dehydration, see page 223.
- And has pain when urinating;
- And a mild febrile seizure;
- And has recently returned from a trip abroad;
- And is breathing faster than normal, or continues to breathe fast even after his fever comes down.

---

more about | Acetaminophen or ibuprofen

Acetaminophen or ibuprofen can be used to reduce fever and treat any aches or pains. Give young children infant acetaminophen or ibuprofen, which are available as an oral suspension or water-soluble tablets and can be used by children under the age of six. Your pharmacist can advise you. Try infant acetaminophen first since it has fewer side effects; if it does not seem to be effective, then try infant ibuprofen. Never exceed the maximum dose. Acetaminophen can be given every 4 to 6 hours. Ibuprofen has a longer interval between doses—6 to 8 hours—so can be useful for controlling fever during the night. Don't give both medications at the same time unless a health professional has advised it.

Never give aspirin to children under 16 years old—it can trigger a serious but rare disease called Reye's syndrome that can affect the brain and liver.

make sure it is well ventilated. If the atmosphere is very dry, hang a damp towel over the radiator to increase the humidity.

If your child's fever is particularly high, keep her as cool as you can. Dress your child in natural fibers (cotton is best) that allow heat to escape. Make sure her bedding is light, too, so that she does not overheat. If your child has a prolonged raised temperature, there is a risk that she could suffer a febrile seizure, (see page 224).

Dehydration

If your child is unwell, she is more likely to become dehydrated, particularly if she has a raised temperature. She will lose fluids through sweating and if she has diarrhea or vomits, she will lose even more. If she has a cough, a lack of fluid can make it worse. Well children need at least 2¾ pints (5½ 8-ounce glasses) of fluid a day (see page 40), and more in hot weather or when they have a fever. If your child is ill, make sure she always has a drink beside her.

Make it fun: use a new or favorite cup or a "special one" that she's not normally allowed to have; try giving her a novelty straw. She may even want a cup that she used when she was younger. While water and unsweetened juice are healthier, it's okay to offer your child her favorite drinks, even if they are fizzy, if she prefers (but not diet drinks because these lack sugar). Encourage her to sip her drink regularly. If she won't drink, tempt her with some salty snacks first; these will replace some lost salts and make her thirsty.

*more***about** | Recognizing dehydration

Children can become dehydrated very quickly, especially when they are unwell and have a raised temperature, vomit and/or suffer from diarrhea. Signs to watch out for are when your child,

- *Says he is thirsty or that his mouth feels dry or appears to be thirsty;*
- *Passes less urine than usual, and the urine is darker in color, and has a stronger smell;*
- *Has eyes that look sunken and may not produce tears;*
- *Has skin that is dry;*
- *Is lethargic or even drowsy.*

How to monitor your child

When you are looking after a sick child, you need to take her temperature and check her pulse rate regularly and keep an eye on her breathing. Make a

TAKING A TEMPERATURE

With an aural thermometer

Place the thermometer in your child's ear until it "beeps"—normally after only a few seconds. Don't use this type of thermometer if your child has an ear infection.

With a digital thermometer

Don't put a digital thermometer in your child's mouth until he is at least six years old. Sit your child on your lap. Raise his arm and place the end of the thermometer in his armpit. Lower the arm over the thermometer and hold it still until the thermometer beeps—about a minute. The reading given will be about 2°F below his actual body temperature.

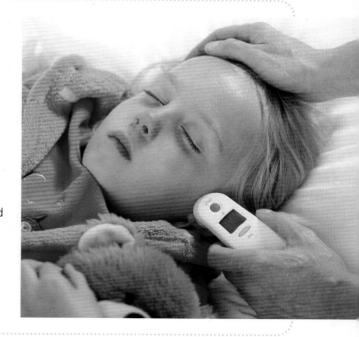

note of any changes (better or worse). If necessary call your doctor—see fever danger box, below.

Checking pulse rate

An adult's heart beats about 60 to 80 times per minute, but a child's heart beats faster and varies throughout the day—it will be faster after exercise and slower when he is resting. A toddler's heart beats around 80 to 130 times per minute, but is generally about 110. By the time your child is six, it will be down to about 100 beats per minute, but can range from 75 to 120. The heartbeat can be measured by feeling for the pulse (a wave of pressure that passes along an artery after each heartbeat) anywhere an artery is close to the skin.

To check your child's pulse, either put the pads of two fingers on the inner side of her upper arm (brachial pulse), or place them just below the wrist crease at the base of her thumb. Count the number of beats you can feel in a minute, and check for strength (is it strong or weak) and rhythm (is it regular or erratic).

Checking breathing

When your child is unwell it's important to monitor the quality of her breathing. A child's normal breathing rate is 20 to 30 times a minute but if she has a fever, she may breathe faster than usual. To check the rate, sit her on your lap and place your hand on her chest so that you can feel for movements and count the number of breaths in a minute. You should also observe the quality. Are her breaths deep or shallow, easy or difficult, noisy or quiet?

If your child is sleeping or in bed, you can leave her there while you do the checks.

Febrile seizure

A high temperature can cause a temporary electrical disturbance in the brain leading to a fit or convulsion in which your child's body becomes stiff, her arms and legs twitch and she loses consciousness. Your child may wet herself. If a child has had one previously, she is more likely to experience another the next time she is unwell. They are more common in children aged six months to three years.

Seizures can be very frightening for you to watch but if correctly managed, they are rarely dangerous. When your child suffers her first seizure, or if she has had previous episodes but this time the convulsions last longer, or are longer than 15 minutes, dial 911 for an ambulance. Otherwise call your doctor.

Treating a febrile seizure

1 Protect your child by placing padding around her so she cannot hurt herself but don't restrain her in any way.
2 To help cool your child down naturally, remove clothing and bedding; you may have to wait until the convulsions stop. Make sure the room is well ventilated.

BE ALERT!

FEVER DANGER

Seek urgent medical help, or dial 911 for an ambulance (even if you have already spoken to your healthcare provider), if your child has a fever:

◆ Of 105°F or higher;
◆ And is lethargic, refuses to eat, has a rash that does not fade when pressed (see page 260), or is having difficulty breathing;
◆ And is having trouble swallowing to the point where he is drooling because he is unable to swallow his own saliva;
◆ And is still lethargic or listless even after being given infant acetaminophen or infant ibuprofen;
◆ Accompanied by a headache, stiff neck, or purplish patches or tiny red spots on the skin;
◆ And has severe pain;
◆ With a febrile seizure lasting 15 minutes or more;
◆ With a febrile seizure followed by difficulty breathing.

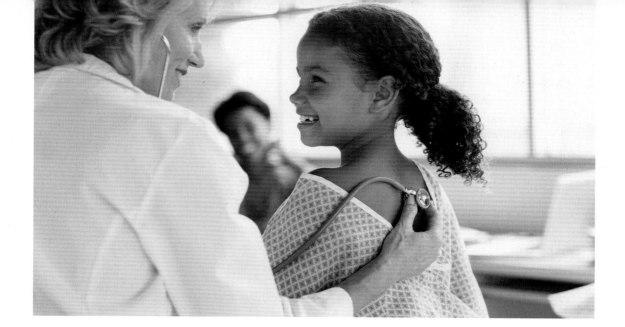

3 When convulsions have stopped, place your child on her side in the recovery position (see page 238) to ensure her airway is open and so that she can breathe.

Doctor appointment

If you need to take your child to your physician, make a list of all of her symptoms. Your doctor will want to know how long she has been ill, what symptoms you have noticed (fever, vomiting, headache), whether she has stopped eating, what action you have taken so far (for example, given medication). In particular, describe anything that has changed (improved or worsened) over the course of the illness. Even if your child is not seriously ill, it can be difficult to take in everything your doctor says during the consultation, so it is worth taking a checklist of questions you want to ask, for example:

- What is the diagnosis?
- How long will the illness last, and is it likely to worsen?
- Is my child contagious?
- What is the prescribed treatment? Is medication needed and what else can I do to alleviate symptoms?
- Should I bring my child in again?

If a long-term condition is diagnosed

If your doctor suspects that your child has a chronic, or long-term condition, it can be especially difficult to take in everything he or she says. Your doctor will probably refer you to a specialist who can confirm the diagnosis, which can involve a visit to the hospital. In these circumstances, it is a good idea to take someone else with you to help you remember the information you are given.

Before you go to the hospital, make a list of the things that are worrying you. It can be very frustrating to come away from a long-awaited appointment only to realize that your particular concerns have not been addressed.

When you get an appointment, you may see one of a team of doctors, led by a consultant. If you need a follow-up, you may not automatically see the same person. Make a note of the doctor's name since it might be possible to request seeing him or her again. Ask about the follow-up arrangements.

How to give medicines

Whether it's tablets, a liquid, or drops, always:

- Check the name of the medication on the prescription and make sure its the right one;
- Measure out the medication exactly as directed;
- Never give medicines prescribed for one child to

another child even if they both appear to have the same condition.

- Count out the tablets or fill the tool (a cup, dropper, or syringe with the quantities marked on them, either in milliliters or ounces) with the correct dosage, before you start. Place on a small clean plate ready to administer.

Oral suspension

Sit your child or your lap or on a chair and give her the medicine. If using a syringe or dropper, let her suck in the medicine while you press the plunger or squeeze the rubber end of the dropper. Have a drink ready in case she does not like the taste.

Ear drops

Lay a young child on the bed on a towel, affected side uppermost. Sit an older child on your lap, facing away from you. Support your child's head, tilting it so that affected ear is uppermost. Pull the ear upward and back slightly to straighten the ear canal and deliver the drops. Rub the base of the ear.

Eye drops

Sit down on a bed or couch and lay your child down with her head in your lap. Pull her bottom eyelid down gently and drop the medication between the lid and ball of the eye. If your child resists, you may need help, or you can wrap a blanket around her arms and upper body.

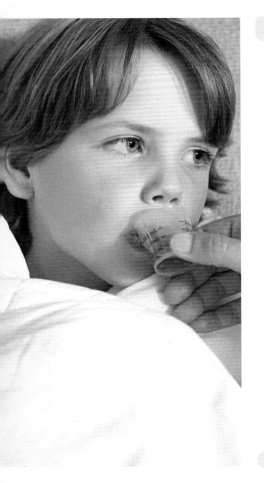

*more**about*** | **Medicines**

If your doctor prescribes a drug for your child ask him or her:

- *What it's for;*
- *How much should be given and when;*
- *Whether it needs to be given before, with, or after food;*
- *What to do if you forget to give a dose, for example, should you double up next time or give the next dose as soon as you remember or after a certain time;*
- *How long to give the medication for. Is it all right to discontinue the medication if your child improves or is the medication an antibiotic, in which case it must be taken for a specific number of days and your child must finish the course even if he appears to have recovered;*
- *What are the side effects, and what to do if any appear;*
- *Will it affect any other medication, for example that given for another diagnosed condition or any over-the-counter medicines you may give the child;*
- *What to do if your child has not completely recovered after he has taken all the medication.*

The pharmacist will also be able to help and can advise on:

- *How long the medication can be kept;*
- *Where to store it; some medications need to be kept in a refrigerator, others need to be put in a cold, dry place.*

Nose drops

Sit your child on your lap and put your arm around his shoulder and support his forehead. Tilt him back slightly and administer the drops.

Nursing your child at home

When your child is unwell, it's best to relax your normal routine. Try not to show your anxiety and be ready to reassure her because she may be a little frightened, especially if she has vomited.

At the beginning of an illness, a child may lose her appetite and want to sleep a bit more than usual. But she does not have to stay in bed, especially in the daytime. If she wants to be in bed, however, make sure you air the bed at least once a day and before she goes to sleep for the night.

A sick child often prefers to be in the same room as her parent. If this is the case with your child, make her comfortable on a couch with her favorite bed covering. Put a table beside her and make sure she has a drink and a box of tissues ready nearby (and somewhere to dispose of the used tissues). If she feels nauseous, leave a bowl within easy reach as well. Offer her snacks of her favorite food if she wants to eat something— small frequent meals are better than large portions which can be off-putting.

Occupying your child

Take your lead from your child. She may be happy to rest on the sofa in front of her favorite television show—and may well fall asleep. When she is not resting, play some quiet games with her or read her stories. Children often regress when they are unwell, and she may want to play with toys you thought she had outgrown or look at books that you haven't read for a while.

You can break the rules to make her feel special; give her pens and paper or a tray of modeling clay and cookie cutters to play with in bed. Keep her indoors when she is first unwell, but as she improves, she will benefit from fresh air by playing outside (as long as it's not cold and wet). Don't let her run around too much because her temperature may go up again. If she is not infectious, you could invite a friend over for a short visit.

HOME MEDICAL KIT

Keep a set of commonly used medications at home. Check the contents regularly and make sure they have not passed their expiry date. Keep all medicines out of reach of your child and make sure they all have child-resistant lids.

- Acetaminophen and/or ibuprofen—make sure it is appropriate for your child's age.
- Antihistamine to relieve mild allergic reactions—make sure it's appropriate for your child's age.
- Oral suspension syringe and stopper for medicine bottle or measuring spoon, depending on which one makes it easier to give medication to your child; your pharmacist may give syringes with prescribed medications.
- Thermometers, both digital and aural; check them regularly to make sure the batteries are working. If your child is prone to ear infections, you need to use a digital thermometer.
- Calamine lotion to soothe rashes.
- Cotton wool or gauze for applying creams.

Going to the hospital

At some point in your child's life, she may have to be admitted to a hospital. This can be very frightening for a parent, but also for your child. The admission may be unexpected, due to an accident or sudden illness, or it may be planned for a specific treatment, surgical procedure, or to administer special medication. Your child may need to be admitted to a hospital not necessarily because she is critically ill but because she needs treatment that can only be given there. However, you still may feel as if you suddenly have little or no control over your child and what is happening to her in the hospital. It will be a new and strange world for you and you may have to place your child's care in the trust of people you have never met before.

If your child has a planned admission, for a minor operation, for example, talk to her about it beforehand. Knowing what to expect before you get there can make things a little easier for you both. Find some storybooks about staying in a hospital or having an operation and read them together. Act out some role-playing games with her. The more familiar she is with what is going to happen, the less daunting it will be for both of you.

Hospital procedures

Your child is likely to be anxious. Everything will be unfamiliar. She may be feeling very unwell or in pain, and there are many different people around; just being examined can appear to be torture for her. If she sees that you are upset or anxious, it can unsettle her even more. Bear in mind that the doctors and nurses who are looking after her specialize in the care of children, so will help you both as much as they can and make your child as comfortable as possible.

Your preschooler may have to undergo tests or have X-rays, and you may not always be allowed to stay in the room with her; make sure she knows where you are. Ask the doctors to explain exactly what is happening beforehand and make sure you are there for her when the tests are over. She may need to have blood tests or needles inserted for intravenous drips and this can hurt.

On the ward

In many cases, your child will be given her own small area on a ward, often in a room with a few other children of a similar age. However, if she has an infectious disease, she may have to be isolated in a room of her own. She will likely have a bed, a bedside table, and a chair.

Many hospitals expect parents to stay with young children, so ask before your child is admitted. You may be given a folding bed beside your child's bed. Or, if she is there for a long stay, there may be a special house where you can stay with the rest of your family. You will need an overnight bag, too, and some money to buy meals and snacks, because these are not normally provided for parents. If you can't stay with your child all the time, make sure she knows where you are, and always return when you promised that you would. Try to share the care with your partner, friends, or relatives so that there is always someone with her whom she knows.

things to take in for your child

1 Favorite cuddly toy or toys;

2 Medical information: your healthcare provider's details and referral letter if you have one;

3 Child's normal medication;

4 2 to 3 pairs of pajamas, a housecoat and slippers, a change of day clothes, socks, and underwear;

5 Toiletry bag with toothbrush, toothpaste, face cloth, soap, shampoo, hairbrush, and hair ties (if appropriate).

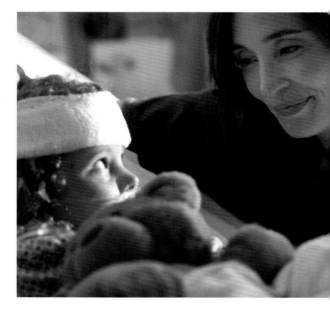

COMMON REASONS FOR EMERGENCY ADMISSION

- Accident resulting in a broken bone that needs surgery;
- Respiratory illnesses or infections such as asthma or pneumonia when oxygen and/or intravenous medications may be needed;
- Dehydration following a severe bout of vomiting as intravenous fluids may be needed;
- Severe infection that requires intravenous antibiotics;
- Febrile seizure that is not followed by complete recovery.

Take some books and games into the hospital with you. Many hospitals also have a playroom where you can take your child in the daytime if she is feeling well enough. Bring in some treats to make her feel special. She may want to listen to story books or music; try loading some onto an Mp3 player for her. If she's old enough, she may like some of the activities on a tablet or laptop. If there is a television, bring in some DVDs. If she's allowed to eat, bring in some of her favorite treats.

What you can do to help

Although you may feel powerless, there is plenty that you can do. You are your child's link to what is familiar and constant. Just being there will help her. Your role is to reassure your child that she will soon feel better and to cuddle her when she's frightened. You should be prepared to:

- Hold her when she is undergoing a painful procedure;
- Find out what tests she will need and tell her about them beforehand;
- Answer her questions as honestly as you can and don't pretend that something won't hurt when you know that it will;
- Find out as much as you can about her illness by asking the doctors and nurses; they will be happy to share with you as much as they know. In particular ask them to "translate" any unfamiliar terms. It can be tempting to research the illness on the internet, but avoid doing so since it can lead to misinformation, worsen your fears, and result in imagined outcomes poorer than reality;
- Try to stick to your child's normal routine as much as you can, although this can be difficult because the hospital day often starts very early.

Going home again

The doctors and nurses will let you know when your child is well enough to be cared for back at home. They will give you information about any necessary ongoing treatments and/or follow-up appointments. Depending on how long your child was in hospital, it may take her a while to settle back into her normal routine. She may wake up much earlier than before and want to eat and go to bed at different times. She may become clingy or accustomed to the attention she was getting while in she was in the hospital and want to continue with it. You will just have to be patient.

One approach is to give her a medical kit of her own and for her to pretend she is the doctor and that you or her teddy bear are the patient. Or you can tell her stories about a make-believe child who had a similar experience. Of course, all the stories will end happily: the child recovers completely and realizes that she much prefers being back at home in familiar surroundings with her family and friends.

INFECTED WOUNDS

If the wounding object was not clean or dirt was left in the wound or entered the body simply because the skin is broken, a wound can become infected. A day or so after an injury the area will begin to appear red and hot, becomes swollen and sore, or has a yellow discharge (pus). Clean around the injury with antiseptic wipes, cover the area with a sterile dressing, and seek medical advice.

CUTS AND GRAZES

Young children frequently incur scrapes and cuts, which are rarely harmful although Infection is a risk whenever the skin is broken (see box, above).

What to do

Wash the injury under cold running water to flush out the dirt or if this distresses your child, use a bowl of tepid water. Dab the injury dry with a sterile cotton gauze pad, wiping from the wound outward and using a new piece of cotton gauze for each stroke. If there are tiny flecks of dirt left behind in the wound, try brushing them off but seek medical advice if there is anything stuck in the wound—it may be plugging the bleeding and the wound could become infected if it is not removed. Do not attempt to "dig" it out yourself.

Press a sterile cotton gauze pad on the wound to stop any bleeding. Cover with a bandage with a pad larger than the injury.

BUMPS AND BRUISES

Bleeding just under the surface of the skin causes bruising that may appear to worsen for a few days after an injury.

What to do

To minimize swelling and reduce pain, sit your child down and raise and support the injury.

Apply a cold pack (see box, opposite page) against the injury for about 10 minutes. Seek medical advice if the pain persists.

SPRAINS AND STRAINS

If your child complains of pain or an inablity to use/put pressure on his hands or feet after running around or violent movement, he may have overstretched or torn a muscle, tendon, or ligament.

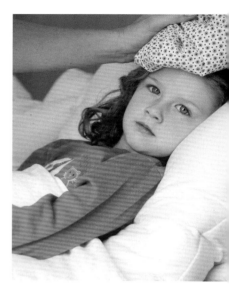

What to do

Have your child rest the affected part (he should sit or lie down) and make sure to support it in a comfortable position. Apply a cold pack (see box opposite page) to help reduce pain and swelling and then apply a thick layer of padding firmly (but not so tight as to affect circulation) around the injured area. Keep the injury elevated.

Seek medical attention if your child is in severe pain or if he is unable to use the injured part.

NOSEBLEED

A forceful sneeze, a bang on the nose, blowing his nose too vigorously, or picking it can lead to bleeding. Seek medical attention if your child loses a lot of blood or if he also has a head injury.

What to do

Sit your child down, tell him to lean forward and pinch the soft part of his nose for about 5 minutes. Release the pressure and check the nose. If it is still bleeding, repeat the pinching for another 5 minutes. Give your child a bowl and tell him to spit out any blood in his mouth; if he swallows it, it could make him feel sick. Once the bleeding has stopped, clean his face with lukewarm water. Encourage your child to sit quietly for a short while, and ask him not to sniff or blow (or pick) his nose.

CAT SCRATCHES

A scratch or bite from a cat or kitten can result in minor bleeding, but may become infected with cat-scratch disease.

What to do

Wash the area thoroughly and cover with an adhesive dressing. If cat-scratch disease occurs, a blister or a small bump called an inoculation lesion (a wound at the site where the bacteria enter the body), will develop several days after the scratch or bite and may be mistaken for a bug bite or blister. Most commonly it is found on the arms, hands, head, or scalp. The lesions are generally not painful. Within a couple of weeks the lymph nodes (glands) in the area nearest the scratch may become inflamed; for example, a scratch on the arm may result in swollen glands in the armpit. Your child may develop a slight fever and feel generally unwell. The symptoms generally last a few days but you should seek medical advice. Your doctor may prescribe antibiotics.

COLD PACK

A cold pack can minimize swelling and relieve pain. Either wrap a small bag of frozen peas in a dish towel (this is ideal because the peas mold to the shape of the injury) or fill a plastic bag with ice cubes, seal it, wrap it in a dish towel, and hold it against injured area.

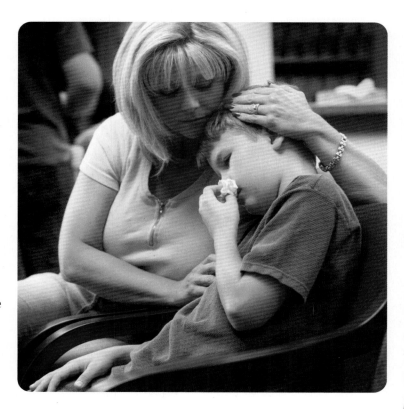

ANIMAL BITES

This type of wound is often dirty because few pets have clean mouths. Treat severe bleeding with direct pressure and elevation (see page 240) and seek urgent medical advice. For minor injuries, clean the area thoroughly with soap and water. Dry it thoroughly and cover with a sterile cotton gauze dressing, if necessary.

TICK BITE

Ticks are minute spiderlike creatures found in woodland and grassy areas that feed on the blood of mammals, including humans. They attach themselves as you walk through the grass, then bury their head in the skin and suck blood. A tick should always be removed as soon as possible because some ticks carry a bacterial infection that causes Lyme disease, which can affect the skin, joints, heart, and nervous system.

What to do

Using tweezers (or a tick remover if you have one), grasp the tick's head as near to your child's skin as possible. Twist firmly and pull the head upward to remove it. Seek medical advice to make sure the head is completely removed.

Monitor your child for signs of Lyme disease—the earliest and most common symptom being a pink or red circular rash that develops around the area of the bite, three to 30 days after the bite. If affected, your child may also develop flulike symptoms, such as tiredness, headaches, and muscle or joint pain.

OBJECT IN THE EAR, EYE, OR NOSE

Young children's natural curiosity and playtime activities often lead them to "experiment" with parts of their bodies, with potentially harmful implications.

What to do

If your child has put something in his ear, tilt his head toward the affected side to see if it falls out. If it's an insect, tilt his head so that the affected ear is uppermost and gently pour some water into it—the insect may float out. If an object remains lodged, seek medical advice.

If your child has poked something in his eye, tell him not to rub his eye. Hold his eyelids apart and look very carefully at the eye to see if you can see anything. Don't touch anything that is on the colored part of the eye; seek medical advice for this. If you can see something on the white of the eye, try holding his eyelids open and pouring water from the inner side outward. If that fails, try lifting it off with the corner of a moistened tissue. If you cannot remove it, seek medical advice.

If an object is lodged in your child's nose, it needs to be removed by a doctor.

SWALLOWED OR INHALED OBJECTS

Many commonly swallowed objects —coins, buttons, or small toys—don't cause any harm but sharp objects can pose dangers.

What to do

If you think your child has swallowed an object, seek medical advice. Don't try to make your child vomit to bring up the object—this could damage his gullet on the way up. In many cases it is appropriate to let nature take its course so that the object passes in the stool but in some cases, X-rays may be used to monitor progress. Occasionally a child will need surgery.

Rarely a small item, such as a peanut, may be inhaled and lodge itself in the lungs. A violent cough may expel it but if it leads to breathing difficulties or choking, see page 239.

BLISTERS

Blisters are often caused by badly fitting shoes but may accompany a burn or sunburn.

What to do

Don't break a blister because there's a risk of infection. Clean it thoroughly with soap and water and gently pat it dry. Cover it with an adhesive dressing, ideally a cushioned blister dressing. Make sure the pad is large enough to cover the entire blister.

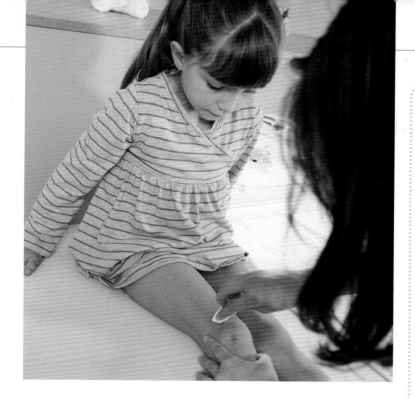

SUNBURN

In spite of your best efforts to protect him (see page 216), your child may develop a sunburn.

What to do

Move your child into the shade or a cool room. Cool the burned area with a tepid sponge, or give him a cool (not cold) bath. Pat his skin dry with a towel and soothe mild sunburn by dabbing the area with after-sun or calamine lotion.

Drape light cotton clothing or a towel over the affected area. Make sure he drinks plenty of water because the sun can be dehydrating, and encourage him to sip and not gulp quickly. Keep your child in the shade until his skin is healed. If any blisters form on the skin call your doctor or take your child to the hospital.

If your child is, or becomes, restless or dizzy, he may be suffering from heat exhaustion. Keep him cool, lay him down, if necessary, and make sure he continues drinking water. Monitor his condition because heat exhaustion can lead to the more serious condition heat stroke (see page 244), which needs urgent medical treatment.

SLIVERS AND STINGS

Your child may get a sliver of wood stuck in a finger from playing with damaged wooden toys or in his foot from walking barefoot on a boardwalk, or may be stung by a bee.

What to do

Clean the area around the splinter with a sterile wipe and pat dry.

TOXIC FUMES

Glue, certain cleaning products, vehicle exhaust emissions, smoke, or gases from defective heaters can produce dangerous fumes. If your child inhales any of these and experiences confusion and breathing difficulties, or if her skin turns a blue-gray color, remove her from the source of any fumes—optimally to where there is plenty of fresh air—and support her in an upright position until her breathing eases. Call for medical assistance.

Using tweezers, try to grasp the end of the splinter and pull it out at the same angle it went in. Don't dig around the wound with a needle to remove it; if you can't get it out easily or the splinter breaks, seek medical advice. Once the splinter is out, squeeze the area slightly to encourage bleeding and to flush out any dirt.

If you can see a bee's stinger in your child's skin, scrape it underneath with a credit card to remove it. Put a cold pack (see page 231) on the site to help reduce discomfort and swelling for up to 10 minutes. Be alert for possible signs of an allergic reaction (see page 244).

FIRST AID IN AN EMERGENCY

As a parent you can make your home safe, but children still have accidents when you least expect it. Most injuries are relatively minor, but there can be more serious incidents, and it's important to know what to do. Enrolling on a first aid course can give you the confidence to deal with an incident, and in particular, help you identify when it's an emergency. It is can be reassuring to know that if you ring an ambulance (911) in an emergency, the operator will guide you through the essential steps.

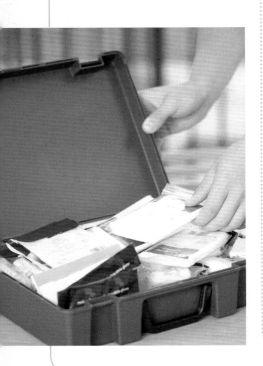

YOUR FIRST AID KIT

Keep a box of first aid equipment at home and one in the car. Both should be out of your child's reach but readily accessible to you. Make sure that anyone who looks after your children, for example, babysitters, knows where to find the box. Check it regularly and replace anything you use as soon as possible. Whether you are making up your own or buying a prepared kit, make sure it contains the following:

- Sterile wound dressings—these are dressings that have bandages attached.
- Sterile dressing pads.
- Selection of bandages: crêpe or self-adhesive bandages for supporting sprains and strains, stretchy open-weave bandages for securing dressings.
- Triangular bandage to use as a sling.
- Adhesive dressings—children love novelty colored ones—but have some hypoallergenic plasters in case a victim is allergic to the other type.
- Blister bandages.
- Antiseptic wipes—ideally alcohol free for cleaning skin around a wound.
- Sterile cotton gauze wipes—for cleaning around a "wet" wound, drying it, or to build up padding around a foreign object in a wound or as a dressing.
- Scissors and tweezers.
- Disposable, latex-free gloves.
- Antibacterial hand gel.
- Calamine lotion or antihistamine spray.
- Safety pins for securing bandages.
- Instant cold packs, especially for your car kit.
- Pocket mask to use for rescue breathing in poisoning situations.

WHAT TO DO IN AN EMERGENCY

Some first aid situations are potentially lethal and knowing how to respond can save a life. It can be very frightening to find that your child has collapsed, or appears unconscious, but stay calm and follow a clear plan.

First, make sure it is safe to approach your child (you cannot help your child if you become a casualty as well). If it isn't safe—there is a live cable, falling masonry, or a fire, for example—keep back and dial 911 urgently.

If it is clear to approach, treat your child where she is. Only move her if her life is in danger

SNAKE AND OTHER BITES

Take the child to ER if you are unsure of the type of snake or if you suspect it may be poisonous. Keep the child at rest. Do not apply ice but loosely splint the bite and keep it at rest, positioned at or slightly below the level of the heart. If you cannot identify the snake but can kill it safely, take it along with you for identification.

For animal or human bites, wash the wound well with soap and water. Seek medical advice: the child may need a tetanus or rabies shot, or antibiotics.

because some injuries can be made worse by wrong handling. Next, deal with potentially life-threatening priorities:
- Check for a response—is your child conscious or unconscious.
- Check if breathing is normal.
- Look for, and treat, injuries that could affect the circulatory system, such as bleeding or burns (see pages 240, 241).
- Finally, assess her for other

injuries. Listen to your child, she may tell you where it hurts. For example, if she fell down the stairs she may tell you that her leg hurts, but there is a risk that she has a head or spinal injury. Look for abnormalities; if she has broken her leg, the injured one may look shorter than the other. Did you or anyone else see what happened, this could help you identify injuries?

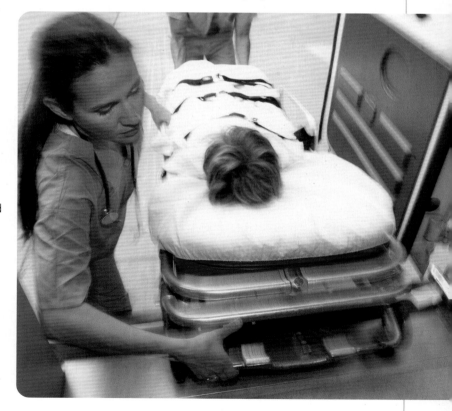

IF YOUR CHILD APPEARS UNCONSCIOUS

What to do

1 Speak loudly and clearly to her—for example, say, "Open your eyes" while you gently tap her shoulder.

If she responds, she is conscious, so attend to any injuries you find, see page 235. If your child does not respond, then she is unconscious. Shout for help and go to the next step.

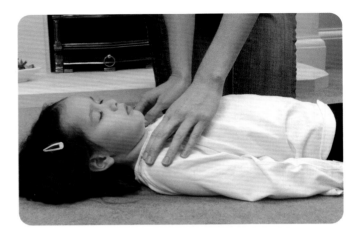

2 Open her airway.

Place one hand on her forehead and tilt her head back, her mouth should fall open. Lift her chin by placing two fingertips on the point of her chin—make sure you don't press on her neck. Ask someone to call an ambulance.

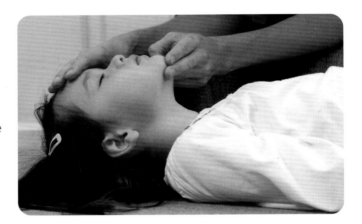

3 Look, listen, and feel for breathing for no more than 10 seconds.

Place your ear as close as possible to your child's mouth and nose, look along her chest for signs of movement, and feel for breaths against your ear. If she is breathing, place her in the recovery position, see page 238. If she is not breathing, begin the next step—rescue breathing and chest compressions (CPR/cardiopulmonary resuscitation) immediately.

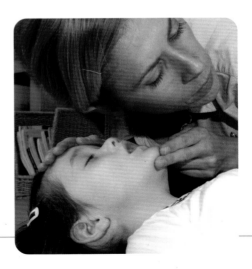

4 Give rescue breaths.

Make sure the airway is still open. Check her mouth
and pick out anything obvious near the front of the
mouth; don't put your fingers in her mouth to
search for obstructions since you may push the item
farther in. Then, keeping the fingers of one hand on
her chin, use your other hand to pinch the soft part
of her nose. Take a breath, place your lips over hers,
and blow steadily until you see her chest rise (about
one second). Remove your mouth and watch the
chest fall. Repeat to give five breaths altogether.

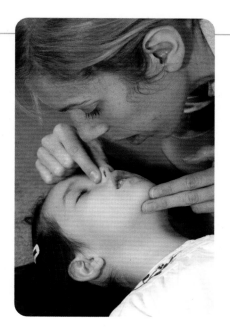

5 Begin chest compressions.

Kneel beside your child level with her
chest and place the heel of one hand on
the center of her chest. Straighten your
arm, lean over your child, and press
down vertically, depressing her chest by
about one-third of its depth. Release
the pressure and let the chest come
back up, but don't remove your hand.
Repeat to give 30 compressions at a
rate of 100 per minute.

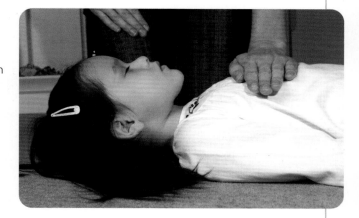

6 Move back to your child's head and give two rescue
breaths this time.

Then give another 30 chest compressions. If you are on your
own, give CPR for one minute before calling for help. Continue
CPR at 30 compressions followed by two breaths until help
arrives or your child shows signs of recovery, such as opening
her eyes, coughing, moving purposefully or breathing normally.

RECOVERY POSITION

If your child is unconscious but breathing, you must place her on her side in what is known as the recovery position. If you leave her on her back, her tongue will fall back and block the air passages to her lungs, or if she vomits, fluid can collect in the back of her throat, also blocking the airway.

What to do

1 Bend the arm nearest you at a right angle to her body, and bring the farthest arm across her body so that her hand is against the side of her face nearest you. Bend her far knee, leaving her foot on the ground. Then pull your child's knee toward you until it is resting on the ground.

2 Adjust her head to make sure her airway stays open. Monitor her breathing and pulse, being alert to quality (fast or slow, shallow or deep) and any changes until help arrives.

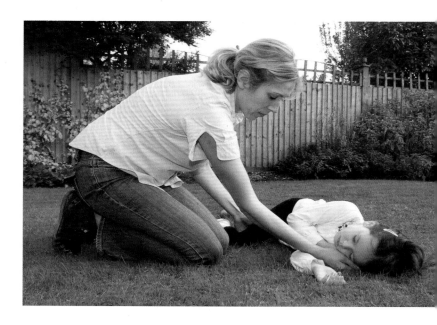

CHOKING

Children often put things in their mouths to "explore" them or can choke on a half-chewed piece of food. If a child is coughing but can still speak, there is only a mild obstruction and it's better to encourage your child to cough and clear the blockage herself. Intervene only when she can no longer speak, cough, or breathe.

What to do

1 Stand beside her and help her to bend forward, supporting her upper body with one hand. With the heel of your hand, give her up to five blows on her back between her shoulder blades. Check her mouth and remove anything obvious, but don't sweep your finger around her mouth.

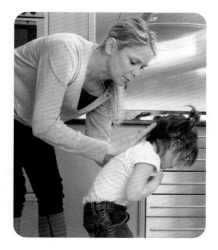

2 If the obstruction remains, give up to five abdominal thrusts. Stand behind your child and put your arms around her upper abdomen. Place one fist between her navel and breastbone and cover it with your other hand. Pull sharply upward and inward. Check her mouth again.

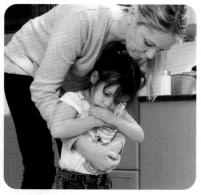

3 If your child is still choking, repeat steps 1 and 2 up to three times, then call an ambulance. Continue back blows and abdominal thrusts until emergency help arrives. If the child loses consciousness, treat as on page 237.

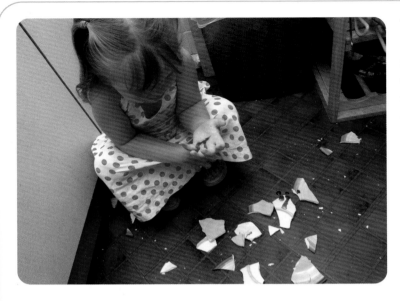

BLEEDING

Severe bleeding can be very distressing for you and your child, and if the blood loss is not stopped, vital body fluids will be lost from the circulation, which can result in a life-threatening condition called medical shock (see opposite page). If a wound is very large, stitches may be needed.

Ideally wear disposable gloves when treating your child.

(see opposite page)

PREVENTING INFECTION

Infection is a risk whenever the skin is broken. Ideally,

- Wash your hands or use sterile wipes or antibacterial foam to thoroughly clean them before and after giving first aid.
- Wear latex-free disposable gloves to prevent cross-infection of germs.
- Check the packaging of any dressing. If the wrapping is damaged it is no longer sterile.

What to do

Place a sterile pad over the wound and press firmly, or use your hands alone if no dressing is immediately available. Raise and support the injured part above the level of your child's heart to slow the blood flow to the area. Use a bandage to secure a dressing over the wound; the bandage should be tight enough to maintain pressure, but not so tight that it cuts off circulation to the limb beyond the injury. Call an ambulance. If the bleeding is very severe, treat as for shock.

2 If there is an object in the wound, do not try to remove it because it could be plugging more severe bleeding. Instead, apply pressure above and below the object then place pads around the object and bandage them.

MEDICAL SHOCK

This is a serious condition that can result from severe blood loss (external or internal), burns, or allergic reaction (see page 244). The fluid part of the blood (plasma) carries nutrients and oxygen to the vital organs of the body. If significant amounts of fluid are lost from the circulatory system, vital organs such as the heart and brain won't receive essential supplies.

Signs of shock include pale, gray-blue, cold, sweaty skin; a rapid pulse that becomes weaker; and shallow, fast breathing. As more fluid is lost, your child will become restless, will yawn and sigh, be very thirsty, and eventually lose consciousness.

What to do

Ask someone to call an ambulance for you. Lay your child down on the floor on a blanket to protect her from the cold. Treat any obvious cause (bleeding or burns). Keep her head low, and raise her legs as high as you can and support them on cushions or a chair. Cover her with a blanket to keep her warm, but don't give her a hot-water bottle. Check her pulse and breathing while you wait for the ambulance.

BURNS

Burns are generally caused by flames or scalding, but some chemicals also cause burns. A burn is potentially serious and there is a high risk of infection.

A burn can affect just the surface of the skin (e.g. sunburn, in which case it is superficial); or there may be damage to some of the skin layers (partial thickness), or it can affect all of the skin layers (deep). Partial thickness burns will often have blisters, and are very painful. Deep burns, however, can be pain-free because nerves are damaged. Some burns can have areas of all three types.

Like bleeding, a burn can cause severe fluid loss from the body and result in medical shock, see above. Always seek medical advice if your child sustains a burn. If in any doubt about the severity, go straight to the hospital or call an ambulance.

What to do

Cool the damaged area immediately by placing it under cold (but not icy) running water for at least 10 minutes: this stops the burning process and will help relieve the pain.

For a chemical burn, put on protective gloves and hold the area under cold running water to wash it off thoroughly. Make sure the contaminated water runs away from you and your child.

Remove any clothing from around the burn because the area will start to swell, but don't touch anything that is stuck to the wound. Lay plastic wrap along the injury (don't wrap it around a limb) to protect it, or for an injured hand or foot, put a clean plastic bag over it. Raising an affected limb can help reduce swelling and pain. Call an ambulance or take your child to the hospital yourself.

Never put lotions or ointments on a burn. If a blister appears as a result of a burn, don't apply an adhesive dressing, because the injury is likely to extend well beyond the blister.

HEAD INJURY

Your child may simply bump her head and have a small bruise and no other sign of injury. However, there is always a risk that a blow literally "shakes" the brain inside the skull; your child may become temporarily dazed and have a headache but will recover completely (this is a concussion)

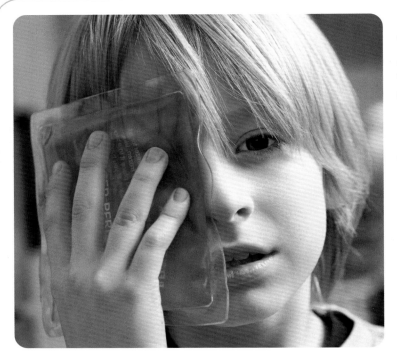

or she may suffer a more serious injury (called compression), in which bleeding occurs within the skull and presses on the brain, or she may even sustain a fracture.

Although symptoms of compression may not appear for hours or even days after an injury, if after a head injury, your child becomes disoriented, drowsy, and/or confused, develops a severe headache, a fever, weakness down one side of the body, and/or unequal-sized pupils, take action immediately.

What to do
Sit your child down, quiet her and hold a cold pack against the bump—she may want to hold it. Reassure her and stay with her. If she does not recover completely within half an hour, seek medical advice. If she recovers initially, but later starts deteriorating, lay her down on the floor—not a chair since she could fall off—and call an ambulance.

DROWNING
A child can drown in as little as 2 inches of water. If yours falls in the bath, remove her from the water immediately. If she falls in water outdoors, rescue her only if it safe for you to do so, otherwise call for help.

Keep her upright as you take her from the water. If the water or weather is cold, there is also a risk of hypothermia (see page 244). Any child rescued from water must be seen by a doctor.

What to do
As soon as your child is out of the water, lay her down and check to see if she is conscious and breathing. If she is unconscious but breathing normally, place her in the recovery position to ensure fluid can drain from her mouth (see page 238).

If she is not breathing, give five rescue breaths initially followed by 30 chest compressions, then two rescue breaths followed by 30 chest compressions (CPR). Continue CPR at a rate of 30:2 until help arrives or your child recovers (see page 237). If she regurgitates liquid while you are giving CPR, turn her onto her side briefly to allow fluid to drain, then restart CPR. If your child opens her eyes, coughs, moves purposefully, or breathes normally, place her in the recovery position. Call an ambulance even if she appears to have recovered completely.

POISONING
If you think your child has swallowed something poisonous, never try to make your child vomit it up. Some poisons burn the gullet on the way down and will burn again on the way back up.

What to do
If your child is conscious, try to find out what she ate or drank. Call an ambulance and give the paramedics as much information as possible.

Save any clues you can find (pill bottles or plant berries, for example) and keep samples of vomit because it can help the medical team plan the treatment. If her lips are burned, give sips of milk to help soothe the burns.

If she is unconscious, treat as on page 236. You may need to wipe the poison from her mouth or use a mask for rescue breaths or try them mouth to nose.

BONE OR JOINT INJURY

Bones can be completely or partially broken in a fall (fracture). Alternatively, the bands of tissue that hold the joints together—tendons—can be stretched or torn, resulting in a sprained joint, or even a dislocated one. It can be very difficult to tell the difference between a break and severe sprain without an X-ray. If in doubt, treat as for a broken bone. If your child sustains a leg injury, don't move her. Make her comfortable where she is and call an ambulance.

What to do

Support the joints above and below the injured area. Use your hands initially, then rolled towels.

If your child has hurt her arm, wrap a folded towel around the injured area to prevent movement and take the child to hospital.

If your child has hurt her leg, suspect a break if the leg cannot bear weight. Support the joints above and below the injury—at

the knee and ankle for a lower leg—and place rolled blankets or towels on either side of an injured upper leg and dial 911.

If you suspect a sprain, see page 230 for the appropriate actions to take.

ELECTRICAL INJURY

Contact with domestic low-voltage electricity, or lightning can cause the heart to stop, and/or result in burns at the point where the electricity enters the body and where it exits.

INCOMPLETE FRACTURE

A young child's bones are much more pliable than an adult's. They have areas both of hard bone and "softer" bone that allows for growth. As a result, an incomplete or "greenstick" fracture may occur where only one side of the bone has broken and the other side is bent.

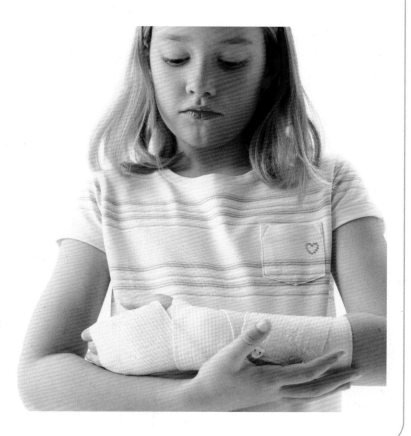

What to do

It is imperative to break the contact with the electricity before you touch your child. Ideally, unplug the appliance at the socket or if this is not possible, stand on a non-conducting surface such as a pile of newspapers, and using a wooden object (broom handle, long wooden spoon), push the appliance away from your child.

If this is unsuccessful, remain standing on the newspapers, and loop a rope, clothesline, or long piece of fabric around your child's feet and pull her away from the appliance.

If she is unconscious, treat as described on page 236. If she is conscious, treat burns as described above.

Call an ambulance; a child with an electrical injury needs to be assessed by a doctor.

HEATSTROKE

Children don't have very effective heat control systems and a life-threatening condition known as heatstroke can occur if a child is exposed to very hot weather for a prolonged period. If the heat control system fails, the body cannot sweat and will be unable to lose heat.

If your child has a headache, is feeling dizzy and restless, has hot flushed skin, and her temperature is above 104°F or, if you do not have a thermometer with you but your child feels very hot when touched with the back of your hand, treat as below. Left untreated, your child will lose consciousness.

What to do

Act quickly. Ask someone to call an ambulance while you move your child into a cool, well ventilated room. Remove as much of her clothing as possible and wrap her in a cold wet sheet, and keep the sheet cool by pouring more cold water onto it.

Leave the sheet in place until her temperature is down to 100.4°F. Replace the wet sheet with a dry one and fan her to keep her cool. Monitor her temperature, breathing, and pulse while you wait for the ambulance. If her temperature starts to rise again, restart the cooling process.

HYPOTHERMIA

Body temperature can also fall too low, for example, if your child is outside for long in poor weather conditions or falls into cold water, Consequences can be serious.

Suspect hypothermia if your child has cold, pale, dry skin and shivers. If untreated, your child will grow confused, her pulse will weaken, and breathing will slow and be shallow until eventually she will lose consciousness.

What to do

It is very important to rewarm your child gradually. Get her inside and replace any wet clothes with dry ones. Wrap her up warmly, cover her head with a hat, and put her gloves on her. Make sure the room is warm.

Never give your child a hot water bottle because this draws vital body heat to the surface away from where it is needed most. Give her warm drinks and high-energy foods, such as chocolate. Stay with her until her temperature has returned to normal. Seek medical advice.

ALLERGIC REACTION

The body's immune system will react to something it perceives as a threat. Common allergens include pollen (the fine powder released by trees, grass, or garden plants as part of their reproductive cycle), pet hairs (especially cat), wasp and bee stings, fungal or mold spores, latex, and foods (especially nuts, eggs, cow's milk, wheat, soy, seafood, and some fruit).

A reaction could be mild and result in a localized itchy rash, a runny nose, and sneezing with reddened, watery eyes, or even abdominal pain or vomiting. An allergic reaction can also trigger an asthma attack (see page 256).

A reaction, however, can be far more severe and result in a generalized itchy rash, swelling of the mouth and throat, difficulty breathing, and even unconsciousness, a condition known as anaphylactic shock. If your child is diagnosed as having a severe allergy, you will be given a special autoinjector pen, known as an Epipen® containing epinephrine (adrenaline) to administer if she comes in contact with the allergen.

What to do

Get rid of the source of the reaction, if possible. For example, remove a bee sting or take your child out of a room where nuts are present.

For a severe attack: If this is the first one, call an ambulance. Help your child into the position she finds most comfortable for breathing—often sitting up.

If your child has a known serious allergy, and she has an Epipen® auto-injector pack, administer it as soon as possible. Take the lid off and press the injector into her thigh (see box). If the symptoms return, repeat the epinephrine injection every five minutes until help arrives.

For a mild attack, talk to your pharmacist or seek medical advice. Keep your child away from likely sources such as pollen. A dose of children's antihistamine may help reduce the symptoms.

EPINEPHRINE AUTO INJECTORS

These are very easy to use. Take the lid off and hold the injector with your fist. Ensure you are putting your thumb over the correct end because if you accidently hold the injector the wrong way up you could deliver the dose into yourself. Hold the injector against your child's thigh (over her clothes if necessary) and push hard for 10 seconds. Rub the injection site gently for up to 10 seconds to make sure the drug begins to circulate.

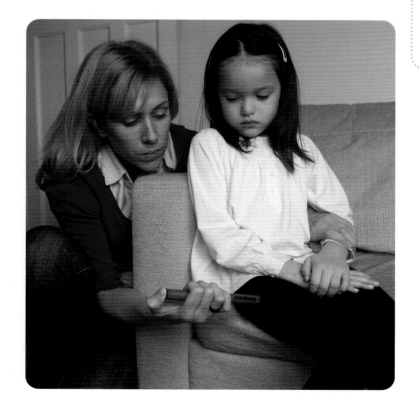

INFECTIOUS DISEASES

These are diseases caused by microorganisms—viruses or bacteria—and are easily passed from one person to another, though some are more contagious than others. Many, like diphtheria and even measles, are now relatively uncommon as a result of successful immunization programs. The diseases are generally spread through contact with the droplets of moisture released when an infected person

DISEASE	SYMPTOMS
MEASLES A potentially serious and highly contagious viral infection. **Incubation** 8 to 14 days. A child is infectious from before the rash appears, to about day 5.	Initially there will be grayish-white (Koplik's) spots in the mouth and throat. After a few days, a red-brown, flat rash will appear; it usually starts behind the ears, and spreads around the head and neck before showing up on the legs and torso. It begins as groups of spots, but after three days the spots join together. Your child will also have a fever, coldlike symptoms, and reddened eyes that are sensitive to light.
MUMPS A viral illness, which is rarely serious in children **Incubation** 14 to 25 days, average is about 17 days.	Possible fever lasting about three days. Characteristic swelling of the parotid glands that sit either side of the face just below the ears; one or both sides may be affected. The swelling can cause pain, tenderness, and difficulty swallowing.
RUBELLA (GERMAN MEASLES) A mild viral infection. **Incubation** 14 to 21 days. A child will be infectious from about a week before the rash appears.	A red-pink rash starts around the ears followed by tiny pink spots all over the body. Your child will have a fever and swollen glands in the neck and may have sore, red eyes. Up to a week before the rash appears she may have had a slight cold, a cough, or a sore throat.

coughs or sneezes. Many of the diseases have similar characteristics, such as a rash and a high fever and most are easily treatable. Some, however, can cause serious complications, so if in doubt, seek medical advice. Ring your doctor or healthcare provider first because he or she may not want a child with a highly contagious illness in the waiting area with other patients.

TREATMENT

POSSIBLE COMPLICATIONS

Symptoms normally last 7 to 10 days. For most children, medical treatment is not needed, but call your doctor for advice. Give your child children's acetaminophen or children's ibuprofen to relieve the fever, along with plenty of rest and fluids. Close the curtains if light hurts her eyes, and bathe them with damp sterile cotton gauze.

Diarrhea and vomiting, conjunctivitis, ear infections, and, more rarely, pneumonia. Hospital treatment may be needed for severe complications. Raised body temperature can cause febrile seizures (see page 224).

Call your doctor to let him or her know you suspect mumps; your child may need to be seen for the diagnosis to be confirmed. GIve your child children's acetaminophen or children's ibuprofen to relieve pain and fever, and plenty of fluids. Offer soft foods if she finds swallowing difficult. Soothe swollen glands with a cold compress.

Possible temporary one-sided hearing loss. Mumps can also lead to meningitis (see page 270) or inflammation of the brain (encephalitis). Older boys can suffer from Inflamed testes, usually only on one side, but this rarely causes infertility problems later.

Symptoms normally last 7 to 10 days. Seek medical advice urgently if you suspect rubella, but don't take your child to the doctor unless he or she asks to see her. Give your child children's acetaminophen or children's ibuprofen to relieve the fever, and plenty of fluids. Keep your child away from playgroup or nursery school. Alert your friends, and never expose any pregnant friends to a child with rubella.

Inflammation of the brain (encephalitis) or joints may occur but these are rare. The main risk is to pregnant women, because contact with rubella infection can cause birth defects in an unborn baby.

DISEASE	SYMPTOMS
WHOOPING COUGH (PERTUSSIS) A highly contagious bacterial infection of the lungs and airways caused by the bacterium bordetella pertussis. If antibiotics (erythromycin) are prescribed, anyone who has been in contact with your child should be given a course as well to prevent the infection from spreading.	A week of coldlike symptoms with a persistent, dry, irritating cough that generally progresses to intense bouts of coughing, which are followed by a distinctive "whooping" noise on inhalation. Your child's face may be very red when coughing. The force of coughing can cause her to vomit and/or burst blood vessels in her nose (causing nosebleeds) and eyes (red spots appear on eyes).
DIPHTHERIA A highly contagious bacterial infection that affects the nose and throat or occasionally the skin.	Fever with temperature likely to be 100.4°F or above, sore throat, and breathing difficulties. Your child may also be exhausted, have a cough, complain of pain when swallowing, and have foul-smelling nasal discharge. A gray-white membrane may form in her throat making breathing difficult. If her skin is affected instead of the throat, there will be pus-filled spots usually on her legs, feet, and hands.
CHICKEN POX A common and usually mild viral disease caused by the varicella zoster virus. **Incubation** 17 to 21 days. A child is infectious until all her spots have crusted over.	Low fever and small red spots that usually start on the trunk and spread to the arms and legs. The spots develop into itchy blisters, which gradually crust over and form scabs that fall off. The spots take about 5 days to appear, then a few more days to form crusts. Some children have only a few spots while others are covered with them.
SCARLET FEVER A mild bacterial infection caused by streptococcus bacterium.	Often starts with a sore throat and fever. A widespread pink-red rash starts in one place but quickly spreads to other parts. The skin feels like sandpaper. Cheeks will be very flushed but the area around the mouth stays white. Your child's tongue may feel furry and be covered in red spots; it may peel after a few days, leaving the tongue sore.

TREATMENT

POSSIBLE COMPLICATIONS

Seek medical advice. If diagnosed within three weeks of it beginning, your doctor may prescribe antibiotics to stop your child from being infectious. In severe cases, your child may need to be admitted to a hospital. Treat fever with children's acetaminophen or children's ibuprofen and give plenty of fluids to prevent dehydration. Clear away excess mucus or vomit during coughing bouts to prevent inhalation. Keep your child away from playgroup or nursery school for five days after she has completed the course of antibiotics.

Pneumonia, severe breathing difficulties, dehydration, weight loss because of excess vomiting, seizures, low blood pressure, and possible kidney failure.

Seek medical advice. Your child will need treatment in a hospital in an isolation ward—sometimes for up to six weeks. If there is a membrane in her throat, some or all of it will be removed surgically. Treatment will include antibiotics and an antitoxin that neutralizes the poisons produced by the bacteria. Anyone who has been in contact with your child will also be given a course of antibiotics.

Permanent lung damage and possible respiratory failure; inflammation of the heart muscle (myocarditis); nervous system complications, which can affect the function of the diaphragm or bladder.

Most children recover without medical treatment but if your child has impaired immunity, she will need intravenous antiviral medication in a hospital. Relieve the itching by applying calamine lotion to the spots. Treat fever with children's acetaminophen or children's ibuprofen. Your child will normally recover completely within 10 to 14 days but seek medical advice if she is particularly unwell.

Possible bacterial infection of spots, more rarely inflammation of the brain (encephalitis).

Seek medical advice; your doctor will prescribe a course of antibiotics. Rash will last about six days, then fade. If it is itchy, dab calamine lotion on the skin. Treat fever and a sore throat with children's acetaminophen or children's ibuprofen and give plenty of fluids. Most children recover 4 to 5 days after starting antibiotics. Skin on the hands and feet may peel for up to 6 weeks after the rash has faded.

Rarely ear infection, throat abscess, sinusitis, or pneumonia may develop, but usually only if antibiotics are not given. If your child is sensitive to the Streptococcus bacteria, it can cause inflammation of the kidneys (nephritis) or of the joints and muscles (rheumatic fever), but this is very rare.

DISEASE	SYMPTOMS
FIFTH DISEASE (SLAPPED CHEEK SYNDROME) This is a contagious viral infection caused by the parvovirus B19. Children are only infectious before symptoms appear	Begins with fever where temperature may be 100.4°F or higher, plus a headache and sore throat. This is followed 3 to 7 days later by a bright red rash on both cheeks, which spreads to the chest abdomen, arms and legs. Rash may last 4 to 5 weeks.
ROSEOLA Common viral illness (especially in very young children), also known as roseola infantum . **Incubation** 10 to 15 days	Sudden fever with temperature 104°F or higher, which lasts 3 to 4 days, then returns to normal. Small pink spots appear as the fever subsides, usually first on the abdomen before spreading to face, arms, and legs, and lasting 12 to 24 hours. Your child may have a sore throat and swollen glands in her neck.
HAND, FOOT, AND MOUTH DISEASE A viral infection.	Fever with temperature around 100.4 to 102.2°F, and a rash of tiny red spots with darkish gray centers most noticeable on the back of the hands and feet. The spots can develop into painful blisters. There may also be blisters in the mouth, which makes eating painful.
TUBERCULOSIS (TB) A bacterial infection caused by mycobacterium tuberculosis. It mainly affects the lungs, and this type is highly infectious. It can affect the bones and nervous system, but this type is not infectious.	Persistent cough—lasting more than three weeks—that typically brings up blood-stained phlegm, weight loss, tiredness, and fatigue with loss of appetite and high fever with night sweats.

TREATMENT

Treat fever with children's acetaminophen or children's ibuprofen and give plenty of fluids. Soothe the rash with calamine lotion. For most children this is a mild disease, which needs no special treatment. Your child can go to playgroup or nursery school because as soon as the rash appears, she is no longer contagious.

No special treatment is required. Treat fever with children's acetaminophen or children's ibuprofen, and don't let your child get too hot. Give her plenty to drink to keep her hydrated.

It is rarely serious, but can be very uncomfortable but usually clears up within 7 to 10 days. Treat fever with children's acetaminophen or ibuprofen and give plenty of fluids—milk and water are best; avoid acidic drinks like fruit juice if your child's mouth is sore. Give her soft foods to eat. Do not attempt to break the blisters because the fluid is infectious. Blisters will usually dry up on their own within a week.

This condition is serious but usually curable with correct treatment. A chest X-ray and sputum and blood tests will be needed to confirm the diagnosis. An infected person will need at least a six-month course of antibiotics, possibly as long as 18 months if it is a variety that is resistant to antibiotics. Anyone who has been in contact with your child will need to be tested for the disease.

POSSIBLE COMPLICATIONS

Very rare. If a woman is pregnant she can pass it to her unborn baby, and there is a risk of anemia and heart failure, which can cause miscarriage. Children with weakened immune systems can develop severe anemia.

Raised temperature can cause febrile seizures (see page 224).

Very rare. Call your doctor if your child is unable to drink any fluids, shows signs of dehydration or is unusually tired.

TB spreads easily within a family who live in the same house. BCG vaccination can provide effective protection against TB and is recommended for groups of people who are at a higher risk of developing TB, and who have been in contact with someone who has the disease.

RESPIRATORY ILLNESSES

The respiratory system is made up of the mouth and nose, throat and windpipe (trachea), which leads to the two lungs each of which is made up of lots of tubes. The larger tubes are called bronchi and they lead to smaller ones called bronchioles that end in tiny air sacs. Children have short passages between the different parts of the system, so infections can quickly pass from one organ to another.

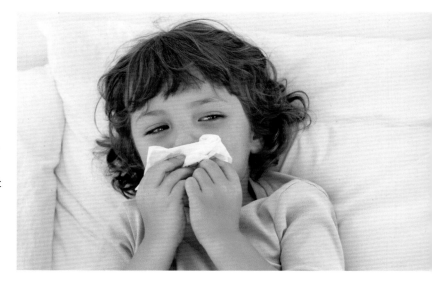

COMMON COLDS

The common cold is a mild viral infection of the upper airways, which causes a runny and/or blocked nose, mild sore throat, and sometimes a cough. There are hundreds of different cold-causing viruses and all children suffer from many colds every year while they build up their immune system. Children often develop colds even more frequently when they start playgroup or nursery school because they are exposed to more children and viruses. Most colds last about a week and don't need medical treatment. A blocked nose, however, can be uncomfortable and prevent sleep.

What to do

Keep your child comfortable and treat the symptoms. For a fever, give children's acetaminophen or children's ibuprofen. Encourage your child to blow her nose as often as possible with a tissue; assist her and make a game of it if it helps. Give her plenty to drink; dehydration can make a cough or a cold worse. Warm liquids such as lemon and honey or an herbal tea may help relax her airways, loosen mucus, and soothe a cough but avoid milky drinks because they can increase mucus production and overly sugary drinks because they can damage teeth. Commercial cold remedies and cough medicines will be of little help and are not recommended for young children.

If the atmosphere is very dry, use a humidifier or put a bowl of water in her room to increase the humidity, which will help to relieve a cough. Or, if you have radiators, putting a wet towel on a warm radiator will release more moisture into the air. If your child is finding it difficult to sleep because of a blocked nose, try putting some decongestant drops on her pillow.

INFLUENZA

Also known as the flu, this is another viral infection, similar to the common cold, but with more severe symptoms. Your child's temperature is likely to be high (100 to 104°F), and she may say that she aches all over. She may feel alternately very hot and then very cold and shivery. She is likely to be lethargic and weak and may feel nauseous.

The flu can be very debilitating, and while antibiotics won't help (because it's caused by a virus), it can leave a child weak and susceptible to other, more serious, bacterial infections that may require antibiotics.

What to do
Treat as you would a cold. Give children's acetaminophen or children's ibuprofen for fever and plenty to drink to prevent dehydration. Your child will need to rest, but she does not need to stay in her bed; she may prefer to be on a couch in the same room as you. Keep the room warm but not too hot, and well ventilated. Check her temperature regularly.

Seek medical advice if temperature stays high for longer than 24 hours or your child develops a chesty cough, an earache, or unpleasant nasal discharge.

SORE THROAT
A sore throat can be the result of a cold or flu virus, or a bacterial infection. Your child may tell you her throat is sore, or you may notice that she can't talk loudly or swallow easily. Look inside her

mouth (you may need to use a flashlight); if she has a sore throat the area at the back of her mouth will be red and inflamed and if there is a bacterial infection, there

may be yellow or white spots on her tonsils (tonsillitis). She is likely to have a cough, a raised temperature, and may complain of a headache.

What to do
Encourage your child to rest. Treat pain and fever with children's acetaminophen or children's ibuprofen, and make sure she has plenty of liquids. Give her soft, mashed food if she is finding it hard to swallow. Seek medical advice if her throat is very sore and inflamed or if the symptoms

don't improve after four days. There may be an infection and your doctor may need to prescribe a course of antibiotics.

SINUSITIS

The sinuses are small, air-filled cavities behind the cheekbones and forehead and a viral or bacterial infection can result in inflammation of the linings of the cavities or sinusitis. Symptoms include pain and tenderness of the face, a raised temperature, and runny and/or blocked nose. It can develop on its own or be the result of a cold or flu, and can last a few days or several weeks.

What to do

Most cases will clear up without medical treatment but seek aid if your child is very uncomfortable or the pain persists. Give children's acetaminophen or children's ibuprofen for pain and fever, and plenty of fluids. Your child may be more comfortable lying down.

COUGHS AND CHEST INFECTIONS

A cough is a natural reflex action that clears the throat and lungs of irritants such as mucus, dust, or even food. It can accompany a cold or the flu and a child may cough simply because mucus is trickling down the back of her throat, or there can be an underlying infection in the chest. A cough can be dry with a hacking sound, or it can be what

is called productive, in which mucus from the lungs (phlegm) is produced. Chest infections can be caused by either bacteria or a virus and vary from bronchitis, an upper-airways infection, to the more serious pneumonia, which affects tissue deep within the lungs.

What to do

If your child is coughing as the result of a cold, but she is eating and drinking normally, there is

nothing to worry about. Give her children's acetaminophen or children's ibuprofen to ease any fever. Over-the-counter cough medicines are not recommended for young children. Drinking warm liquids, such as lemon and honey or an herbal tea may help relax the airways, loosen mucus, and soothe a cough but avoid milky drinks, which can increase mucus production. If your child has a persistent cough, has lost her

---

*more **about*** | Chest infections

Bronchitis

This is an infection of the upper airways. A child will have a productivecough that sounds "wet." She is likely to cough up yellowy-gray or green mucus. Like most respiratory tract infections, the cause can be viral or bacterial. Most cases will clear up without medical help, but if your child has a persistent cough, or the mucus is green, seek medical advice because antibiotics may be needed. There is a risk that bronchitis can develop into pneumonia.

Bronchiolitis

This is a viral infection of the lower respiratory tract that can be serious in babies, but rarely affects children over two years old.

Pneumonia

This is inflammation or swelling of the tissue in one or both of the lungs. The tiny air sacs within the lung fill up with fluid, making breathing difficult. A chest X-ray will confirm the diagnosis and your child will need to be treated in hospital. Pneumonia can be caused by a viral infection, in which case the treatment aims to relieve the symptoms; if the cause is bacterial, antibiotics will be given. Children are routinely vaccinated against streptococcus pneumoniae, the bacterium that most commonly causes the disease, as part of their immunization program (see page 218).

appetite, and has a fever and/or there is any sign of wheezing, seek medical advice. Likewise, see your doctor if the cough is worse at night and/or brought on by running around—this could be asthma (see below).

LARYNGITIS

This is an infection of the voice box or larynx. It is mostly caused by a viral infection and may follow a cold or sore throat. A child will have a fever and sore throat, but significantly will have difficulty speaking, sound very hoarse, or may not be able to talk at all. She will have a constant tickly cough.

What to do

Most cases of laryngitis clear within a week without medical treatment. Treat a fever with children's acetaminophen or children's ibuprofen. Give plenty of liquids to soothe the throat and prevent dehydration. Warm drinks such as lemon and honey or an herbal tea can help; avoid milky drinks because they increase mucus production. Over-the-counter medications are not recommended for young children. Seek medical advice if your child is in discomfort, has a prolonged high fever, or has lost her voice.

CROUP

A condition that affects young children, croup is an infection of the windpipe, the larynx

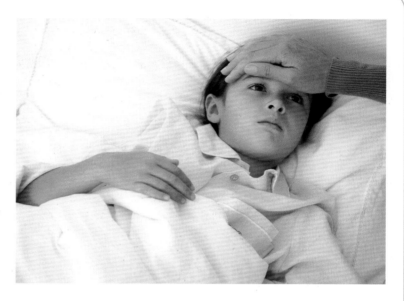

(voicebox), and the main air passages into the lungs. It is generally caused by a virus. A child with croup has a distinctive short, barking cough and may make a rasping sound, known as stridor, especially when she inhales. She may be hoarse and develop breathing difficulties.

What to do

Most cases of croup get better without medical assistance. During an attack, sit your child on your knee supporting her back. Stay calm, and reassure your child because an attack can be worsened if she panics. Create a steamy atmosphere because moisture can help breathing. For example, take her into the bathroom and sit her on your lap beside a bath filled with hot water. If she does not improve, call an ambulance.

HAY FEVER

This is a common condition that results when a person has an allergic reaction to pollen—the fine powder released by plants as part of their reproductive cycle. Symptoms include sneezing, a runny nose, and watery, itchy reddened eyes. It generally erupts during spring and into summer, because different children are sensitive to different pollens, for example, it could be trees (early spring) grass (spring into late summer), or wheat (later summer). Hay fever often runs in families, especially if there is a history of asthma (below) or eczema (see page 257).

What to do

There is no cure for hay fever and many children who develop it when young will grow out of it in time. In the meantime, you can only treat the symptoms and try to avoid the triggers, though this can be difficult especially if grass is the cause. Antihistamine medication can alleviate most symptoms. Eye drops may help if your child's eyes are very red and uncomfortable; it can help to wear sunglasses too.

If your child suffers from severe hay fever, ask your healthcare provider to arrange for tests to ascertain exactly what the trigger is so you can try to avoid it.

ASTHMA

This is a long-term or chronic condition that affects the tubes that carry air in and out of the lungs. When a child comes into contact with something that irritates her airways (a trigger), the muscles around the walls of her airways tighten narrowing the airways and their linings become inflamed and start to swell. The linings make sticky mucus, which can further narrow the airways and can cause coughing.

Symptoms include a persistent cough, often with a wheezing sound in the chest. Your child will be short of breath and may say her chest feels tight.

Unlike other coughs, this type is often brought on by exercise. Other triggers include house mites, dust, a smoky atmosphere, or pet hair. Asthma can also be brought on by a chest infection.

There is no cure for asthma, but with a combination of medication and lifestyle changes, it is possible to keep the condition under control. Children often outgrow their asthma by the time they reach their teens.

What to do

If your child has never had an asthma attack before and she develops breathing difficulties, take her to a hospital, or call an ambulance. She will probably need oxygen, and may be given a short course of steroids. She will be assessed and likely to be prescribed inhalers, one to use everyday that helps prevent attacks and another to ease the symptoms when they occur. Children are given inhalers with a "spacer." You place the inhaler in the bottom of the spacer and add the medication to it. The child then puts her mouth over the mouthpiece and breathes in and out normally. A spacer helps ensure that more of the medication gets into the lungs and not just into the mouth or lost in the air.

4 steps to take if your child has an asthma attack

1 Give your child the recommended dose of the reliever inhaler.

2 Sit him down in the most comfortable position for breathing and encourage him to take slow, steady breaths.

3 If the attack is not easing, repeat the dose of the inhaler.

4 If the attack is still not improving, call an ambulance.

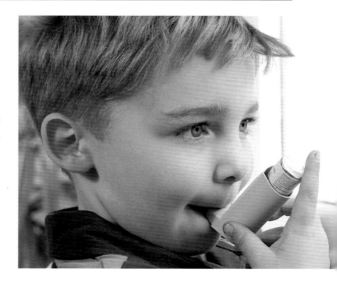

SKIN CONDITIONS

Because your child's skin is far more sensitive than an adult's, it is more susceptible to skin disorders. These can vary from irritation by sun, detergents, skin infections, or rashes caused illnesses or fever. Most of the skin problems are not serious and will clear up on their own. If in any doubt, always seek medical advice.

ECZEMA

This is a long-term condition that causes the skin to become itchy, red, dry, and cracked. Atopic eczema, which mainly affects children, is the most common form (about one child in 20 develops it), and those affected by it often have a family history of eczema, asthma (see page 256), or hay fever page (see page 255). However, it may also be a result of intolerance to certain foods.

Atopic eczema commonly appears in areas with folds of skin such as, behind the knees, the inner side of the elbows, on the side of the neck, and around the eyes and ears. It can vary in severity but most children are only mildly affected and have periods where it is not noticeable, and flareups where additional treatment is needed.

Severe eczema can cause cracked, very sore skin that's red and oozing fluid, and may even bleed if the child scratches the skin. Eczema can be very irritating for a child at night and cause her to scratch more. Very cold or very hot conditions can bring on a flareup.

What to do

If you suspect that your child has eczema talk to your doctor. Use emollient creams on her skin and put some in her bathwater, too. While some eczema develops for no particular reason, sometimes there is a trigger. Your doctor will work with you to find out the possible cause. If the problem persists, your child will be referred to a dermatologist for more tests.

Try to dress your child in clothes that are less likely to irritate the skin, for example, cotton. Keep your home fairly cool since heat can aggravate the condition.

If the eczema is severe, your doctor may prescribe the weakest effective corticosteroid cream to rub onto her skin to reduce the redness and swelling in flareups. In very severe cases, your child may need special bandages and dressings to keep her skin moist and stop her from scratching it. If the skin becomes infected, a course of antibiotics may be required. Other medication such as immunosuppressants may also be prescribed.

Keep your child away from anyone who has cold sores.

CONTACT DERMATITIS

This is a type of eczema caused by an irritant such as the adhesive on bandages, rubber, metal from a bracelet, some plants, bubble bath, scented soap, laundry soaps, and fabric softeners. Symptoms may take a few days to appear. Your child's skin will be red and inflamed and there may be a scaly rash. Her skin will be itchy and may blister, or even break, especially if she scratches a lot. Depending on the trigger, the rash may be localized or widespread.

What to do

Relieve the symptoms by applying calamine lotion to the affected area. If it is widespread, an antihistamine may be needed. If you know the cause, restrict your child's exposure to it.

If you are not sure of the cause, think about any recent changes you have made, for example, to washing routines. If the rash started after you changed your detergent and/or fabric softener, it may be worth changing back to the previous one. If the symptoms persist and you are unable to identify the cause, seek medical advice: tests may be needed identify the cause.

IMPETIGO

This is a highly contagious skin condition that causes large fluid-filled blisters and sores to develop on the skin—mainly around the mouth and nose. Bacteria enter and infect the skin where it is broken by a cut, an insect bite, or a preexisting skin condition, such as eczema (see page 257) or scabies (see page 258). The most infectious type results in sores that burst and leave a distinctive yellow crust on the skin. It is rarely serious, and would heal on its own, but the condition is generally treated with antibiotics because it is so contagious.

What to do

Take your child to your doctor or healthcare provider to confirm the diagnosis. Your child will probably be prescribed an antibiotic cream to apply to the sores. Your child will remain infectious until the sores have dried and healed or for 48 hours after starting treatment. In the meantime, keep her home from nursery school or away from her playgroup and encourage her not to touch the sores (this will stop the infection from spreading). Make sure she uses her own towels and facecloth and showers or bathes daily. Keeping her nails short may discourage the infection from spreading.

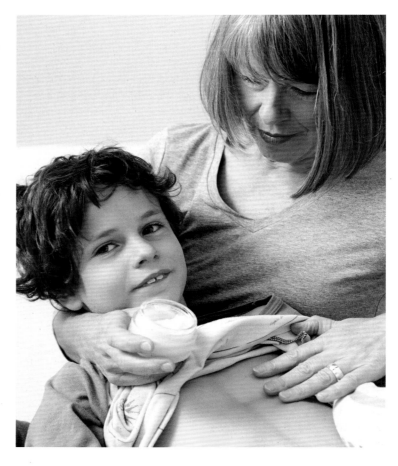

URTICARIA

Also known as hives, or nettle rash, urticaria is a raised itchy rash that may be limited to one body part, or it can spread over the entire body. It is caused by an allergic reaction to something a child has touched (for example, a nettle), or eaten. The trigger causes high levels of histamine and other chemical messengers to be released in the skin, so the blood vessels in the affected area open up (causing the redness or pinkness) and become leaky. The extra fluid in the tissues causes swelling and sometimes itchiness.

Urticaria normally subsides in a few hours, but occasionally lasts for a few weeks.

What to do

Apply calamine lotion to the affected part of the skin or give your child a coolish bath to soothe her skin. If the rash persists, your child may benefit from some antihistamine medication suitable for children; your pharmacist should be able to advise you. Contact your doctor immediately if the rash affects your child's face because it could cause her mouth to swell resulting in breathing difficulties.

If your child has frequent attacks, try to identify the cause to prevent the attacks occurring.

WARTS
These are small, brown or flesh-colored rough lumps that often develop on the skin, in particular the hands (warts) and the soles of the feet (plantar warts). They are caused by the human papilloma virus and are not serious, but they are contagious. They can be spread directly by skin-to-skin contact, or indirectly from contact with a contaminated surface, for example, the area around a swimming pool, or even the bathroom floor. Warts and plantar warts can appear singly or in clusters and while not usually painful, plantar warts can be uncomfortable to walk on.

What to do
Most warts and plantar disappear without treatment, but this can take a couple of years.

You can treat them with an over-the-counter medication; ask your pharmacist for advice. If the warts are on your child's genital area, seek medical advice immediately; never use proprietary medicines on this part of the body. If your child has a plantar wart, she should wear a special rubber swimming sock on her foot at the pool to prevent the infection from spreading.

MOLLUSCUM CONTAGIOSUM
This is a highly contagious viral infection that causes small, raised, itchy spots. It usually affects children under the age of five, or those with a weakened immune system, as a result of cancer treatment, for example.

What to do
Seek medical advice to confirm the diagnosis. Treatment is not normally recommended since molluscum contagiosum clears up on its own, although it can take 12 to 18 months. If your child has the virus, keep affected areas of her skin covered and avoid sharing towels, facecloths, clothing, or baths. Make sure your child does not scratch the spots because this may lead to other areas of skin becoming infected and prolong the infection.

SCABIES
Scabies is a contagious, intensely itchy skin condition. It occurs when tiny parasitic mites (Sarcoptes scabiei) burrow into the skin. There may be a rash where the mites have burrowed. It spreads by close contact with an affected person: children are especially at risk if there is an outbreak at their playgroup or nursery school, as are their parents.

Scabies mites can survive outside the human body for between 24 and 36 hours, and an infestation can spread quickly because people are usually unaware that they have the condition until two to three weeks after exposure.

What to do
Seek medical advice because, without effective treatment, the scabies mite life cycle can continue indefinitely—mites are resistant to soap and hot water and cannot be scrubbed out of the skin. Your doctor is most likely to prescribe permethrin cream, or if that does not work, malathion lotion. The lotion or cream is applied to areas where the scabies mites often burrow, such as the wrists, elbows, armpits, and under the fingernails, then left in place for a few hours. Treatment is repeated every few days. Wash your child's bedding, nightwear, and towels after each treatment.

To prevent reinfection, all members of your household and any close contacts, should be treated, even if they do not have any symptoms.

RINGWORM
This is a highly contagious and common fungal infection that causes round, reddish gray, scaly, and sometimes itchy, patches on the skin (or bald patches if it appears on the scalp). It is not serious and in spite of its name, it

has nothing to do with worms. There may be only one patch or several and they spread outward as they progress.

What to do

Consult your doctor. He or she will prescribe an antifungal cream if the skin is affected or shampoo, and possibly medication, if the infection is on the scalp.

It is important to prevent the ringworm from spreading to other members of the family; don't share towels, or let other children share the affected child's bath water. Your child does not need to avoid playgroup or nursery school, but let the caregivers know she has the condition. You may be asked to cover the affected area with a bandage.

BOILS

Pus-filled painful lumps can arise if bacteria infect hair follicles. Generally a boil will clear up on its own in about two weeks but there are things you can do to make the boil drain itself of pus and to make your child more comfortable.

If the boil lasts for more than two weeks or is very painful or large, take your child seek medical aadvice. Oral antibiotics may be prescribed and/or a cut made in the boil to release the pus.

What to do

Apply a warm compress several times a day to the affected area.

Infections or allergic reactions are responsible for most rashes and spots, so suspect this is the case with your child if a rash or spots appear and she is otherwise well. If, however, your child is under the weather, and/or the rash is itchy or sore, seek medical advice. Your doctor may need to see it to confirm a diagnosis and even if it's not serious, he or she can suggest ways to soothe discomfort and calm the rash.

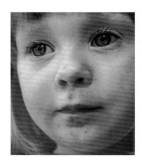

Many infectious diseases (see charts on pages 246–251) are characterized by different types of spots, some of which can be uncomfortable. Applying calamine lotion to the affected area can cool the spots and relieve itching.

If you suspect an allergic reaction, try to work out the cause. For example, have you started using a different soap on your child's skin or a new detergent to wash her clothes? This could be contact dermatitis, see page 257. Has she brushed against a leaf or cuddled a new household pet (see urticaria page 258)?

One disease in particular—meningitis, which is inflammation of the layers around the brain (see page 270)—can result in blood-poisoning, or septicemia, which causes a rash that begins as red or brown pinprick marks, and develops into larger red or purple blotches in the late stages. This is a very serious condition, which can be identified with the glass test.

Glass test

If your child has been unwell with flulike symptoms and a fever and develops a rash, press the side of a glass against the rash. This rash is caused by bruising under the skin and, unlike other rashes and spots, will not disappear if pressed. If you can see the rash through the glass, call an ambulance, even if you have already spoken to your doctor.

When it does drain, carefully wipe the pus away using sterile cotton gauze soaked in antiseptic solution. Cover the affected skin with a bandage. Don't poke or squeeze the boil to make it burst because you may spread the infection. If your child gets frequent boils try using an antibacterial soap.

GASTROINTESTINAL PROBLEMS

Children often get infections that cause diarrhea and vomiting. These infections are very easily transmitted from person to person, and very young children are especially vulnerable because of their tendency to put everything into their mouth. One of the major risks is dehydration from the loss of fluid.

GASTROENTERITIS

This highly contagious infection of the stomach and bowel (large intestine) can be caused by a virus, bacteria, or parasite. If affected, your child may begin by vomiting, and then have diarrhea (several loose, watery stools in a 24-hour period). She may also have a fever. If she is suffering from "food poisoning," she will probably also have stomach cramps.

What to do

Most cases of gastroenteritis suffered by children are mild and pass within three to five days without the need for treatment, but it is best to seek medical advice for your preschooler if she suffers from persistent vomiting or diarrhea that lasts longer than 24 hours, or eight hours if she has not been able to hold down any fluids—there is a serious risk of dehydration. Rarely, children need to be hospitalized and given fluids intravenously. Always consult your doctor if your child has been abroad recently (the cause may be a parasite); there are symptoms not usually associated with gastroenteritis, for example headache or stiff neck; of if there is blood or mucus in her stools.

Don't give your child over-the-counter antidiarrhea medications (they are not recommended for

5 ways to prevent spread of gastrointestinal problems

1 **Encourage your child to wash her hands properly** after going to the bathroom and before eating.

2 **Clean the toilet thoroughly** using disinfectant after each episode of diarrhea and/or vomiting, making sure that you also clean the handle and seat, and then wash your own hands.

3 **Don't let other members of your household share** your child's towels, facecloth, cutlery, or eating utensils.

4 **Keep her at home** for at least 48 hours after she has recovered.

5 **Don't take your child to a swimming pool** for at least two weeks after the last episode of diarrhea—rotavirus (the most common cause of severe diarrhea in young children) can be spread in water.

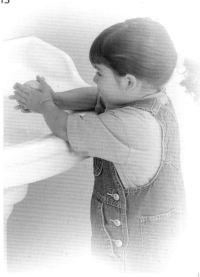

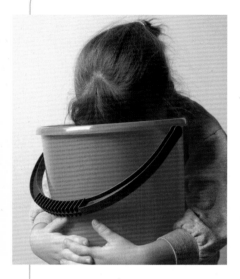

children under the age of 12), or medicines that prevent vomiting (antiemetics) because of the risk of side-effects, such as muscle spasms or allergic reactions.

Provide your child with a bowl to throw up into just in case she can't get to the bathroom on time. Wipe her mouth when she has vomited. Give her water, diluted fruit juice, or semiskim milk to drink and encourage her to sip it often. If she is feverish, give her children's acetaminophen. Bedrest is not essential but make sure she has easy access to the bathroom.

Initially your child may not have much of an appetite, but when she feels hungry again start her off with bland foods that won't upset her stomach, such as toast or rice, and gradually introduce other foods. Don't send her back to nursery school or playgroup until at least 48 hours after the last episode of diarrhea and vomiting.

TODDLER DIARRHEA

Some children (more commonly boys) up to the age of five suffer from persistent diarrhea, even though they are not unwell. Sometimes called chronic nonspecific diarrhea, affected children may have soft stools several times a day and pass recognizable pieces of food, for example, vegetables. Some children complain of mild stomache pain as well.

Diet, especially one that contains too much fruit juice and sweet drinks, is often the cause; one theory is that the balance of fluid, fiber, undigested sugars, and other foods that reach the large bowel (colon) becomes upset. Children outgrow it as the bowel becomes more efficient. It is not caused by food intolerance.

What to do

The condition is not serious but your healthcare provider will want to eliminate other causes or infections. He or she will measure your child to make sure she is growing normally. A change of diet often helps. Offer fewer sweetened drinks, and make sure that your child eats foods containing fat, such as whole milk and cheese, and easily digested fiber (broccoli, carrots, or sweet potato). If necessary, mash foods that she finds hard to digest.

CONSTIPATION

If your child passes stools infrequently and they are hard and dry, she may be constipated. This can happen if she becomes dehydrated following an illness, such as fever or vomiting, or due to dietary reasons, for example, her diet has changed recently, or if she is not eating sufficient fiber-rich foods, such as fruit, vegetables or wholewheat bread. It can also result from withholding stools while being toilet trained.

What to do

Children do vary in their toilet habits and some children go for two to three days without passing a stool. If you are concerned, however, encouraging your child to drink more fluids and adding more fiber-rich foods to her diet may solve the problem but consult your doctor if constipation persists for more than a week, or your child is in pain when she tries to defecate.

Your doctor will ask about your child's diet and if a change has not made a difference, he or she may prescribe stool softening medication or a laxative.

Encouraging your child to go to the bathroom ane have a bowel motion at the same time everyday can establish a more regular habit, but this can take a couple of months. If the problem persists, your child should be referred to a gastrointestinal specialist.

PINWORMS

These are tiny parasitic worms that look like little pieces of white thread. They infect the large intestine and lay their eggs around the anus.

Pinworms are very common and spread easily from person to person as a result of poor hygiene. You may see them in your child's stool or around her bottom. They often cause itching around the anus, especially at night, which may disturb your preschooler's sleep. When she scratches, the eggs get stuck on her fingernails and are transferred to her mouth or clothes.

What to do

Your doctor can prescribe medication in the form of tablets or oral suspension, or it can be bought over-the-counter from the pharmacy. If any member of the household has pinworms, everyone needs to be treated. Pinworms have a six-week lifecycle so it is essential to follow a very strict hygiene regime for at least six weeks to prevent reinfection. The day after the family has been given the medication, wash everyone's night clothes and bedding. Clean the house thoroughly, and insist that everyone wash their hands frequently, particularly before eating and always after going to the bathroom. Keep your child's fingernails short, and discourage your child from putting her fingers in her mouth. Put underwear on your child at night, and change it every morning. Make sure everyone in the house uses a separate towel and facecloth.

APPENDICITIS

This is inflammation of a small fingerlike pouch connected to the large intestine called the appendix. The condition starts as a pain in the center of the abdomen, which then travels toward the lower right-hand side, gradually worsening as it moves. Appendicitis is a medical emergency and the appendix needs to be removed surgically; if left untreated, it can burst and cause potentially life-threatening infections. Appendicitis is more common in children over the age of 10.

What to do

If your child complains of a severe pain in the abdomen that is worsening, call your doctor immediately. Appendicitis can be difficult to diagnose and there may be another cause of the pain, such as a bladder infection. If in doubt, take your child to the hospital, or call an ambulance.

---

more *about* | Causes of gastroenteritis

Rotavirus is the leading cause of gastroenteritis in children. It is often spread when an infected child does not wash her hands properly after using the toilet. The first infection by rotavirus tends to be the most severe because the body has no resistance. After being infected with the virus once, the body starts to build up immunity to it. This is also why rotavirus infection is extremely rare in adults. All young babies are currently immunized against it as part of their routine vaccination program.

Norovirus is sometimes known as the winter vomiting bug and it affects people of all ages. It is highly infectious and will last a couple of days. It develops 12 to 48 hours after contact with an infected person and you are infectious during that period.

Food poisoning. Food may be contaminated with bacteria such as salmonella or E.coli, as a result of poor food hygiene or insufficient cooking. Or it can be contaminated with a virus.

MOUTH AND TOOTH CONDITIONS

The skin around the mouth is even more delicate than the skin that covers the rest of the body. The soft lining of the mouth and the tongue is easily damaged by a sharp tooth, or food or drink that is too hot or too cold. Children commonly put lots of things—from fingers to toys in their mouths—so this area is very exposed to a variety of potentially damaging infections.

COLD SORES

These are small fluid-filled blisters that appear around the mouth, generally on the lips. They are secondary infections caused by the herpes simplex virus, which has entered the body as a result of an earlier illness. Cold sores often start as a tingling, or even burning sensation at the site of the infection, and a few days later, the blisters appear. These will burst forming a weeping sore with clear fluid oozing out. As the fluid dries, a crusty scab will form, under which healing takes place.

Cold sores are highly contagious.

What to do

Cold sores usually clear up without treatment within 7 to 10 days but antiviral creams can help alleviate the symptoms and may speed up healing. Ask your pharmacist for a cream suitable for young children; always wash your hands after applying the medication. Encourage your child not to touch or pick at the sore.

Your child may not want to drink if her lips are very sore and so risks becoming dehydrated. In this case, try letting her drink through a straw.

Cold sores are at their most contagious when they burst, and remain so until they are completely healed. To prevent family and friends from becoming infected, make sure no one shares a towel or facecloth and that you don't come in contact with the sore through kissing.

MOUTH ULCERS

Commonly called canker sores, these are small open sores in the lining of the mouth or on the tongue. They are not serious and will normally heal on their own within four to 10 days, but they can be very painful and if your child has one, she may be reluctant to eat. Ulcers mostly appear for no apparent reason, but can occur because a child has a very sharp tooth, or as a symptom of gingivostomatitis (see opposite); rarely, they may be caused by an underlying disorder.

What to do

If the ulcers are painful, give your child children's acetaminophen or children's ibuprofen to relieve the pain. You can buy anesthetic gels suitable for young children at a pharmacy. Give your child bland and soft food to eat and make sure she continues brushing her teeth properly (use a softer brush

---

more about | The herpes simplex virus

After an initial infection (symptoms include swollen gums, sore throat, producing more saliva than usual, fever, or even dehydration, headache, or feeling nauseous), the herpes simplex virus remains dormant in the nervous tissue, but triggers such as strong sunlight, colds, or stress may cause it to be reactivated.

if necessary). Seek medical advice if the ulcer has not healed after 10 days, your child has repeated ulcers, or she has a fever as well.

GINGIVOSTOMATITIS
This is a viral infection accompanying the first infection by the herpes simplex virus—the same one that is behind cold sores (above). Gingivostomatitis generally affects children under the age of three.

Your child will develop a fever and a sore mouth, which is followed by small, yellowish painful ulcers that rupture, and red swollen gums. Her neck glands will be swollen, and she may have bad breath. She'll find it difficult to chew or swallow, and may be reluctant to drink.

What to do
Call your doctor. He or she will prescribe pain relief and possibly antiviral medication. If your child is very unwell, she may need to be admitted to a hospital so that fluids and antiviral medication can be given intravenously.

GINGIVITIS
Not to be confused with gingivostomatitis, this is an inflammation of the gums that is caused by not brushing teeth and gums properly. The bacteria in the plaque that collects around the base of the teeth and in the gum margins irritate the gums. The first sign you may see is that your

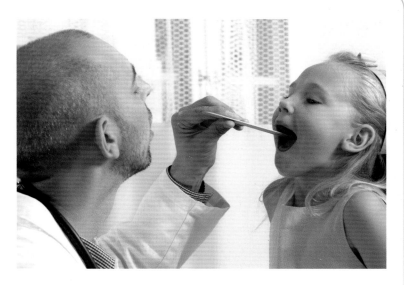

child's gums bleed when she brushes her teeth; she may tell you her gums are sore. If left unchecked, gingivitis can cause the teeth to loosen.

What to do
Take your child to the dentist for a checkup. If the attack is mild, then just a better dental hygiene routine may be sufficient.

If the condition is severe, an antibacterial mouthwash may be recommended.

Once the gums have recovered and are less tender, the dentist may want to scrape away the plaque to prevent another attack.

TOOTH DECAY AND DENTAL ABSCESS
The same bacteria that contribute toward gingivitis can cause tooth decay. They break down the sugars in food and drink to provide them with energy and in

so doing create acids, which, if left on the teeth, will de-mineralize the hard outer tooth enamel (cause loss of calcium and phosphate). This eventually breaks down the enamel and the layers beneath, causing decay.

If bacteria enter the teeth through the decay, the tooth can become infected (an abscess). Pus will collect beneath the tooth and can enter the tooth's sensitive core, damaging the nerves and blood vessels beneath it.

What to do
Good dental hygiene (see page 65) can prevent tooth decay and routine dental checkups can pick up signs of problems early.

If you see a blackened area on one of your child's teeth, or she complains of a toothache, take her to the dentist.

If the decay is at an early stage, the dentist will scrape away

LIP LICKER'S DERMATITIS

Some young children who still suck their thumbs or excessively lick their lips are prone to a rash around the mouth caused by saliva. Saliva can be irritating; it makes the lips dry and chapped while inflaming the surrounding skin, which becomes scaly.

Applying a moisturizing lip balm frequently and treating the adjoining skin with petroleum jelly is the best way to deal with the problem. The problem resolves as soon as the lip licking stops.

any plaque, allowing the surface of the tooth to come into contact with saliva. The saliva helps re-mineralize the tooth, allowing it to heal over time. If decay is severe, the dentist may need to remove the damaged area of tooth and insert a filling.

If an abscess has developed, take your child to the dentist immediately. The dentist will need to drill into the tooth to relieve the pressure and then remove the damaged area. If the damage is severe, the tooth may have to be removed altogether.

MALOCCLUSION

Ideally, all upper teeth sit directly over the lower teeth and the points of the molars fit the grooves of the opposite molar. A malocclusion is a misalignment of upper and lower teeth and the condition tends to run in families.

Treatment may be needed eventually if the teeth are so crooked or out of position that a child finds eating and talking difficult. Malocclusion can also interfere with speech development.

Malocclusion can be caused by a difference between the size of the upper and lower jaws or between jaw and tooth size (especially in adult teeth), which can result in overcrowding of teeth or in abnormal bite patterns. However, it can also result from early childhood habits such as thumb sucking, use of a pacifier beyond three years of age, and continuing to use a bottle for a prolonged period.

What to do

Very few people have perfect teeth alignment and most problems are so minor that they do not require treatment.

If there is a family history of malocclusion that needed treatment, your dentist will check your child as she grows, because early detection and treatment may optimize the time and method of treatment needed.

Many types of malocclusion are not preventable but you can help by discouraging thumb sucking or the use of dummies. Treatment will not be carried out until your child is much older (normally 11 to 13 years), and may include extraction of some teeth, and/or wearing of braces.

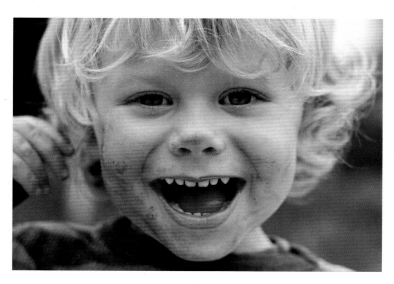

EAR AND EYE PROBLEMS

Ear and eye infections are very common in young children and need prompt treatment. If left untreated, persistent ear infections can result in short-term hearing impairment. Some eye problems can cause impaired vision. Other problems with hearing and vision are often present from birth and these, too, may impact on a child's development.

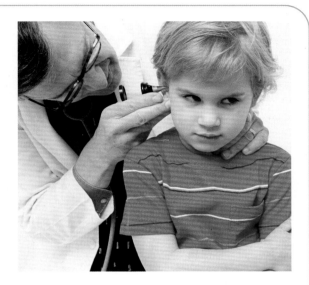

EAR INFECTIONS

Infections can occur in the outer (otitis externa) or inner ear (otitis media) and can be painful. The latter is often a complication of a virus such as cold or throat infection, but can also be caused by a bacterial infection. A young child's Eustachian tube, which connects the nose to the middle ear, is short and horizontal, so infections can pass easily from one area to another. Many children suffer from recurrent ear infections.

Suspect that your child has an infection if he has a fever and feels generally unwell. If young, he may pull at his ear but if older, he may tell you it hurts. His hearing may be temporarily impaired.

What to do

Take your child to your doctor. He or she will examine the ear with an auriscope and is likely to recommend the appropriate dose of children's acetaminophen or children's ibuprofen to reduce pain and fever.

If your doctor suspects a bacterial infection, a course of antibiotics may be prescribed.

Occasionally an eardrum will burst; if this happens, the pain may ease because pressure on the eardrum is relieved, and mucus will weep from the ear.

A perforated eardrum will heal within a few weeks, but you should not take your child swimming until it does.

EXCESSIVE WAX

Earwax protects and lubricates the ear canal and is made up mainly of dead cells, hair, and dust. A child's earwax is generally wet and soft but if he has too much or the wax is hard, it can block the ear canal and cause temporary hearing impairment, so may need to be removed.

What to do

Seek medical advice. You may be advised to wait and see if the wax clears on its own or, if your child's hearing is affected, you may be prescribed eardrops to soften the earwax and encourage it to clear more quickly.

GLUE EAR

If your child becomes unable to hear, either his middle ear may be filled with fluid or it's the result of a persistent cough or cold.

What to do

Take your child to your doctor who will refer your child for a hearing test either at the hospital or child health clinic. The tests may be repeated over a few months since most cases clear up within three months. If there is no improvement, you will be referred to an ear, nose, and throat (ENT) specialist for further assessment; intervention is normally only recommended if symptoms are prolonged and/or the hearing loss is significant enough to interfere with a child's language and speech development. Treatment involves minor surgery. Small tympanostomy tubes, also known as grommets, are inserted in the eardrum, which allow the fluid to drain from the middle ear. Hearing will improve immediately. The tubes normally fall out as the eardrum heals. Sometimes this operation needs to be repeated.

CONJUNCTIVITIS

Also known as pink eye, the layer of tissue that covers the surface of the eye—the conjunctiva—can become inflamed. One or both eyes will be red and itchy and there may be a thick yellow discharge that dries and crusts over the eyelashes, most noticeable after your child has been asleep. Conjunctivitis can be caused by a viral or bacterial infection or be the result of an allergy. It is very common and infectious conjunctivitis is easily passed on to others.

What to do

Conjunctivitis often clears up without medical treatment. Wipe the sticky discharge away with sterile cotton gauze pads and water. Use a separate piece for each stroke, and always wipe from the inner side of the eye outward. If the symptoms persist, seek medical advice. Your doctor may take a swab of the discharge to determine the cause. If it is a bacterial infection, an antibiotic eye ointment will be prescribed. If your child attends a playgroup or nursery school, you need to keep him at home until the infection has cleared up.

STYES

A stye, or hordeolum, is a small, often painful lump, or abscess (collection of pus), which develops on the inner or outer eyelid and is caused by an infection. The eye may also be red and watery.

What to do

Most styes get better without treatment within a few days. An external stye may turn into a yellow spot and release pus after three or four days. One on the inside of the eyelid will be more painful and may last slightly longer. Try placing a warm compress (a cloth warmed with warm water) against the eye to encourage the pus to be released. If the stye does not improve in a few days, consult your doctor; he or she may want to drain it. You should never attempt to burst a stye yourself.

CATARACTS

This is a clouding in the lens of the eye that can impair vision. Although more common in the elderly, and occasionally present at birth, cataracts can develop during childhood. One or both eyes may be affected. If a child has a cataract in one eye, his vision is likely to be fine in the other one. If the cataract is large and central, the effects will be more noticeable than if it is small and away from the center.

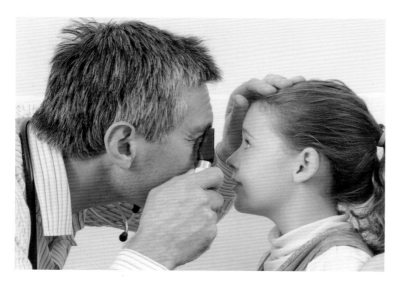

What to do

If you notice your child's eyes jerking quickly from side to side (a condition known as nystagmus, which may be associated with cataracts), tell your doctor who will arrange an appointment with an ophthalmologist.

Your child may need surgery to replace the cloudy lens with an artificial one. The timing of surgery will depend on the degree of cloudiness and visual impairment. If the cataract is only moderately severe, surgery may be delayed until your child is older. He may also need to wear glasses and, sometimes if one eye is weaker than the other, the stronger eye will need to be covered with a patch so that the weaker eye will work harder, reducing the possibility of a lazy eye (see below).

LONG-SIGHTEDNESS

Hypermetropia is a common condition whereby a person is able to see things better far away than close up. It may be picked up at a routine assessment or you may notice that your child has problems looking at books, squints, or says her eyes or head hurts.

What to do

Get in touch with your doctor. He or she should arrange for your child to be seen by an optometrist, who may recommend glasses if there is a vision problem.

Many children grow out of hypermetropia by the time they are adults.

SHORT-SIGHTEDNESS

Myopia is not as common as long-sightedness, but a young child may be able to see things better close up than far away. It often runs in families.

What to do

Talk to your doctor, who will refer you for tests. Diagnosis of the condition requires an assessment by an optometrist, who may prescribe glasses.

SQUINT (STRABISMUS)

When the eyes are not aligned correctly, they can appear to be looking in different directions, and this is sometimes more noticeable in photographs. Squints can be the result of a lazy eye (see amblyopia, below), long-sightedness, or even a cataract.

What to do

Seek medical advice. Your doctor should refer your child to an ophthalmologist for an assessment because squints should be treated as soon as they are detected to prevent them from becoming permanent. The recommendations depend on the severity of the squint, but may include glasses, possibly with an eye patch, botulinum toxin (botox) injections, eye exercises and, less commonly, corrective surgery. Treatment is very effective in young children.

LAZY EYE (AMBLYOPIA)

This occurs if the vision in one eye does not develop properly so a child relies on his "good" eye. It arises because light does not focus correctly on the light-sensitive retina at the back of the eye. Normally the retina translates the images into signals for the brain to interpret. If the retina in one eye is not sending the correct signals, the brain will rely more heavily on the better eye for information. There are a number of causes, such as a squint or the difference in quality of vision in your child's eyes, or one long-sighted eye. Children with a lazy eye usually have problems judging the distance between themselves and objects accurately, which can make tasks such as catching a ball more difficult, but are generally unaware that anything is wrong.

What to do

Seek advice from your doctor. Most cases of lazy eye can be treated, usually by correcting the underlying problem, such as a squint. Glasses may be recommended, and often the use of an eye patch to cover the good eye and encourage the weaker eye to work harder.

NERVOUS SYSTEM PROBLEMS

The nervous system is made up of the brain, spinal cord, and nerves, which between them control many body functions. Any injury or infection that affects this system can have long-lasting consequences.

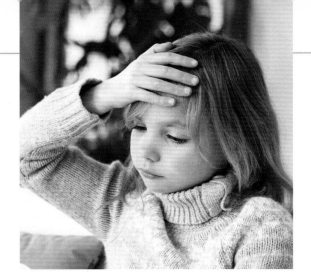

HEADACHE

Most children complain of occasional headaches. However, some children suffer from recurrent headaches that interfere with their everyday activities.

A tension headache is one resulting from emotional stress, for example, a problem at nursery school or an event that the child is worried about, or it can even be caused by him clenching or grinding his teeth.

A headache can also be a symptom of a migraine, which is often felt as a throbbing pain on one side of the head, and may be accompanied by vomiting, sensitivity to light (your child may say lights are sparkling), or noise.

A migraine can last for anything from a couple of hours to a couple of days. Attacks can be triggered by emotional stress, but some foods, in particular chocolate, oranges, and cheese also trigger attacks, as can tiredness or too much sun.

What to do

Try to establish the cause of the pain; sometimes children say they have a headache when they mean an earache or a toothache or an ache they can't explain.

If you suspect a tension headache, give your child the recommended dose of children's acetaminophen or children's ibuprofen. If the headaches are frequent, discuss this with your healthcare provider so that he or she can eliminate other more serious causes, though these are very rare.

If you think the problem is a migraine, give your child the recommended dose of children's acetaminophen or children's ibuprofen and encourage him to rest in a darkened room. When you are able, take him to the doctor. He or she will want to identify trigger factors and may offer an antiemetic to minimize vomiting during an attack as well as prescribe other medications in case of repeated attacks.

MENINGITIS

This is a serious infection, as a result of either a virus or bacteria, which causes inflammation of the meninges, the layers, or membranes around the brain and spinal cord. Bacterial meningitis is particularly serious as the same bacteria also cause septicemia (blood poisoning), which can be fatal. The most common disease-causing bacteria are Neisseria meningitidis and Streptococcus pneumoniae but there are also several others. Meningitis can develop very quickly, however, with prompt medical attention in a hospital most children make a full recovery. However, some will suffer after effects, which can range from mild to more serious, and occasionally disabling, because the infection damages an area of the brain.

What to do

Call your doctor immediately if you notice any of the symptoms (see box opposite page). If you have already seen the doctor and any of the symptoms worsen, do not hesitate to call again, and if you notice a rash developing call an ambulance; tell the control that you suspect meningitis. Your child will be admitted to hospital and given intravenous antibiotics.

The diagnosis will be confirmed by blood tests and a lumbar puncture (fluid taken from around the spinal cord). Anyone who has been in contact with the affected child should also be given a short course of antibiotics as a precaution.

EPILEPSY

This is a life-long condition in which a person has a tendency to suffer from seizures (a disturbance in the electrical activity in the brain); it can develop at any age. (See box on page 272 on types for help in diagnosis.)

Sometimes epilepsy develops after a child has sustained a head injury or has had an illness that affects the brain, such as meningitis; some children have a family history of epilepsy. In many cases, however, the cause is unknown. Neither are all seizures the result of epilepsy. The condition will not be confirmed on the basis of only one seizure; specialized tests, such as an electroencephalogram (EEG), and possibly brain scans such as a CT and/or MRI are needed. If your child has had seizures as a result of a raised temperature, he does not have epilepsy although he has a slightly higher chance of developing it than children who have never had one.

What to do

Call an ambulance if this is his first seizure, or if he's had them before and the seizure lasts more than five minutes, if he is having repeated seizures, or if he is unconscious for more than 10 minutes. Call your doctor for advice in any other circumstance. If possible, ask someone to video the seizure so that your doctor can see the seizure pattern.

Your doctor will want to know what your child was doing

In focal seizures, only part of the brain is affected but in tonic–clonic seizures, the whole body is involved; both follow a pattern. A focal seizure can be followed by a tonic-clonic seizure.

Focal, or partial, seizures

In these seizures, the epileptic activity starts in part of a child's brain. They normally only last a couple of minutes. A child may appear fully conscious and alert, or he may be unaware of what is happening. He may have unusual sensations or feelings, his skin may be hot and flushed or even very pale, he may start chewing, swallowing, or smacking his lips, scratching his head for no reason, or may wander off into another room.

Tonic–clonic or generalized seizures

In the first (tonic) phase, the child loses consciousness and, if he is standing, will fall to the floor. His body stiffens as all the muscles contract; he may let out a loud sound at the same time because the muscle contraction forces air out of the lungs. His breathing pattern changes, so there is less oxygen than normal in his lungs, and in his blood, causing his skin to look bluish (cyanosis). This will be most noticeable at his mouth, ears, and fingernails. He may bite his tongue and the inside of his cheeks.

In the second (clonic) phase, convulsions begin. His limbs begin jerky movements as groups of muscles tighten and relax in turn. He may clench his jaw so breathing may be noisy. If he bites his tongue, the saliva may be blood-stained. He may also lose control of his bladder and/or bowel.

After a few minutes the convulsive movements will stop and he will regain consciousness, but may be completely unaware of what happened. He may say that he is very tired and fall into a deep sleep.

immediately before a seizure because it may help identify what triggered it—fatigue, lack of sleep, and stress are common triggers, and for a few children, flashing or flickering lights.

If epilepsy is confirmed, your child will be monitored carefully. He may be given antiepileptic drugs to help control his tendency to have seizures; with the right medicine, many children have few or no seizures. If a trigger is identified, avoiding it can help, although this can be difficult. An epilepsy specialist will review your child regularly, and his medication will be adjusted as he grows. Surgery or a special diet may sometimes be recommended.

FIRST AID FOR EPILEPSY

It is not possible to stop a seizure, and never try to control your child's movements during one. Never put anything in his mouth because he could choke but make sure he cannot hurt himself.

If it is a focal seizure, sit him down somewhere quiet. Clear a space around him and move any objects, such as hot drinks, well out of reach. Stay with him until he recovers.

If it is a tonic–clonic seizure, clear a space around him, removing any objects that could hurt him or place rolled-up towels or cushions around him, especially by his head, to prevent injury. Take note of when the convulsions start.

When the convulsive movements stop, he may be unconscious for a short time. Open his airway and check breathing (see page 224). Once he is breathing, place him in the recovery position. Monitor him until he has completely recovered.

GENITALS AND URINARY SYSTEM PROBLEMS

Most conditions that affect the genitals or the urinary system are minor and clear up quickly with treatment. Some conditions, however, are caused by underlying structural defects and may not be picked up on during regular health checks.

URINARY TRACT INFECTION (UTI)

An infection can occur in any part of the body used to make and get rid of urine—the kidneys (pyelonephritis), ureters, bladder (cystitis), or urethra (urethritis); the urethra is most commonly infected. Bacteria can easily pass from the rectum to the urethra and result in urethritis.

UTIs are not usually serious, but must be properly diagnosed and treated to prevent scarring of the kidneys, which can cause problems in later life. Girls tend to suffer more UTIs than boys.

Suspect one if your child is passing urine more frequently than usual (especially if he is bed-wetting having previously been dry at night), and complains of pain or a burning sensation when he is passing urine. He may be irritable and/or appear lethargic, vomit, have a temperature of 100.4°F or above, and tell you that he has a pain in his lower back or abdomen.

What to do

Always seek medical advice as soon as possible (within 24 hours) if you think your child has a UTI. A urine sample from your child will be tested and if an infection is confirmed, your child will be given a course of antibiotics. If the infection is serious, he may need to be admitted to a hospital, but usually can be treated at home. Another urine sample will be needed a few days after treatment to demonstrate the infection has cleared. If your child is prone to recurrent infections, he may be given a low dose of antibiotics for a few months, and may even require surgery. While your child is unwell, make sure he drinks plenty of fluids because they dilute the urine and ease discomfort while urinating; they also help flush out the bacteria. Teach your child to always wipe his bottom from front to back to prevent bacteria from spreading.

TIGHT FORESKIN

At birth the inner surface of the foreskin is attached to the head of the penis (glans). From about the age of two, the foreskin begins to separate naturally from the glans until it can be pulled back—you should never attempt force it. In some boys, this does not happen until they are about four years old. If the tissue that holds a baby's foreskin in place remains for longer than normal a tight foreskin can result. A tight foreskin can also occur if there is an abnormally narrow opening in the penis (phimosis).

What to do

If your son is more than four years old and having trouble urinating or cannot retract his foreskin, take him to your doctor. If left untreated he is at greater risk of UTIs. Circumcision to remove the foreskin, or surgery to separate the tissues may be recommended; both operations would be performed under anesthetic.

BALANITIS

This is an inflammation of the foreskin and the head of the penis (glans) and it can be caused by a fungal or bacterial infection. It most commonly results from not cleaning the penis properly, but a tight foreskin (see page 273) can also increase the likelihood of balanitis. It can also be a reaction to chemicals used in soaps and detergents. Suspect balanitis if your child has a red rash at the tip of his penis (it may be scaly or ulcerated) or there is tenderness, pain, swelling, itching, and discomfort, a discharge or pus from underneath the foreskin (this may smell foul), and he is unable to pull back his foreskin.

What to do

Take your child to your doctor so the cause can be identified. You will be prescribed either an antiviral or antibiotic ointment and be advised to keep the head of the penis and foreskin as clean as possible using only warm water and nothing that might irritate

the area, such as soap or detergent. Occasionally, especially if there are recurrent infections, circumcision will be advised

VULOVAGINITIS

This is a common condition that causes minor inflammation or irritation of the vagina and vulva. The linings of both can be quite thin in young girls, making the area susceptible to irritation especially from some soaps and detergents, or even wearing underwear that is too tight. Poor hygiene can also contribute.

You may notice your child scratching her vaginal area. There may also be a vaginal discharge (greenish yellow if it's a bacterial infection; white if it's a fungal infection), redness of the skin between the labia majora, and burning or stinging on passing urine. Threadworms (see page 263) may also be to blame.

What to do

Good hygiene, avoiding possible irritants such as bubble bath, and changing to looser cotton underpants will clear up most mild cases. However, take your child to the doctor if she complains of pain when passing urine, is very uncomfortable, or symptoms persist for more than two weeks, because other causes will need to be eliminated. If there is an infection, an antifungal or antibiotic ointment will be prescribed.

GLOMERULONEPHRITIS

This is a potentially serious kidney disorder that affects the tiny filters inside the kidneys. Your child may have a rash, complain of pain in his lower back and possibly in his joints, and exhibit tiredness or breathing problems. But often there are no noticeable symptoms and this infection of the glomeruli may only be picked up as a result of urine or blood tests done for another reason.

What to do

If your child complains of any of the above symptoms, see your doctor. If glomerulonephritis is suspected, your child will be referred to a kidney specialist and put on a low-sodium low-protein diet to ease the strain on his kidneys; his fluid intake may be restricted. If a bacterial infection is suspected, he will be given antibiotics. Glomerulonephritis normally clears up within a week.

BONE, MUSCLE, AND JOINT DISORDERS

Any serious or long-term problems must be treated in order to prevent problems with muscle development and mobility. If your child has started limping, find out if she has injured her leg or foot or trodden on a sharp object. Inspect the soles of her feet and look between her toes for a wound. If she complains of joint pain, pain in her bones, or develops a limp for no apparent reason, always take her to see your doctor.

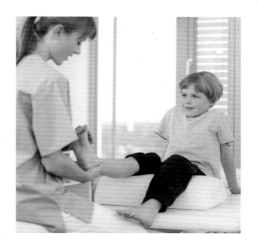

IRRITABLE HIP

Also known as transient synovitis, this is a condition in which the lining around the hip joint becomes inflamed and fluid accumulates within the joint. It can be very painful and your child will find it difficult to walk.

It may follow a hip injury, but in some instances it develops after a minor viral infection of the chest, throat, or digestive system. It is more common in children over the age of four, and it affects boys more than girls.

What to do

If your child complains of severe pain in her hip, groin, thigh, or knee, and/or is limping for no apparent reason, take her to your doctor. He or she will examine her leg and hip and ask her to try and walk on it and order an X-ray, blood test to rule out infection, and possibly an ultrasound scan to confirm the diagnosis and rule out Perthes disease (see page 276). The recommended treatment is anti-inflammatory medication such as children's ibuprofen, and bed rest (or on the couch) until the pain is resolved— normally 7 to 10 days. If there is an infection, fluid may need to be drained from the joint, and antibiotics will be prescribed. It can help to massage your child's hip and hold a covered hot-water bottle against it. Your child should not to be too active too soon because the problem may return.

BONE INFECTION

Children are forever getting superficial cuts and grazes, which usually heal on their own. In deeper wounds, however, dirt can be carried farther internally and bacteria can more easily travel to other parts of the body. If bacteria, most commonly Staphylococcus aureus, reach bone they can cause a serious infection called osteomyelitis. A bone can also become infected when the blood supply to that area is disrupted, but this is rare in children. Osteomyelitis most commonly affects the long bones of the arms and legs, but can affect other bones too. If your child has the condition, she will complain of severe pain in the infected bone and may be generally unwell. She may have a fever and feel tired or nauseated. The skin above the infected bone may be sore, red, and swollen.

What to do

If your child complains of bone pain and has a fever, take her to your doctor urgently. Blood tests to confirm the diagnosis will be needed and she will be given antibiotics to treat the infection. If the infection is caught early, she should make a complete recovery but rarely, infected bone may need to be surgically removed.

RICKETS

This is a condition that affects bone development in children. It is caused by a lack of vitamin D and calcium, the vitamin and mineral needed for healthy bone growth. Without them, developing bones become soft and malformed, which can also lead to deformities such as bowed legs and curvature of the spine. A child can become deficient if her diet is lacking in vitamin D or calcium or if she cannot absorb one or both nutrients.

What to do

If your child has bone pain, delayed growth (as measured against the appropriate developmental chart), or skeletal problems, take her to your doctor. A routine checkup may not pick up the changes because older children are not routinely undressed to be examined. Rickets can be successfully treated in most children by ensuring they eat calcium- and vitamin D-rich foods and/or take the appropriate supplements. If your child has problems absorbing vitamins and minerals, or cannot take supplements, she may be given a yearly vitamin D injection. Sunlight also contains vitamin D, which is absorbed by the skin, so try to increase the amount of time your child spends outside.

If your child develops a bone deformity, your doctor may suggest treatment to correct it.

For example, she may need to wear a brace to support the affected area while her bones grow, or she may need surgery.

PERTHES DISEASE

This is a childhood condition that affects the head, or top, of the femur (thigh bone) where it fits into the pelvis. Occasionally the blood supply to the growth plate in the top of the femur becomes temporarily inadequate, causing softening of the surrounding bones. When the supply returns, the tissue reforms and remodels itself over a few years. With early diagnosis, most people with Perthes disease heal without intervention, but some children need a temporary cast to prevent deformity. Perthes disease affects boys more than girls and tends to develop around the age of four.

What to do

If your child complains of hip pain or develops a noticeable limp, take her to your doctor as soon as possible. An X-ray will be needed to confirm the cause of the problem. For less severe cases, pain relief and bed rest for 7 to 14 days, or until the pain subsides, will be recommended. If there is a risk of deformity, your child may need to wear a temporary cast as a preventive measure. Regular X-rays or scans will monitor your child's recovery and bone growth. Treatment is aimed at promoting the healing process and ensuring that the head of the femur remains aligned in the pelvis. In very severe cases, deformity is not preventable and the child may develop arthritis later on in life.

ARTHRITIS

Your child may suffer pain, redness, and swelling and stiffness in one or more of her joints due to one of three types of juvenile idiopathic arthritis (JIA). Oligo-articular JIA is the most common and affects up to four joints in the body, generally the knees, ankles, and wrists. Polyarticular JIA, or polyarthritis, affects five or more joints—often the small joints of the hands and feet. Systemic onset JIA affects the whole body and symptoms such as a fever, rash, lack of energy, and swollen glands, may develop some time before the joint becomes painful.

What to do

If your child complains of severe joint pains or stiffness, or starts to limp, or you notice a rash with a fever, take your child to the doctor. Your doctor will arrange for blood tests to identify the cause. Anti-inflammatory drugs such as children's ibuprofen will be prescribed; if they do not help there are stronger medications. There is no cure for arthritis, but regular physiotherapy and exercise, especially swimming, can help maintain your child's mobility and strength.

BEHAVIORAL PROBLEMS

It's important to separate "normal" disruptive behavior (see page 139) from that which might have a genetic or medical cause. It's also vital that the problem is correctly identified so it can be treated effectively; some higher-functioning autistic children will often be diagnosed with other conditions such as Attention Deficit Hyperactivity Disorder (ADHD), Attention Deficit Disorder (ADD), Developmental Coordination Disorder (CDD) dyslexia (see box, page 281), or epilepsy.

Autism

Also known as ASD (Autism Spectrum Disorder), this is a lifelong developmental condition that impairs a child's ability to interact socially, understand social situations, and communicate successfully with others. Children with autism find it difficult to pick up on social cues that other children understand intuitively and need to be taught basic social skills and helped to make sense of the world around them.

Autistic children have difficulty interpreting facial expressions and tone of voice, which prevents them from understanding how other people feel. An autistic child may also not appreciate the reciprocal nature of conversation, so he will appear to behave eccentrically and insensitively to others. A child with autism will usually have some form of language delay and when he does talk, he will take speech literally and struggle to understand jokes or figures of speech. He may also speak in a stilted manner or at

length about a topic of special interest to him, and will be oblivious to his listener's level of interest.

Autism is a spectrum condition. This means that even though there are common traits in all children with autism, each child will be affected by the condition in different ways and to different degrees. Children with classic or lower-functioning autism, defined as lower by reference to the child's IQ, may also have learning disabilities but there also exist autistic children with normal to above-average IQs who are able to function competently.

It is a popular misconception that autistic children are savants with special or prodigious talents and abilities. Although savants are more common among autistic people, in fact, only ten percent of the autistic population exhibit these traits as opposed to one percent of the normal population.

The causes of autism are currently unclear except that there

is no link between the MMR vaccine (see page 217) and autism. The fact that the MMR is given to children at around 18 months, when the first signs of autism can appear, is coincidental rather than causative. A combination of genetic and environmental factors is probably responsible for the condition. There is currently no single test available that can determine whether or not a child has autism.

About one in a hundred of the population are on the autistic spectrum and autism is more common in boys than girls. About four times as many boys are diagnosed with autism as girls but in higher-functioning forms of autism, such as Asperger syndrome (see page 278), this figure is thought to be as high as 16 boys diagnosed to every girl. It is not known whether boys are genetically predisposed toward having autism or whether autism is underdiagnosed in girls. The traditional view of high-functioning autistic boys as social misfits who obsessively collect useless information does not take into account the fact that a girl's special interests may extend to subjects such as fairies, horses, or fashion instead. Girls may be less commonly diagnosed with higher-functioning autism or Asperger Syndrome because they are better at masking their difficulties than boys. It appears, though, that girls with lower-functioning autism are more severely affected than boys, with a ratio of two to one.

Diagnosing autism

A diagnosis is not usually made before the age of 18 months because it is very difficult to assess a child's level of interpersonal skills before this age. A child with higher-functioning autism will usually not be diagnosed until he is about three years old, when the difficulties in relating to others become more obvious. Talk to your doctor if you are concerned about your child and you observe any of the traits detailed below. In some cases, a child will be assessed by a specialist developmental pediatrician acting as part of a multidisciplinary team, which may be made up of speech and language therapists, occupational therapists, family workers, and psychologists. As part of the assessment, the team will take a full developmental history, usually interview you in detail as well as talk to your child,

and may want to visit his nursery school or playgroup and home.

You may be concerned that a diagnosis of autism will affect your child adversely by labeling him as different. In fact, the diagnosis of autism can be beneficial to you and your child because he can make significant progress with the right help. Adjustments can be made to your home and nursery school environment to enable your child to cope better.

Recognizing the signs

Some of these characteristics are common in young children with or without autism and it is important to remember that none or all of these signs on their own or together necessarily mean that your child has autism. But if you are concerned that your child is not reaching his developmental milestones, ask your healthcare provider if a developmental pediatrician can assess your child.

- Speech is delayed or nonexistent or your child talks in an eccentric way that may sound robotic or monotonous.
- Difficulty understanding simple directions, instructions, or questions.
- Doesn't make eye contact or appears to look straight through people.
- Sensitivity to smells, bright lights, and loud noises such as vacuum cleaners, motorbikes, and hairdryers.
- Soothes self by flapping hands, rocking, spinning wheels on toy cars, or switching lights on and off.
- Doesn't like being touched, cuddled, or picked up.
- May have a blank facial

expression and doesn't pick up on other people's (including parents') facial expressions or tone of voice.

- Little interest in playing with toys; may only be interested in organizing toys or groups of objects in a repetitive way, for instance by lining up cars or grouping toy soldiers in strict order of rank.
- Obsessions with objects or topics, such as train timetables, makes of cars or a favorite DVD.
- May have problems with sleep—either getting to sleep initially or staying asleep once settled.
- Suffers severe temper tantrums that are especially difficult to control.
- Exaggerated interest in visual stimuli, especially television screens, computers and DVDs.
- Prefers rigid routines and finds change difficult.

What to do

There's no known cure for the condition but special educational programs, lifestyle strategies, and speech and language therapy could help your child improve and gain a level of independence

ADHD

Attention Deficit Hyperactivity Disorder leads to problems with attention and/or hyperactivity and impulsivity that are inappropriate for your child's developmental level and are impairing her

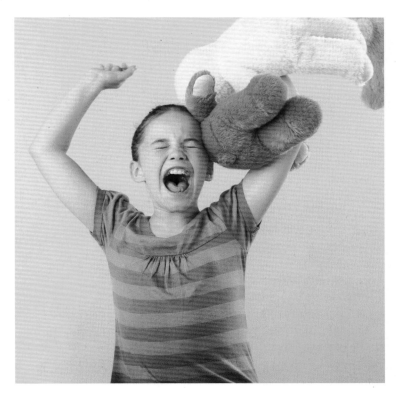

MEDICATION FOR ADHD

If your child is diagnosed with ADHD, medication may make a big difference, helping her focus her thoughts better and ignore distractions. This will enable her to pay more attention and control her behavior, with the aim of improving her school performance and ability to succeed in social activities. The medications most often prescribed are stimulants; the most common is methylphenidate, such as Ritalin®. Such medications help children focus attention, control impulses, organize and plan, and stick to routines. They are prescribed in a variety of doses and schedules. Some children respond to one type of stimulant but not another. In addition, there are some nonstimulant medications that are used to treat ADHD. It may take some time to find the best medication, dose, and schedule for your child. The pediatrician or child psychiatrist will follow your child closely and adjust the medication as needed.

performance. There are three common types:

- **Inattentive only:** Children with this type (formerly known as ADD) are not overly active. They do not disrupt the classroom or other activities, so their symptoms may not go noticed. This is the most common form found in girls.
- **Hyperactive/impulsive:** Children with this type show both hyperactive and impulsive behavior, but are able to pay attention.
- **Combined inattentive/ hyperactive/impulsive:** Children with this type show all three symptoms; this is the most common type.

A child with ADHD is on the go all the time, has difficulty concentrating, and is impulsive (does things without thinking). Since most preschool children normally show these symptoms, the diagnosis is often not made before the age of six, and three to six more boys are diagnosed than girls. ADHD may be problematical for parents, and if untreated, can significantly affect learning and progress in school.

ADHD is one of the most common chronic conditions of childhood. A report published by the Centers for Disease Control and Prevention in November 2013 showed that up to 11 percent of children aged 4 to 17 have been diagnosed with ADHD at some point in their lives. It is important that you get help if you suspect your child is affected. The cause is unknown but genetics may be a factor. While there is no specific test for ADHD, a diagnosis can be made following an appropriate clinical assessment. If you think that your child has ADHD, consult your doctor, who should check if there are other conditions present that may account for the symptoms and, if not, should involve a pediatrician and/or a child psychologist to assist in obtaining a diagnosis.

SYMPTOM	BEHAVIOR
Inattention	Has a hard time paying attention, daydreams, and forgets things. Does not seem to listen. Is easily distracted from work or play. Does not seem to care about details, makes careless mistakes. Does not want to do things that require ongoing mental effort. Does not follow through on instructions or finish tasks. Is disorganized. Often loses important things.
Hyperactivity	Is in constant motion, as if "driven by a motor"; cannot stay seated but squirms and fidgets. Runs, jumps, and climbs when this is not permitted. Cannot play quietly. Talks constantly.
Impulsivity	Acts and speaks without thinking. Has trouble taking turns and cannot wait for things, such as calling out answers before a question is complete or interrupting others. May run into the road without looking for traffic first.

Because it is very common for children to exhibit behavioral problems, parents, teachers (if appropriate), and other caregivers need to provide information on the core symptoms, their duration, and the degree to which they interfere with the child's ability to function. Special checklists are often used to identify the key symptoms, which the diagnostician will use, and he or she may observe your child's behavior in different settings as well as taking a careful history.

Diagnosing ADHD
The behaviors on page 280 must:

- Occur in more than one setting, such as home, school, and social situations, making it difficult for your child to function in these settings;
- Be more severe than in other children the same developmental age;
- Start before your child reaches age seven. (However, symptoms may not be recognized as those of ADHD until your child is older);
- Continue for more than 6 months.

Once the diagnosis is made, management of the behavior will be discussed. The possible modes of treatment include medication, behavior therapy, dietary changes, and support in school. In addition to the above, education, parent training, and counseling may all

more **about** | DCD and dyslexia

Developmental Coordination Disorder (DCD), also called dyspraxia, affects about 5% of children, most commonly boys. It is a motor learning problem demonstrated by a child's inability to plan and produce smoothly coordinated movements, such as those needed for sitting, crawling, and walking initially and then later on to hop, skip, peddle a bike, tie shoelaces, or fasten buttons. Although occupational and physical therapy can help, and most children improve with age, it often goes unrecognized and can lead to educational, social, and emotional problems.

Dyslexia is a learning disability where a child has trouble reading and spelling because while she is able to recognize individual letters, she is unable to put them in the right order. A child may also have difficulty recognizing specific sounds, processing language at speed, and with short-term memory. The problem affects between 4 to 10% of children but is not generally diagnosed until a child starts learning to read at school. Once the problem is recognized, special programs and strategies should help her develop the necessary skills to learn effectively. Most children with dyslexia are still able to reach their full academic potential.

be needed. You may also be able to get help from a hyperactive or ADHD support group.

TICS AND TOURETTE SYNDROME
Tics are rapid, repetitive involuntary body movements. They usually affect the facial and neck muscles and may appear as grimaces, twitches of the eye, or shoulder shrugging. Tics tend to run in families and affect more boys than girls. Tourette syndrome is a tic disorder that is frequently associated with ADHD.

What to do
Tics often appear during stressful periods, so it's important that your child's life has minimal pressure—not too many commitments, for example. Discuss the problem with your child if he is old enough to be aware of it in order to suggest ways of dealing with any of his playmates who may comment derogatorily on the behavior or make fun of him.

INDEX

ACKNOWLEDGMENTS

The publisher would like to thank

Jemima Dunne for supplying text for the health and medical section.

Rachel Nixon for supplying text on autism.

St. John's Ambulance Brigade for the loan of first-aid pictures on pages 236, 237, 238, 239, 240 and 245.

Getty Images for supplying cover photograph.